PLAZA

The Hormonally Vulnerable Woman

WRITTEN BY GEOFFREY REDMOND, M.D.

The Good News About Women's Hormones

EDITED BY GEOFFREY REDMOND, M.D.

Androgenic Disorders
Lipids and Women's Health

The Hormonally Vulnerable Woman

Geoffrey Redmond, M.D.

ReganBooks

An Imprint of HarperCollins*Publishers*

This book contains advice and information relating to health care. It is not intended to replace medical advice and should be used to supplement rather than replace regular care by your doctor. It is recommended that you seek your physician's advice before embarking on any medical program or treatment. All efforts have been made to assure the accuracy of the information contained in this book as of the date of publication. The publisher and the author disclaim liability for any medical outcomes that may occur as a result of applying the methods suggested in this book.

FIRST EDITION

Designed by Kris Tobiassen

Printed on acid-free paper

Library of Congress Cataloging-in-Publication Data has been applied for.

ISBN 0-06-082553-7

05 06 07 08 09 QWF 10 9 8 7 6 5 4 3 2 1

To my patients, who by openly sharing their
experiences have taught me so much
about the human side of hormones.

CONTENTS

PART I: HORMONES AND WOMEN'S LIVES   1

1. Are Your Hormones Ruining Your Life? Recognizing Hormonal Vulnerability   3
2. What Your Hormones Do and Why   26

PART II: MONTHLY CHALLENGES   43

3. Is My Period Normal? When Your Cycle Needs Help—and When It Doesn't   45
4. Birth Control for the Hormonally Vulnerable: Finding a Method That Respects Your Body's Sensitivities   59
5. The Week from Hell: PMS and Other Hormonal Miseries   82
6. The Comprehensive Program for Overcoming Your PMS   96

PART III: WHEN HORMONES HURT   129

7. Female Pain: Cramps, Endometriosis, Fibromyalgia, and More   131
8. When Hormones Go to Your Head: Migraine and Other Headaches   150

PART IV: HORMONES MAKE SEX POSSIBLE—OR NEARLY IMPOSSIBLE   161

9. Why Have So Many Women Stopped Enjoying Sex?   163
10. Sex and Women's Lives   172
11. Sex Is Much More Than Hormones   182
12. What the New Research Has Discovered About Testosterone and Women's Sexuality   189

13. Testosterone: The Decision   198

14. How to Use Testosterone *Now* to Get the Zest Back in Your Sex Life   201

15. Getting the Most from Your New Sexuality   214

PART V: THE MOST VISIBLE PART OF YOUR BODY MAY BE THE MOST VULNERABLE: WHAT HORMONES CAN DO TO SKIN AND HAIR   225

16. The Most Heartbreaking Hormone Problem: If You're Starting to Lose Your Hair   230

17. Peach Fuzz and Worse: Hormones and Facial Hair   265

18. Acne: Not Just for Teenagers   276

19. Making Sense of Your Testosterone Results   288

20. Effective Treatments for Hormonal Skin and Hair Problems   297

21. The Hormone Problem That Affects Nearly Everything: Polycystic Ovary Syndrome (PCOS)   310

PART VI: MENOPAUSE: STRAIGHT TALK ON THE TOUGH QUESTIONS   347

22. The Great HT Scare: What They Didn't Tell You About All Those Studies   349

23. What Menopause and Perimenopause Feel Like   363

24. Menopause: The Decision   381

25. How to Feel Good Without Estrogen: Alternative Treatments   389

26. If You've Decided to Try Estrogen: Choosing the Best Preparation for You   396

27. Planning for Your Bones' Future: Preventing Osteoporosis   418

PART VII: HORMONES AND THE SOUL   425

28. Hormones and Spiritual Healing   427

A Bill of Rights for Women Who Are Hormonally Vulnerable   442

Information Resources   445

Books   445

Organizations   447

Medical Information Online—Some Comments   447

Acknowledgments   449

Index   455

PART I
Hormones and Women's Lives

1.

Are Your Hormones Ruining Your Life? Recognizing Hormonal Vulnerability

You probably picked up this book because you have noticed that your body is changing, and you suspect hormones are to blame. Your skin may have started to break out again, or your menstrual cycle may have lost whatever predictability it once had. Perhaps you put on twenty pounds in less than a year—or had to resort to extreme dieting just to maintain weight. Or you may be one of the 30 percent of women whose sex drive goes into hibernation. Showering may have become a terrifying ordeal because clumps of hair clog the drain. Or your mood may have a life of its own, which clashes with your own life.

Perhaps you recognize yourself in what some of my patients have said about how they feel when their hormones start to assert themselves:

"Something has happened; I'm not the same me."

"I don't feel like I'm living in my body anymore."

"I cry every time I wash my hair because so much falls out."

"I'm never sure when to schedule an important event because I never know if I'll be in control of my emotions when that day comes."

"Sex used to be very important to me but now I couldn't care less. Except for my husband, I wouldn't mind if I never had it again."

"Lately my joints ache, and it even hurts to comb my hair. My doctor told me I'm just getting older. But I don't think forty-eight is old, and I felt perfectly fine until a few months ago."

"I spend twenty minutes every morning plucking hairs from my face."

"I'm tired of all the jokes about hormones. They are not so funny when you are struggling with them every day."

"Please help me. I don't want to live the rest of my life feeling like this. You are my last hope."

Each of these women had a different problem, but there was a common factor: *hormonal vulnerability*.

Each was in good health and, according to conventional medicine, had no disease. Yet they did not feel well and were not able to enjoy their lives. Most dispiriting of all, each had sought desperately, but unsuccessfully, to find an explanation for what was happening and a way back to being normal. Some were told dismissively by their doctors, "There's nothing wrong with you." Or they went through an elaborate workup, only to be told, "All your tests are normal; there's nothing that can be done." Some were put on medications that did not help. The treatments did not work because the cause—*hormonal vulnerability*—was not understood. Several sought relief from herbs and supplements without success, not because herbal medicine does not work—it often does—but because they did not have reliable information about what herbs to use and how to use them.

The result of this massive disregard of hormone problems by the medical establishment is the nearly terminal discouragement of many affected women. Yet there is no reason for the widespread pessimism about women's hormones. Medicine has learned a lot about how these body chemicals affect health and well-being. A few doctors now recognize that some women are particularly sensitive to their own hormones, even when levels are supposedly normal. This condition I term *hormonal vulnerability*. Sadly, most in the medical establishment are still unaware of this condition, even though there are new and excellent treatments for its various forms. Information is scattered in bits throughout thousands of medical journal articles and too often presented in technical language of extreme obscurity.

Showing how biochemical research about hormones can be used to bring joy back into the lives of hormonally vulnerable women is the task I've set for myself in writing this book. Here you will find complete, up-to-the-minute findings on all the major hormonal conditions. However, this book goes beyond the abstractions of scientific research. Because hormones are not only chemicals but also feelings and experiences, I will emphasize how they affect women's lives. I've learned a lot about this, not only from my formal medical education but also from listening carefully to the stories of the nearly ten thousand women who have consulted me about these conditions. I will also speak frankly about the problems women have getting help. Part of the burden of hormone problems is massive denial by a medical establishment that is quite often unsympathetic. If you have been thwarted in your efforts to get help, you will learn that you are not alone. To empower you to get the help you need, I will give you practical tips on how to navigate the labyrinthine health care system.

My experience in caring for hormonal problems for more than twenty-five years has shown me that there is almost always a solution. The most important thing is not to give up hope. *No matter how discouraged you may be, no matter how many health care professionals you have seen, how many medications or herbs you have taken, or how many times you almost gave up, you can feel yourself again.* This book will show you how.

WHAT ARE HORMONES?

All women know something about hormones because they experience their fluctuations every month. Sometimes hormones speak in a whisper and mostly leave you alone. Other times they shout and tiresomely demand your complete attention. In an ideal world, hormones would do their important work of regulating bodily functions unobtrusively and leave you free to live your life as you want. Alas, this is not always the case. If hormones are making their presence known in your life, it is best to give them the attention they want. Step one is to know what they are.

Quickly defined, hormones are chemicals released into the blood by structures called endocrine glands; their job is to coordinate processes throughout the body. Hormones regulate such essential functions as metabolism, the sleep-wake cycle, energy, mood, response to stress, the structure of the bones, and, of course, the menstrual cycle and reproduction. The most important glands are the ovaries, adrenals, pancreas, thyroid, and pituitary. (I explain more about these glands in later chapters.) Though hormones are released in extremely minute quantities, they have the power to profoundly alter body processes.

Most of our knowledge about hormones is fairly recent. Because the amounts in blood are infinitesimal, technology capable of measuring them dates back only to the 1970s. Unlike many other blood chemicals, *hormone levels are not constant but fluctuate in complex patterns as they regulate the body's rhythms*. Without these fluctuations, there would be no menstrual cycle and no new human beings entering the world. But there would be no hormonal discomforts either. The basic difficulty is that hormones travel to all parts of the body and do different things in different places. The same hormone's effects may be wanted in one place, but unwelcome in another.

Consider estrogen, the main female hormone. It has an essential nurturing effect on the body, widening blood vessels so that more blood flows to cells to deliver nutrients and cleanse them of toxins. Estrogen also soothes the walls of arteries, making them less vulnerable to scarring that can eventually lead to heart attacks. The second female hormone, progesterone, prepares the body for pregnancy, protects against uterine cancer, and sometimes helps with sleep. Testosterone—yes, women have it too—strengthens muscles and bones and has some role in keeping a normal sex drive.

But for women who are vulnerable, hormones can wear another face. Their estrogen may surge without warning, bringing on sore breasts, nausea, or irritability. Or it may just as suddenly plummet, precipitating an agonizing migraine. Progesterone can cause bloating and the blues. Testosterone can help keep sex exciting, but too much can spoil the complexion and make hair grow where it is unwanted.

Hormones must stay in balance or be gently corrected when they don't. As all women know, hormones are intimately connected to feelings. They are the bloating many women feel before their periods and also the weepiness and irritability. They are the facial blemishes that keep coming long after their teen years, the struggles with weight, the sapping of energy, and many other frustrations that will all be covered in detail in later chapters. I see the mission of my medical specialty of endocrinology as understanding the connection between these two aspects: hormones as complex molecules made up from carbon, hydrogen, and oxygen and hormones as life experiences.

Many women come to feel that doctors do not understand their hormones, and often they are right. Except in the subspecialty training of endocrinologists, hormones are covered only briefly in medical education. While the reproductive role of hormones is taught, their effect on well-being is not. Hence, many excellent doctors in other specialties have only limited knowledge of hormones.

Why do hormones get short shrift? There are several reasons. We live in a materialistic culture, and hormones cannot be seen nor touched. Their effects usually do not show on endoscopy or MRI scans. They can be measured with tests, but interpretation of these tests is complex because normal ranges are not fixed. The proper levels of hormones vary with age, phase of the cycle, even the time of day. During the menstrual cycle, estrogen levels ebb and flow more than tenfold. Testosterone levels fluctuate too, so that a woman may have a high level in the morning but a normal one in the afternoon when her blood is drawn. The word "hormone" comes from the Greek word meaning to stir up or provoke, a derivation that well captures what these chemicals do.

Interpretation of hormone tests requires a knowledge of these vagaries. Often a considerable measure of intuition is needed over and above purely scientific knowledge to figure out what hormones are up to because a level that's right for the "average" woman may not be for one who is hormonally vulnerable. The elusiveness of hormones makes some physicians feel uncomfortable when dealing with their convolutions. It is much easier to assess the heart with an echocardiogram or look at the stomach through a gastroscope. Too, hormones affect both mind and body, and mainstream medicine still tends to be uncomfortable with problems that involve both. Of course there are doctors who are fascinated by hormones and adroit at figuring out what is happening when they go awry. It is this sort of doctor you need to find if you are having hormone problems.

IS IT MY HORMONES?

Women usually suspect when their hormones are misbehaving, often before their doctors do. I've provided a chart which lists the common symptoms that result when hormones come unhinged. If anything on this list gives you a jolt of recognition, look to hormones as the likely basis. A quick word of caution, however. Symptoms can have many different causes, and only a medical workup can pinpoint the exact basis in an individual case.

This list is to help you, not alarm you. All women have some of these symptoms occasionally. Although they can have serious causes, most often they do not. (At least not serious as the medical profession defines it—potentially life threatening.) It's when they become so persistent and severe as to interfere with your life that they need medical attention.

COMMON SYMPTOMS CAUSED BY HORMONES

Changes in thoughts and feelings

Mood swings, whether they are premenstrual or not
Crying for no reason
Irritability—flying off the handle easily
Fatigue/lack of energy
Sluggishness
Decreased memory
Trouble concentrating
Dizziness, light-headedness
Anxiety
Feeling anxious or "wiped out" an hour or two after eating—
    "hypoglycemia"
Hot flashes and night sweats
Loss of interest in sex

Weight problems
Difficulty losing weight
Food cravings

Changes in skin and hair
Dull complexion; loss of feminine glow
Increased oiliness
Acne
Rosacea (redness on nose and "butterfly area")
Thinning of hair on the scalp (alopecia)
Increased hair on face or body (hirsutism)

Bodily discomforts
Headaches
Breast fullness or pain
Pain or discomfort when combing hair
Unpleasant sensation when touched
Cramps
Bloating
Excessive fluid retention
Aches in muscles or joints
Generally feeling terrible

Changes in the menstrual cycle
Infrequent periods (usually more than five and a half weeks apart)
Too frequent periods (usually less than three and a half weeks apart)
Spotting
Very heavy periods
Prolonged bleeding
Cramps that are more than mild
Difficulty becoming pregnant

Changes in the pelvic region and vagina
Loss of pleasure with sex
Dryness
Chronic pain or pain with intercourse
Vaginal infection that never quite goes away

All these symptoms—and what you can do about them—are fully explained in later chapters. (It may be helpful for you to copy this list and use it to organize your information in preparation for a visit to a health professional. With this aid, you can be secure that you will not forget anything important.)

After reading this list, you may feel you have more than your share of problems. Sadly, there is no limit on how many hormonal symptoms a woman may have. If you have several hormonal disturbances, you need help for all of them together. Getting your skin cleared up is nice, but what if you still have no energy? Being rid of menopausal hot flashes is a great relief, but what if your hair is still falling out? For this reason, I emphasize a holistic approach.

HORMONES AND HOW YOU LOOK AND FEEL

If looks and feelings are particularly important to women, it is ironic that female hormones can have such powerful adverse effects on mood and appearance. Yet they do. (Men worry about how we look and feel also, but our hormones usually don't cause us problems until much later in life.) Unfortunately, our contemporary Western culture is hypocritical about appearance. The media fill pages and airwaves with perfect-looking women, but when people admit an interest in their own looks, they are stigmatized as vain. This double bind is getting worse, not better. Studies have shown that a few decades ago most women were satisfied with their appearances, but now a majority fear that their faces and bodies are not attractive enough. In the face of this mass insecurity, hormones often won't cooperate—they can decide for themselves if your hair will be oily, your skin blemished, or your waist widened. Too often, fashion wants women to look one way, hormones, another.

Interest in how one looks is a positive trait, a way of caring about yourself. Styling hair, applying makeup, and choosing clothes are ways a woman expresses her freedom to decide how she will present herself to the world. (She still exerts this freedom if she chooses not to wear makeup or pay attention to how she dresses.) To want to look good does not mean thinking appearance is everything. While I do not endorse society's judging women by their appearance, I do endorse being honest about the situation and recognizing that women deserve help when hormones change grooming from self-expression to self-concealment.

Just as women feel their appearances should be pleasing, they often believe their moods must be also. When hormones make being happy impossible, women often feel guilty because they do not want to seem ungrateful for the good things they have in their lives: family, home, career. But it's not fair to blame yourself when hormones have made being cheerful impossible.

Hormones do a lot of good things for a woman—until they take over and rule her life. Something happens—it's hard to put into words but very real. A woman's body just does not feel the same. The main event may be PMS, it may be chronic fatigue, it may be the beginnings of hair loss, it may be menopause, or it may not fit any of these overly neat medical categories. Feeling good seems to be a thing of the past. This truth is both simple and sad: *Hormones can interfere with happiness*.

If reading this is making you feeling discouraged, don't be. *The first step in solving a problem is admitting it and taking it seriously*. Once you have recognized that hormonal vulnerability is the source of your problem, you will be able to understand what is happening and find help. This book is devoted to helping you do this.

HORMONES AND AGING

One of the ways women's problems are often dismissed is by the statement, "You're just getting older." True, we're all getting older, but this does not mean that feeling bad is inevitable. As medicine advances, we are starting to understand that what used to be called "aging" is actually the result of specific biological processes, many of which can be favorably modified. Exercise and proper nutrition can maintain our bodies in good condition for many more years than used to be thought. While it is true that as we get older there may be a greater tendency to loss of energy, mood swings, hot flashes, sleep problems, and hair and skin changes, these adverse tendencies can be corrected. The forty-eight-year-old of today is not like an eighteen-year-old, but neither is she like the forty-eight-year-old of her mother's or her grandmother's generations. She is likely to be much more actively in-volved, and for this she needs—and can have—a higher degree of physical well-being. That attractively healthy glow need not go away at forty or fifty. Nor does menopause mean having to slow down. Maintaining the right balance of hormones can do much to prevent the supposedly inevitable effects of aging on skin, hair, bones, energy, and overall well-being. A holistic approach, such as I employ, recognizes that our minds and bodies are not static but continuously changing. With proper attention to hormonal health, the challenges of each new stage of life will lead to new satisfactions.

THE HORMONALLY VULNERABLE WOMAN

Medicine is finally recognizing what women have known all along: Some women are simply *hormonally vulnerable*. Their bodies are more finely tuned and particularly sensitive to hormonal shifts that other women may not even notice. It's not fair, but it's reality. Basi-cally, hormonal vulnerability is a state in which a woman's body does not respond as it should to the chemicals that are supposed to smoothly coordinate bodily functions. Women who are hormonally vulnerable need—and deserve—particularly close attention to their hormones. Their bodies may need special pampering when hormones fluctuate.

Being hormonally vulnerable does not necessarily mean being vul-nerable in other ways. Many of my patients with hormonal vulnerabil-ity are actively engaged in life, with careers, children, or both. I've had patients who are athletes who manage peak performance, despite the lack of support from their hormones. Another is an attorney able to stay cool in court even when her hormones are doing their best to dis-tract her. Some are single mothers managing stressful jobs while par-enting their teenage children. There are millions of women like these and, usually, no one else knows the extra effort they must make every day just to do what others take for granted.

Up to now, there has been no overall name for the female experi-ence of hormones being out of kilter. Yet, in my experience, women who are hormonally vulnerable usually know that they are; they just did not have a word or phrase to convey the myriad problems set off

by their hormones. These women are more aware of their bodies because they have to be; they feel subtle biochemical changes that others
might not even notice. If you are hormonally vulnerable, paying careful attention to what your body is telling you will help you identify the
causes of your problem. This book will help you interpret your body's
internal language to work out what is causing your difficulties. I am
not suggesting that you go it alone; you will still need help from health
care practitioners. However, with today's rushed medical consulta-
tions, if you do not have some idea of what might be wrong and what
the treatments might be, you may leave without getting much help.

WHAT IT'S LIKE TO BE HORMONALLY VULNERABLE

Hormonally vulnerability can take many forms. One of the most distressing is alopecia—female hair loss. Men are supposed to lose hair,
though of course we don't like it. But it's not normal for a woman, and
it's devastating when it happens—as it does to about 20 percent of
women before age fifty and at least 40 percent after that. First, you
may notice that more hair appears on your clothes and in the drain.
Then your part gets wider, or your ponytail thinner. Some scalp may
show. You may undergo medical tests and, more often than not, all are
normal. But of course something is wrong—the vulnerability of the
hair follicle to hormones. The trigger may be a sudden dip in estrogen,
the hormone that is hair's best friend. Or it may be that the years of
exposure of the follicle to testosterone, hair's worst enemy, have finally taken their toll. Some women's hair follicles are not so sensitive
to these hormones; they never get alopecia. Other women's follicles are
hormonally vulnerable; slight changes disrupt their function. The result: thinning hair.

PMS is another example. All women have major swings in estrogen
and progesterone during their cycle, and both hormones can affect the
function of neurons in the brain. While these effects are tolerable for
most women, those with PMS have a nervous system that's hyperresponsive to these hormonal oscillations. The result: incapacitating
mood swings. Though the hormone levels are normal, a more delicately tuned constitution feels the changes too acutely.

Hormonal vulnerability may involve only one hormone or several.

Some women have multiple vulnerabilities, though most of the medical profession will not admit this. Instead they are dismissed as neurotic because their tests are normal, ignoring the question of how their bodies respond to these so-called normal levels. Hormonal vulnerabilities are affected by age, nutrition, stress, and many factors in the environment. They may involve the entire body—the woman who feels bad all over before her period—or specific parts. Because the breast is one of the most delicate areas of the body, many women experience pain there, either premenstrually or throughout their cycles.

Just as hormonally vulnerable women's bodies overreact to their own hormones, they are often highly sensitive to medications. Consider birth control pills. Most women feel fine on them and appreciate the lighter, more comfortable periods. But for a vulnerable few, oral contraceptives (OCs) can bring on nausea or mood swings. For most women with pill vulnerability, there is at least one that will cooperate with their bodies. Unfortunately, most physicians who prescribe OCs were never taught how to match the pill to the woman. In chapter 4, I discuss how to select a preparation that will respect your personal hormonal sensitivities.

If you are hormonally vulnerable, medication can usually help, but it must be started and adjusted with particular care. One-size-fits-all medication is not for you because doses intended for "average" women don't work if you are not average. A woman's endocrine system is a delicate mechanism and must be approached gently. For this reason, later in this book I not only discuss treatments but also explain how they can be modified for sensitive constitutions.

WHY HORMONAL VULNERABILITY IS IGNORED BY DOCTORS: THE DISEASE HANG-UP

Let's admit it: The health care system is not exactly user-friendly. Women with hormone problems ask only for a reasonable explanation and to feel their normal selves again. However, when there is no official medical term for what is wrong, it can be hard to find help—or even sympathy—from the health care establishment. Too often a woman's expectation that she should feel good and look good is dismissed as if it were unreasonable. Some doctors still do not accept diagnoses that women know are real—PMS or chronic fatigue, for example. Or they may recognize that a hormonal problem—such as hair loss—is real but think it does not matter. Many women feel diminished after interactions with such physicians. They feel that they were not taken seriously or that the doctor implied that his or, sometimes, her, time has been wasted. Unfortunately, some doctors, when they do not understand or do not know how to help with a problem, respond by denying the validity of the problem altogether.

One reason for these physician attitudes is what I call the *disease hang-up*—by which I mean the assumption that what is to be treated is a disease rather than a person whose body is no longer working quite right. *Effective healing must acknowledge that what is treated is not a disease but a person who happens to have a disease.* Someone with diabetes is more than a "diabetic;" someone in menopause is more than a "menopausal woman."

Once we let go of the disease hang-up, we can recognize that *if someone does not feel well or, to be more direct, cannot enjoy life, she is entitled to help—even if her condition is not defined in a textbook and even if her lab results are normal.* Usually in this book I use terms like "condition" or "problem" because although the women with them definitely do not feel well, they are not diseased. PMS is not a disease, nor is menopause. But they interfere with quality of life, which is a fancy way to say that life stops being pleasurable. Ultimately, *the function of healing is to bring back the joy of life.*

HORMONAL VULNERABILITY CAN BE OVERCOME

Let's look now at the process for overcoming hormonal vulnerability. Here I will give you an overview; details will be filled in later as I discuss each condition.

The first step is what I call *biochemical self-understanding*—learning the ways hormones influence how you look and feel. Better knowledge of your own hormonal biochemistry will prepare you for the important first step of organizing your thoughts so you will know better what you need from the health care system. Being able to identify what is actually happening with your hormones will guide your search for a physician who really has the expertise to help you.

The next step is getting help from a particular physician. To help you with this, I'll give you inside advice on how to deal with doctors by revealing how they feel about women with hormone problems. I hope that a peek at physicians' beliefs and emotions will help you avoid the sort of adversarial relationship that has become all too common. I've worked within the health care system for more than thirty years and in later chapters will reveal some secrets that can make your encounters with it less frustrating.

GETTING WORKED UP FOR HORMONE PROBLEMS: WHAT'S INVOLVED

Medical evaluation for a hormone problem should involve a very thorough medical history and physical examination (remember that hormones have effects all over the body) and, usually, blood tests. In later chapters, I discuss in detail which tests are helpful for each condition and give some guidelines on how to make sense of your results. I'll also explain why seemingly normal results sometimes are not really normal.

At any doctor visit you are entitled to a specific treatment plan. This is more than a hurriedly spoken diagnosis and a stack of prescriptions. What your plan should include is itemized in the sidebar.

MIDDLE WAY MEDICINE

If I did not have great admiration for modern scientific medicine, I would not have spent so many difficult years studying it, but I also think it is a mistake to ignore the older ways of healing that have served humanity for thousands of years. When I was in medical school, I came to realize that I needed something more than pure science and so came to study Eastern philosophy and meditation. This taught me that spiritual approaches are a valuable complement to physical ones. In my practice, I have developed what I call *Middle Way Medicine,* which integrates the best of each approach while avoiding extremes. In chapter 28, I suggest simple spiritual practices that people of any religious belief can use to aid the healing process.

Middle Way Medicine is open to unconventional approaches. Some

WHAT YOUR DOCTOR'S TREATMENT PLAN SHOULD INCLUDE

- What is the likely diagnosis *and why*

- An explanation of the diagnosis *that makes sense to you*

- What tests or other steps will be taken to establish the diagnosis

- How your condition will affect your future and overall health

- What you need to be concerned about—and what you don't

- Presentation of all reasonable treatment options, *including alternative remedies*

- Information on how prescribed medications work and their side effects

- Plans for monitoring your response and options to consider if the first treatment does not work

- Adequate time for you to reflect on the information you have received

- Respect for your right to make your own choices

of my colleagues will be shocked when I state my opinion that alternative remedies are usually not the last things to try, but the first. When they work, they are usually safer and better than prescription medications. At times, however, alternative methods may be a poor choice because they delay effective treatment or have safety problems of their own. As I discuss each condition in later chapters, I'll make suggestions on how to safely and effectively use alternative medicine. Choosing an alternative practitioner can be even more difficult than choosing a doctor, but I'll make some suggestions on this too. My approach in this book is to weave together all the effective forms of healing to provide guidance for you to develop a holistic program for yourself.

Something from you is also required: Being willing to trust and to try different approaches until you find what works. With luck, the first medication, or the first supplement, will solve your problem. But often it takes longer; patience is a necessary resource for healing. Trust does not mean not asking questions or doing whatever a doctor tells you; it does mean pondering a doctor's suggestions and, if they make sense to you, giving them a chance.

The very power that hormones have over women makes many afraid that treatment might make matters even worse. As one of my patients recently put it, "The word on the street is, 'Don't let them mess with your 'mones.'" In the past, this has sometimes been justified because medicine did not understand hormones well enough, and some early forms of treatment were too crude for women's delicately balanced biochemistry. Unfortunately, I still see women who were treated improperly and would have been better off if no one had "messed with their 'mones." Usually, but not always, the effects of poorly conceived treatment are reversible. Yet overall, care for women's hormonal conditions is much better than it used to be. We have very sensitive tests for measuring levels and forms of medication that permit precise dosing of these potent substances. *Properly done, hormonal treatment can be life-changing for the millions of women who are hormonally vulnerable.*

IS TREATMENT FOR HORMONAL CONDITIONS SAFE?

Recently, a woman whom I was seeing for hair loss—probably the most distressing of all hormone conditions—told me that the previous doctor she had consulted, although he had acknowledged that her condition was treatable, told her the treatment was so dangerous that it was worse than the condition itself. She wanted to be sure and so consulted me for a second opinion. In fact, treatments for this condition rarely cause side effects, and when they do, they are mild. Admittedly, there is not a drug known to humanity that does not sometimes have side effects; nevertheless, most, when used properly, are not dangerous.

Why then do doctors sometimes scare patients this way? There are several reasons. One is simply misinformation; they are not very familiar with the medication and do not know enough about its safety. A second is that they do not think the condition is important enough to justify taking medication. This happens frequently with "cosmetic" conditions such as alopecia—as if appearance did not matter at all.

The irony is that these are often the safest to treat. A third reason, the least excusable, is that the doctor does not want to bother treating the condition and knows that scaring the patient is a quick way to get rid of her.

You should not make a decision to have any treatment—or not to have it—until you are fully informed about possible adverse effects. Nor, however, should you allow yourself to be put off with vague remarks. There may be times, of course, when you decide not to take a medication because you think the possible risks are not worth it. However, this should be based on facts, not scare talk.

Not all the scares come from doctors. Some come from friends or anonymous Internet postings. Again, before you are discouraged by talk such as, "That can make you gain weight" or "I've heard that's really dangerous" or just "I don't think you should take that," get the details. Friends are usually well-meaning but not necessarily well informed about your health issues. This even applies if they are nurses or doctors whose expertise is in a different area. On the Internet, rumors regularly make their rounds. A recent one is that spironolactone, a testosterone blocker, can affect your liver. While spiro certainly can have side effects, liver toxicity is almost unheard of, based on my review of the National Library of Medicine database. Like any important life decisions, those regarding medical treatment should be based on facts. When you read a post on the Web, you have no idea about the poster at all. She or he might be a truly knowledgeable authority or completely off the wall. More medical information is available than ever before but much is contradictory, placing the burden on the consumer to figure out whose advice to follow.

In this book, I've done my best to give the reasons behind my advice and to give options so that you will have the information you need to make decisions that you will be comfortable with. I've also given additional information sources in the Resources on page 445.

WHAT HORMONES HAVE TO TEACH US

While I would never suggest that having hormone problems is good for someone, many women discover that in cultivating awareness about their particular hormonal vulnerabilities, they have come to understand themselves better. This self-understanding is both chemical and spiritual. We tend to think of ourselves as made of our thoughts, emotions, and experiences. And we are. But we are also made up of chemicals, including hormones. To experience our inner chemistry—quite different for men and women—is to appreciate more fully our own humanity. Admitting that our chemicals affect how we think and feel does not deny free will. On the contrary, we can better control our destinies when we are more conscious of the chemical tides of our bodies.

For some women, the education they acquire through researching their hormone problems is satisfying in itself. And in the process of applying what they have learned to helping themselves, they develop a closer relationship to their own bodies. By recognizing their bodies' special susceptibilities, they can change their lifestyles to protect themselves. Some, realizing the power of the mind to heal the body, are led to meditation or yoga or to a renewed commitment to prayer and devotion. What they started in desperation to alleviate an unbearable situation led them to new activities whose benefits flowed into other areas of their lives.

Some women find, as they learn more about their hormones, that they do not need medical treatment. Subtle changes in thought and lifestyle, sometimes enhanced by meditation, may ward off hormonal upheavals like mood changes or migraine. My own migraine stopped after I began meditation, as I discuss in chapter 8.

Before I go on, I want to acknowledge the role of these women who have told me their stories and have honored me by their trust. They have been my greatest teachers and deserve much of the credit for what follows. Many of their stories are in this book, though I have, of course, changed their names and details so that none will be recognizable.

MOLECULES AND FEELINGS

Doctors are supposed to be detached and objective, and when we write, we are supposed to be impersonal as well. I hope you have noticed by now that this is not my approach. Scientific objectivity and detachment *are* very important when figuring out diagnoses and pondering the benefits and risks of different treatments. Medical journal articles also must be written in an unemotional way. But the limits of objectivity must, in my opinion, be recognized to a far greater extent than they usually are. Patients are not experiments. Laboratory results are data, but they are also statements about actual people. When people seek help from a doctor, they want their lives and health to be returned to a happier state. One hears little about human happiness in medical school, yet it seems to me that this is the real goal of medicine. Life offers many ways for us to be happy but, unfortunately, also many ways that our abilities to be happy can be impaired. Illness is paramount among these.

In medical training, we are taught to regard disease as a derangement of bodily function that can be understood in terms of chemistry and physics. One learns to employ a dazzling array of technologies to translate a person's symptoms into anatomical and biochemical abnormalities. This is the methodology of scientific medicine, and it has, beyond doubt, markedly reduced the amount of suffering caused by disease. Just consider, for example, what it must have been like to have a toothache when there was no dentistry. Yet, we must guard against the technology becoming an end in itself so that we forget its ultimate purpose is to help people to feel better.

SOMETHING ABOUT MYSELF

This book is certainly not an autobiography, but since I view medicine as a human undertaking, it is only fair that I tell you something about myself. For the past two decades, the focus of my medical practice has been the treatment of women's hormonal disorders. I've now treated nearly ten thousand women with these conditions, one of the largest experiences of any physician in the world. Often I am the last resort for women who have seen as many as fifteen different doctors without their problems being solved. They now come to my New York City facility from all over the United States and sometimes from abroad. I am proud of this, of course, but also saddened that it is so hard to find help for these common problems.

It took me many years to reach this point. My specialty of women's hormone problems is an uncommon one, and I came into it from an unusual direction. Looking back, I can see that my fascination with hormones began in my early teens. Of course, my curiosity was in part related to the changes in my classmates and me as we progressed through puberty. But beyond that, it was a dream I had even then of understanding life in chemical terms. My favorite book in those days was one published by *Scientific American* called *The Chemistry of Life,* which I bought with my one week's allowance. I reread the chapter on hormones many times; some of what I learned stayed with me until medical school.

The dream I conceived in my teens—that biochemistry can help us to better understand ourselves—has been mostly fulfilled. Although I never imagined that our emotions are simply chemicals, it seemed to me then, as it does now, that hormone biochemistry offers us essential insights into how our minds and bodies are interconnected. Endocrinology, the science of hormones, can be applied to rectify the subtle internal chemical derangements that so often detract from the joy of life.

As I have lived longer, my dream has evolved. I still think well-being requires a harmonious relationship with one's own hormones, but I have come to further appreciate the spiritual aspects of being human that science has not so far illuminated. Hormonal problems, such as PMS, are also spiritual crises; the most effective healing addresses biochemical causes without neglecting the soul. Because I am a physician, not a guru, my first responsibility is to help restore physical health, but this does not mean neglecting the role of mind and spirit.

I'd always wanted to be a scientist as well as a physician and so, after completion of my medical at Columbia College of Physicians and Surgeons, I went on to research training at Rockefeller University, an institution that is to science as a remote Himalayan temple is to religion. Its tranquil campus and lack of bustle provides the ideal setting for scientists to remove themselves from the trivia of daily life and to focus on making discoveries. Practicality is hardly thought of. Though the pure science I learned there has been of immense value in my later work, I gradually came to recognize that spending my days at the lab bench was less satisfying to me than applying science to solve the problems of actual people. Since then I have continued to do research, but it has mostly concerned treatment rather than theoretical knowledge.

For me, it is the challenge of applying biochemical knowledge to solving the difficulties of ordinary life that is most exciting.

My research has been in the areas that most concern women: acne, excessive hair growth, hair loss, oral contraceptives, mood swings, polycystic ovary syndrome, pubertal development, menopause, and sexual problems. I've also done clinical research on important general health issues such as high blood pressure and diabetes. I am particularly proud of my study establishing the birth control pill Ortho Tri-Cyclen, which is as effective for the treatment of acne. I say more about what the pill can do for acne—and what it cannot do—in chapter 4. More recently, my research has focused on reproductive safety—being sure that new pharmaceuticals do not adversely affect delicate hormonal balance.

I initially chose pediatrics over internal medicine as my specialty, for two reasons. First, pediatricians seemed to take into account the impact of medical conditions, and their sometimes invasive treatment, on the lives of their young patients. Second, I've always found the developmental approach one of the best ways to understand human problems, whether medical, psychological, or spiritual. About 2,500 years ago, philosophers in Greece, India, and China simultaneously drew attention to the fact that everything in the world, including ourselves, is constantly changing. That is obviously true of children, and so of all medical specialties, pediatrics has been most aware of the importance of development. Internal medicine seems to take less account of the obvious fact that adults develop too. Our bodies—and our expectations of them—are different at thirty-five than at twenty-five and different at fifty than at forty. Some of the most fundamental of these changes are orchestrated by hormones, and so a developmental perspective seems to me essential in endocrinology. The changes of adult life had tended to be viewed negatively as "aging," a process of decline. While it is obvious that some physical functions decline—at fifty we cannot run as fast as we did at twenty—this misses the point that as we mature, though we lose some abilities, we gain others.

My early interest was the endocrinology of puberty. This difficult passage is one of life's greatest challenges, particularly in our culture. I soon discovered, however, that the problems related to female and male hormones hardly end with the teens. Hormones continue to change throughout our lives. Yet this developmental perspective tends to be lacking in endocrinology. The fields of psychiatry and psychology, although more aware of development, have tended to get caught up in their elaborate theories and to disregard how organic conditions affect the mind. Often physical problems are mistakenly interpreted as neurotic. Just yesterday, for example, I saw a young woman, Anne, for hair loss whose therapist had suggested that her distress over her thinning hair meant that she had body dysmorphic disorder. This term refers to thinking one's body is abnormal when it is not. The best-known example is anorexia nervosa, in which girls who are too thin think they are too fat. This term definitely does not apply to someone who is distressed because of a *real* change in her body. Anne did not have body dysmorphic disorder at all—her hair really was falling out, and her reaction was that of a normal woman responding to the loss of an important part of her body. The answer for her was not years of expensive psychotherapy, but hormonal treatment to help grow her hair.

Perhaps I am particularly aware of the human aspects of medicine more because my education was not exclusively in the sciences. I majored in English literature as an undergraduate at Cornell University and went on to get an M.A. in the same subject from the University of Virginia. Some years later, I became fascinated by the ancient cultures of Asia, particularly those of China and India, and began to make use of some of their spiritual techniques, since discovering them amid the stresses of med school. I've visited Asia many times and taught in medical schools in China, Taiwan, Hong Kong, Thailand, Korea, Japan, and India. I've also lectured on the relation of Asian philosophy and religion to science in several Asian countries as well as at Oxford University and UNESCO in France. My articles on Buddhism have been published in several Buddhist journals as well as *The Encyclopedia of Biomedical Ethics*. All this has, I believe, given me an approach to healing that embraces technology but does not limit itself to it.

As medicine tries to be more and more objective, it tends to exclude those aspects that are art rather than science. This is not entirely unreasonable; healing does need objectivity to sort out what works from what doesn't. The pitfall to this approach is that it too easily forgets that healing involves more than prescribing medications. The effort to base medicine as much as possible on evidence is commendable; the tendency to ignore anything that cannot be objectively measured is not. The function of medicine, in my view, is not simply curing disease but also restoring health and happiness. Science is necessary for this but is not sufficient by itself.

A Chinese palm reader once told me that my most important knowledge was what I had taught myself. This is not entirely true— without advanced formal training in endocrinology, I could not practice as I do. Although I ground my practice on scientific information as presented in medical texts and journals, much of the knowledge I apply in treating patients was acquired by listening to the women who consulted me describe their experiences with their hormones. Gradually, I learned to recognize hormonal vulnerability, the many ways in which hormones can interfere with women's lives.

This is my fifth book on medical subjects. Three were medical texts that I edited, including *Lipids and Women's Health* (Springer-Verlag, 1990) and *Androgenic Disorders* (Lippincott-Raven, 1995); the other was a book for women themselves, *The Good News About Women's Hormones* (Warner Books, 1995). I have come to feel that the greatest need is not for textbooks but for information hormonally vulnerable women can use themselves. One of my aims in writing this book is to serve as a "consumer advocate" for hormonally vulnerable women by empowering them with the background they need to raise their doctors' consciousness about hormones. Reluctantly, I've concluded that this may be the most effective way to educate the medical profession. Although I've lectured on the subjects of this book to tens of thousands of doctors over the past two decades, it is pressure from patients that will finally convince them to address hormonal vulnerability.

2.

What Your Hormones
Do and Why

You already know a lot about hormones—maybe even more than you want to know—because of their effects on your own body. Puberty, menstruation, conception, pregnancy, childbirth, nursing, and menopause are all hormonal events, as are the many subtle changes in body and mind that women feel but for which medicine may or may not have a name.

Hormones can be looked at from two vantage points: as a part of women's experience or, scientifically, as chemicals that can be measured and studied. The latter is what is taught in medical school. Part of my task in writing this book is to bring these two ways of looking at hormones together, to show how the chemical events cause changes in body and mind, and how these subjective changes can be understood in biochemical terms. This is not because I consider the scientific explanations to be more real or important than feelings, but because when properly applied, scientific medicine can be an extremely powerful way to relieve the problems that hormones too often create.

Let's consider the main female hormone, estrogen, as an example. In biochemical terms, estrogen is described as a four-ring steroid molecule with the A-ring aromatic. The term "aromatic" here has nothing to do with aromas but rather a certain sort of organic chemical structure.

(This term is a useful one to know because conversion of other hormones to estrogen is referred to as aromatization; medications that prevent estrogens from being formed are termed aromatase inhibitors.) Humans have three forms of estrogen: estradiol, estrone, and estriol. (Chemically, these differ only slightly, in how many so-called hydroxyl groups they contain.) This technical terminology by itself seems remote from estrogen as a part of women's experience: a girl's body becoming a woman's, the good feelings at the beginning of each new cycle, but also the breast tenderness, migraine, and some of the other cyclic discomforts later in the cycle. Yet, it is scientific knowledge of the structure of estrogen that has made it possible to recognize its diverse effects on a woman's body and to devise treatments for when these effects are uncomfortable. Looking at a chemical diagram—or a lab report—does not tell what estrogen *feels* like. The scientific and subjective aspects of estrogen—as with other hormones—seem far apart. This is one of the reasons women have difficulty getting help with hormone problems. When women are with their doctors, there is a frequent disconnect: Women concentrate on how they feel, while doctors are thinking about hormone levels. Sadly, our medical education system leaves many doctors more comfortable with molecules than with emotions. Yet, doctors are not completely wrong in this. They do need to understand the biochemistry because it is the basis of treatment.

In this chapter, I'll cover some biochemistry as a background to connecting laboratory knowledge to women's experience. (Much of the science was discovered by women, such as Dr. Rosalyn Yalow, who won the Nobel prize for discovering the method that made modern hormone tests possible.) Developing a feel for your own biochemistry is useful for all women, but an absolute necessity if you are hormonally vulnerable. To help you develop this biochemical self-understanding, this chapter discusses what hormones are, how they function, and why some women's bodies have difficulty sorting out the effects of rapid hormonal shifts. My focus will be the three key hormones that are most important in a woman's life: estrogen, progesterone, and testosterone. In later chapters, I'll cover less familiar ones that nevertheless play a crucial role: the prostaglandins, for example, which make childbirth possible but also cause menstrual cramps, and serotonin, which regulates mood and energy. Finally, I'll provide essential new information on insulin, usually associated with diabetes but also the PCOS and antiweight loss hormone.

WHAT IS A HORMONE?

The medical definition of a hormone is a chemical released in one part of the body that travels through the blood to influence processes in other parts of the body. Hormones serve to signal and coordinate body processes. They share this orchestrating function with the nervous system. Indeed, the two systems interact extensively. The so-called "master gland"—the pituitary—is actually controlled by the part of the brain just above it, the hypothalamus. Hormones in turn have profound effects on the way the brain functions. This is obvious in the hormonal storms of puberty, the mood changes of the menstrual cycle, and the hot flashes of perimenopause and menopause.

The problem is that this coordinating system does not work as smoothly as it should. Hormones fluctuate beyond what is comfortable. Physicists tell us that this is characteristic of all control systems, which, when they go too far in one direction, they tend to overcompensate in the other. To be fair to hormones, they do manage to keep us going. Yet, I think most women would agree that the system leaves a lot to be desired.

Most of the hormones we'll be concerned with here belong to the chemical family referred to as steroids. Many now associate the term "steroid" with " 'roids" taken by some athletes to bulk up and improve their performance. However, anabolic steroids, to use their full name, are just one category of steroid. They are actually synthetics designed to mimic testosterone's muscle-building effects. Steroids are actually a very diverse group of hormones that include estrogen, progesterone, testosterone, cortisol, and the blood pressure raising hormone aldosterone.

Because they are involved in reproduction and gender differences, estrogen, progesterone, and testosterone are often referred to as sex steroids. However, some of their most important effects, such as the bone-protecting effect of estrogen, have no clear relation to either sexuality or reproduction. Too, these hormones can also have effects that are anything but sexy: cramps, sore breasts, facial hair, and acne, to name a few.

HOW HORMONES WORK

Hormones seem like powerful substances with a will of their own. Their effects on both body and brain are dramatic and, seemingly, inescapable. But they bring out what is potential in our genes. Breasts develop at puberty because they have a built-in capacity to grow in response to estrogen. Of vital importance for the theme of this book, there is much individual variation in how a person's body responds to hormones. This is why breasts vary so much in size: Some are more responsive to estrogen than others. It is also why some women tend to have sore breasts and others do not. Testosterone, too, elicits a variable response. It turns on the sex drive at puberty but does not determine how strong it is, nor its direction. Whether a man or woman is gay or straight, for example, is something residing in the brain; it has nothing to do with testosterone levels.

There are really two aspects to hormone action: the level of the hormone, which can be measured in a clinical lab, and how vigorously the cell responds when the hormone attaches to its receptor, something that tests do not tell us. The level of a hormone is determined by the interaction of the pituitary and the gland which secretes it—ovary and adrenal for the sex hormones. Response to hormones is mediated by molecules called receptors. Steroid receptors are mainly located in the cell's nucleus, where they influence expression of the genetic potential stored in DNA. The receptors determine what is referred to as "end organ response." The "end organ" is the part of the body that responds to the hormone. Thus, breasts and uterus are end organs for estrogen and progesterone, while the skin is an end organ for testosterone's tendency to increase hair growth.

The great limitation of our ability to understand individual differences in hormonal effects is the gap between blood levels, which are easily and routinely measured, and what the hormone is actually doing to the body. Hormonal vulnerability is mainly a matter of end-organ response; lab tests may be normal while your symptoms clearly are not normal.

A skilled clinician can infer end organ response pretty accurately—the timing of cyclical or premenstrual mood swings provides a clue as to the relative roles of estrogen and progesterone, for example. More facial hair indicates hair follicles that overreact to testosterone, and so on. With women's hormone problems, there is no substitute for the physician taking a careful history and doing a complete physical examination. Despite being unfashionably low tech, these traditional procedures can give clues to hormonal events that will not show up in blood tests or high-tech imaging procedures. The latter are of vital importance too; my point is that neither takes the place of the other.

One reason women have so much trouble getting diagnosed for hormone problems is physicians' tendencies to rely entirely on tests and ignore the mental and physical effects of the hormones. Hormones reveal themselves in the sensations and emotions they evoke and the slight traces they leave on the body. Correct inference regarding receptors requires both a knowledge of endocrine biochemistry sufficient to make sense of test results and the ability to detect the end organ effects of the different hormones. (Receptors can actually be measured, but this is a research procedure requiring samples of tissue. They are available only for very few conditions, such as breast cancer. In most situations it is not practical to do such measurements. No woman with PMS, no matter how badly her life is disrupted by it, will be willing to have a bit of her brain tissue removed in order to study why it overreacts to the hormone swings of her cycle.)

ESTROGEN

Estrogen makes the feminine areas of a woman's body feminine. It stimulates breast development at puberty and widens the hips. Internally, it causes the uterus to enlarge to the point of being able to bear a child and the vagina to be moist and resilient enough for comfortable sexual intercourse. During the initial half of the menstrual cycle, estrogen causes the lining of the uterus (the endometrium) to thicken so it will be able to support a pregnancy.

These effects of estrogen have been known for nearly a century. Recently attention has turned to more subtle but equally important effects, such as its action on bone. Despite its apparent solidity, bone is a dynamic tissue; old bone is always being broken down, and new bone is formed to take its place. Because estrogen is needed for this new bone formation, when levels drop at menopause, bones start to weaken. The obvious question: If estrogen is needed for strong bones, why don't men get osteoporosis more often than women? The answer is another of those yin-yang situations in which the sexes are less distinct than imagined. Men's testicles make estrogen as well as testosterone; they continue to do so throughout a man's life. After menopause, unless they are on hormone therapy, women have less estrogen than men. So it seems that both sexes need estrogen, and, though the evidence is less clear, both probably need testosterone.

Another important effect of estrogen is vasodilatation, which simply means that this hormone causes blood vessels to open up wider and carry more blood into tissues. In this sense estrogen has a nourishing effect. Some discomforts of menopause probably result from reduced blood flow due to the absence of estrogen. This is an area of active research, and we don't yet have a complete picture of how estrogen affects the circulation.

Estrogen is also important for brain function. Women in perimenopause/menopause often report brain fog that happens with estrogen replacement. The cognitive benefits of estrogen are probably the result both of improved brain blood flow and direct action on nerve cells in the brain.

Another organ that is greatly affected by estrogen is the liver. Estrogen's effect on the liver is in a sense related to its nurturing function—it enables the liver to make larger amounts of a great variety of proteins. Liver proteins boosted by estrogen include those that carry hormones in the blood and clotting factors.

Estrogen, then, is far more than a sex and reproduction hormone. A general lack of appreciation of the overall positive effects of estrogen is one reason women find a deaf ear turned to their problems at menopause. It is assumed that because estrogen is a "sex hormone," its effects will be limited to reproduction and sex. In fact, estrogen seems to maintain health and comfort at many levels, not only the vagina, uterus, and breasts but also the bones, muscles, circulation, and brain.

THE KINDS OF ESTROGEN

Estrogen is actually a general term for a family of hormones, which includes three made in the human body, some made only in animals, and a variety of synthetics. The main human estrogen is estradiol. (I emphasize human because of the bizarre practice, which should have ended decades ago, of prescribing horse estrogen for humans.) Estradiol begins to be made in large amounts at puberty and is the main form of estrogen until menopause. During pregnancy, another estrogen, estriol, is also made in large amounts. There is a very old theory that estriol may be protective against breast cancer, but recent research has found women with breast cancer actually have higher levels of estriol.

The other important estrogen is estrone, which is made not only in the ovaries but also in fat tissue. For this reason, overall estrogen levels tend to be higher in heavier women. After menopause, the ovaries make less estrogen, but fat cells continue to make estrone so that this form of estrogen makes up a greater portion of the total amount. This is more than a biochemical detail because there is another old theory that estrone may be a factor in the development of breast cancer. The idea is that estrone is the main estrogen after menopause, when breast cancer risk starts to go up and that levels are higher in overweight women, who also have an increased breast cancer risk. This evidence is only circumstantial. Though an estrone-breast cancer connection has never been proven, it has never been refuted either.

For this reason, many, myself included, think forms of estrogen containing estrone are less desirable than ones containing only estradiol. But there is a catch here. Oral estradiol is largely converted to estrone when it is absorbed into the blood and passes directly through the liver. This means that after you swallow an estradiol pill, much of it ends up as estrone. You can prevent your liver from tampering with estradiol by using it in patch or gel form, as detailed in chapter 26.

When estrogen is measured as a lab test, usually only estradiol needs to be tested. After menopause, it is sometimes helpful to determine estrone as well. An older test called *total estrogen* measures all three forms, but in my experience, it's less informative because it lumps all three kinds of estrogen together.

IS ESTROGEN GOOD OR BAD?

Essential as estrogen is for healthy functioning of a woman's body, the sad fact is that estrogen can be too much of a good thing. When levels surge, especially in women whose bodies are vulnerable to it, a variety of symptoms can be triggered. Menstrual flow may be heavy, and vaginal mucus may be more than is comfortable. Breasts may swell and become tender to even light pressure. The normal widening of hips and rounding of thighs that began at puberty can turn into embarrassing bulges. To try to control these with exercise is often a struggle because it cannot fully counteract the powerful action of estrogen.

For the most part, however, it is not estrogen itself that causes problems but sudden fluctuations in its level. For the hormonally vulnerable, the ups and downs of estrogen often bring on personal ups and downs: generalized discomfort and sore breasts when levels rise, then irritability, mood swings, lack of mental focus, migraine, hot

THE ESTROGEN SCORECARD

Estrogen gets points for:
Turning girls into women
Making sex possible
Making pregnancy possible
Enhancing blood flow
Nurturing bones, brain, and other tissues

But points off for:
Fluctuating uncomfortably during the cycle and at menopause
Sensitizing breasts
Triggering mood swings
Causing the nausea of morning sickness
Possibly playing a role in the development of breast cancer

flashes, vaginal dryness, and insomnia when levels fall. Tests are of no help because by the time symptoms have appeared, the change in estrogen is long past.

However much estrogen is disrupting your life, you can't do without it; all you can do is negotiate peace terms with it. This book will guide you in these negotiations. Before that, however, the estrogen scorecard I've provided as a sidebar on page 33 may help you refine your awareness of the role of this hormone in your life.

PROGESTERONE

Although progesterone is just as essential as estrogen, its functions are more limited. The roots of its name describe its role: *pro-gest*ation—progesterone produces the changes in a woman's body necessary for her to become pregnant and maintain the pregnancy. Progesterone is made by the ovary only during the second half of the cycle and during pregnancy. If your cycle is regular, and you're not approaching menopause, you probably ovulate nearly every month and so progesterone will be measurable in your blood from a day or two after ovulation to a day or two before menstruation. During the rest of a cycle, and at all times if a women is not ovulating, progesterone levels in blood are very low. After menopause, all women have progesterone levels close to zero. I emphasize this because I see many women who became worried when they were told that their progesterone was too low. Usually it was because their blood was taken at a phase when progesterone is *supposed* to be low.

The good news about progesterone is that it makes pregnancy possible; the bad news is that it also makes PMS possible. Here individual differences are important. For some women, progesterone has mood-soothing effects. For others who are vulnerable to this hormone, it contributes to the all-too-familiar monthly miseries: bloating, puffiness, mood swings, and irritability.

Progesterone, especially as a cream, has been heavily promoted for virtually every woman's problem. Much of what you may have heard about progesterone is, unfortunately, myth. Progesterone does great things—protects the uterus against cancer and makes pregnancy possible—but it is far from the cure-all for women's problems. What progesterone can mean in your life is covered in chapters 5 and 26.

SYNTHETIC PROGESTERONE

Although natural progesterone is readily available, synthetic forms are prescribed far more often. Artificial versions of progesterone are called progestins. These can have undesirable effects, especially in women who are hormonally vulnerable. Most notorious is Provera (medroxyprogesterone acetate, MPA), which can produce truly major PMS. Bizarrely, this is still the form of progesterone most commonly prescribed as part of hormone therapy for menopause. Fortunately, natural progesterone is readily available by prescription under the name of Prometrium. The progestins in oral contraceptives have fewer problems, especially the newer ones, as discussed in chapter 4.

TESTOSTERONE

Women's testosterone comes from the ovaries and adrenal glands. While the ovary contributes more on average, this is highly individual. Levels begin to rise at the beginning of puberty, peak in the late teens or early twenties, then gradually fall. Even at their peak, however, women's levels are not more than 10 percent of men's. By menopause, testosterone levels in most women are barely measurable.

Like estrogen and progesterone, testosterone belongs to the steroid hormone family. Hormones with testosterone-like activity are referred to as androgens. The most important of these in humans are androstenedione and DHEA-S. Both are inactive but can be converted to either testosterone or estrogen. There are also many synthetic androgens, among them the drugs abused by athletes to improve their performance. These are usually referred to as anabolic steroids, a term that emphasizes their ability to build up muscle. Some women athletes use anabolics; the result can be a decidedly unfeminine appearance. Because the use of anabolics is not only illegal but also unhealthy, it does not need to be further covered here.

For women, testosterone is the most problematic of the three main sex hormones. It is blamed for those men's traits that aggravate women, but its effects on women's bodies are welcome or not, depending on individual patterns of vulnerabilities. Testosterone does do some good things for women. It strengthens muscle and bone and seems to play some role in cognitive function. Most conspicuous is its role in sex drive. In chapter 12, I'll have much more to say about how it can be used to restore flagging interest.

Enthusiasm for the sex-enhancing benefits of testosterone should not remove scrutiny from the unwelcome effects testosterone can exert on a woman's body: oily skin and scalp, acne, unwanted facial and body hair, loss of scalp hair, and, possibly, insulin resistance. Fortunately, pronounced masculine-like changes, such as voice deepening or complete baldness, are exceedingly rare in women, as is enlargement of the clitoris, thought it is commonly mentioned in medical texts as a consequence of high testosterone levels. These effects are rare in women because the average female testosterone level is about 40 ng/dL. In contrast, men's levels are usually between 400 and 800—10 to 20 times the female level. Even women with the high testosterone levels found in conditions such as polycystic ovary syndrome rarely have levels much above 100. Testosterone becomes a purely male hormone only at the very high levels that occur in men.

DHT (DIHYDROTESTOSTERONE)

Some of the effects of testosterone, such as building up muscle, are direct effects of testosterone itself. Others are due to conversion in the tissues to its more active form, dihydrotestosterone, more easily referred to as DHT. The conversion of testosterone to DHT is brought about by an enzyme called 5-alpha-reductase. DHT is thought to be particularly important in the wilting of hair follicles, which causes hair thinning in both men and women. For this reason, it receives much attention in Internet postings about women's hair loss. Actually, in most circumstances, it is a moot point whether testosterone itself or DHT is causing the problem because treatment is usually the same. A group of medications called 5-alpha-reductase inhibitors can block the production of DHT in hair follicles. These are explained in chapter 20.

PHARMACEUTICAL FORMS OF TESTOSTERONE

As with progesterone, testosterone used to be given in synthetic forms that had undesirable effects. Orally active synthetic forms can adversely affect cholesterol and even, in some cases, cause liver damage. Newer ways to get natural testosterone into the body have made the synthetics obsolete. Some oral contraceptives contain progestins that have testosterone-like activity. I'll discuss this in chapter 4; here I'll just point out that better OCs are available that do not have this problem.

THE YIN-YANG OF ENDOCRINOLOGY

According to ancient Chinese metaphysics, everything in the world is formed by interaction of yin and yang, which are, among other things, the feminine and masculine principles. The famous yin-yang diagram in which each flows into each other is familiar to nearly everyone. More than 2,000 years ago, the Chinese recognized that nothing is purely masculine or purely feminine. Endocrinology has at last confirmed that this is true on the most fundamental biochemical level. We will encounter this principle over and over as we extend our understanding of hormones. Their yin-yang nature shows in many ways. The female hormone estrogen is actually derived from androgens. In men, estrogen comes from the most male organ, the testicle, and is also derived from testosterone, just as in women testosterone comes from the ovaries. Some of the brain effects of testosterone, possibly including male sex drive, are due to testosterone being converted to estrogen in the brain.

Some confusing things can result from this mixed, yin-yang nature of hormones. Mentally, most think of themselves as all woman or all man. Yet men's estrogen can sometimes lead to slight breast development, and women's testosterone can sprout facial hair. Since the mainstream of society basically offers only two kinds of gender—male and female—these gender-discordant changes are quite distressing. Though on a philosophical level we may appreciate our dual yin-yang nature, very few want to look like a mixture of male and female. Fortunately, there are effective treatments to block or reverse these effects of hormones.

Because gender is so basic to our existence, it is endlessly fascinating, hence the media preoccupation with transvestism and other forms of cross-gender behavior. Only a very few really want to be gender-ambiguous. Gays, even if they mimic female stereotypes, still consider themselves men. Similarly lesbians, even those who affect a masculine manner, have no doubt that they are women. Men or women who actually want to cross gender are a tiny, if visible, minority. Their concerns are important but beyond the scope of this book.

WHAT CAN BE DONE ABOUT HORMONES?

This leads to what is the core of this book: What you can do to fight back when your own hormones turn against you. As you will see, when you and your hormones are at odds with each other, you can make peace, and on your own terms. In this chapter, I'll cover some general principles; in later chapters, I'll spell out the practical details.

In principle, treatment of hormonal conditions is simple, though the details are not. Basically, hormones cause problems in three ways. Either the level is too high or too low, or fluctuations are too extreme. How high is too high and how low is too low depends on individual vulnerabilities. If hormone levels are below what the body needs, therapy aims at increasing hormone levels or enhancing their effects. If the hormone is too high, or the body is vulnerable to it, the treatment strategy is too lower the level or block its effect, or both. There are also treatments that can smooth out hormonal swings, for example with PMS. There is a lot more to straightening out hormones, of course, which is why it takes a whole book to explain.

You may be wondering, can men be hormonally vulnerable too? The answer is yes, but men's hormone problems tend to be less individual than women's. All men, for example, eventually develop enlarged prostates, due to the action of testosterone on the prostate. Erections get less hard with age, though many men retain reasonable erectile function through old age. Perhaps the classic example of male hormonal vulnerability is male pattern baldness, which is caused by overreactivity of the hair follicles to testosterone.

HOW HORMONES ARE MEASURED

The stack of lab reports has all but replaced the stethoscope as the symbol of the physician. The immense increase in what we can measure in the lab is mostly a good thing but has brought some new problems with it. Lab tests are so routine in medicine today that it is easy to forget how new they are. As a child, so far as I can remember, I never had a single lab test—though I do vividly remember getting injections.

Two sorts of technology have made today's proliferation of tests possible. First, immunoassay, invented by Rosalyn Yallow and Solomon Berson, uses the extreme specificity of antibodies to measure minute levels of hormones and other biologically potent substances. Most modern lab tests use a variant of this procedure. The original procedure was quite labor-intensive. During my postdoctoral research training at Rockefeller University, I spent untold hours manipulating thousands of tiny test tubes by hand to measure hormone levels. The second advance is laboratory automation; huge machines can now do thousands of tests with minimal human effort.

Like most advances, however, the new laboratory technology has brought a new set of problems. Accuracy is often not as great as both patients and doctors assume. The availability of so many tests also means that sometimes they are misinterpreted, creating a situation in which results confuse rather than clarify. This is particularly true with hormone problems, which tend to be subtle and elusive. When so many tests are done, false positives can occur just by chance. In my practice, I frequently see women who have been needlessly alarmed by test results that looked abnormal but really represented only normal variation.

When hormone assays are done by hand, one gets a sense of whether the test is giving accurate results or not. With an autoanalyzer, this intuitive feeling is lost. The serum sample is put in at one end of the machine, and the result is printed out at the other. What happens in between is hidden from view. In the old hands-on days, if a lab result did not look right to me, I could call the lab person who actually did the test and discuss my concerns. Usually they would do the test over, and if a problem was found, they would thank me for drawing their attention to it. Other times, they would call back and say, "We've rechecked our assay, and it's working fine. We reran your patient's test, and it came out the same." Then I'd have to go back and figure out how the test fitted with the other findings to arrive at a diagnosis.

The relationship between physician and lab used to be a collaborative one. No more. Economics has changed all this. The large health insurance companies give their business to the low bidder. These large commercial labs give a level of service comparable to that provided by telephone companies or banks. All send out sheets covered with numbers. Most of the time, these numbers are correct. But when they are not, trying to get them corrected is all but impossible.

Now when I call because I think I have noticed a problem, the answer is always that everything is fine and nothing could possibly be amiss. Just last week I received a report on a patient for whom, due to someone's careless reading of the requisition, the testosterone level was done twice. One result was 54 ng/dL, and the other was 17—*on the same specimen*. Now no lab is absolutely accurate. If the second result had been 49, say, or 57, I would have chalked this off to acceptable measurement variation. But in this case, the difference was beyond what is acceptable. For a woman, a testosterone of 54 is mildly elevated while 17 is quite low. So depending on which number I believed, this patient's testosterone might be high or it might be low; hardly a helpful result. To help you avoid such false alarms, I've listed some lab test pitfalls in the sidebar on page 41.

It's now hard to choose a specific lab because insurance restricts choice. The best is still Esoterix (formerly Endocrine Sciences), but to get your tests done there takes extra effort, and may be expensive, if not covered by insurance. (Tests can be sent to Esoterix through Lab Corp.) Fortunately, most of the time, tests give the answers we need, but when they do not, never forget that labs are fallible.

Some doctors use tests as a crutch. When they don't know what is wrong, they order every test they can think of in the hope that the laboratory will figure out the diagnosis for them. This is a fallacy. Labs don't make diagnoses. Health care professionals who are human beings do. Correct interpretation requires experience with the condition under consideration. A doctor who has seen results of a particular test in thousands of patients with a condition will have a better idea of its vagaries than one who spends most of his or her time on other conditions.

LAB TEST PITFALLS

If a result does not make sense to you, consider several possibilities.

Reference ranges (approximate normals) listed on the report form may be incorrect. This is commonly the case, for example, with testosterone and also with TSH, the most common thyroid test.

The reference range may not apply to you. What is normal can be affected by age, gender, time of day, phase of the menstrual cycle, medication, and many other factors. The doctor interpreting the test may not be aware of the effects of all these factors.

The interpretation may not be what is obvious. The common thyroid test, T4, can be high because the thyroid is overactive—or because you're on birth control pills.

A test result outside the normal range is not necessarily significant. To give one example, a low CO_2 on a chemistry profile usually means only that the person was breathing rapidly because he or she was nervous during the blood draw.

The lab result may simply be wrong. If the result does not seem to fit your situation, the lab should be willing to repeat it at no additional charge.

HORMONAL VULNERABILITY AND TESTS

When you are frustrated by problems for which the cause is elusive, it is easy to get a little obsessed with tests in the hopes that repeating them, or finding a new one, will provide an answer that has so far not been found. While there is no doubt that improvements in technology have made the lab an immensely powerful aid in medicine, labs still cannot always provide a clear answer. In my practice I sometimes see hormonally vulnerable women who, in their frustration at getting no answers, have had as many as fifty tests without their problems being solved. Almost always, what was lacking was not the right test, but the right interpretation of tests they'd already had.

SALIVA TESTS

Recently there has been a fad for measuring hormones in saliva instead of blood. Actually, saliva measurements have been around for a long time. Despite the hype, the only reason to do saliva testing is to avoid repeated sticks and excessive blood loss when multiple measurements are needed. Saliva tests are accurate only when samples are collected under careful research conditions. As tests for diagnosis, most are worthless. First, the normal ranges are not standardized. Second, they do not tell anything that blood tests would not tell. Third and most important, they tend to be inaccurate. Though I have see many patients who bring saliva tests ordered by another doctor, I have never seen these tests clarify a diagnosis. At this time, saliva tests for hormone levels are at best a waste of money and at worst a cause of incorrect diagnoses.

I've been open about the problems with labs and hormone measurements, but I do not mean this to be discouraging. Tests have transformed my speciality of endocrinology from being mostly guesswork to being highly scientific. Correctly used, tests can make it possible to determine the cause of problems that until recently were totally baffling. Tests tells us how much of a hormone is present in the blood, but they do not always tell what it is doing elsewhere in the body. Tests are one of the first steps toward getting a diagnosis, but the next step is their interpretation by a skilled clinician.

PART II

Monthly Challenges

Is My Period Normal? When Your Cycle Needs Help and When It Doesn't

Menstruation is inherently mysterious. Blood suddenly appears from structures hidden deep in the body; the bleeding recurs regularly but not entirely predictably; emotions tend to slip from control. From early in human history, superstitions have grown up around this normal biological event, some of which persist to this day. At the very least, these myths cause needless worry; at worst they can cause harm. The sidebar on page 46 lists some common beliefs about menstruation, none of which is necessarily true.

IS MY PERIOD NORMAL? WHEN YOUR CYCLE NEEDS HELP AND WHEN IT DOESN'T

Human life is based upon regularities. Day and night, the seasons, weekends following upon five days of work, all help us attune our bodies to the demands of life. The problem is, of course, that external demands rarely coincide with biological rhythms. Especially for women whose cycles present challenges, relative predictability makes these easier to allow for. If mood is likely to be a problem or cramps limit physical activity, it helps to know when to expect them and when they will end.

SOME MENSTRUAL CYCLE MYTHS

Myth: You have to have a period every single month to be healthy.
Fact: Most women miss an occasional period.

Myth: Periods remove toxins that would otherwise stay in the body and harm it.
Myth: A missed period may back up into the body and cause internal damage.
Fact: Not menstruating is not harmful in itself, but the underlying cause may be.

Myth: If your periods are irregular, you cannot become pregnant.
Fact: Becoming pregnant may just take longer.

Myth: Not having periods does not matter, unless you are trying to get pregnant.
Fact: Periods coming six or more weeks apart may indicate a hormonal disorder.

Myth: Not getting your period may be due to stress.
Fact: Only severe stress, such as being in a combat zone, affects the cycle. Ordinary life stresses, such as the demands of school or a job, do not.

Myth: Exercise is a common reason for missing periods.
Fact: Only extreme exercise, such as running thirty or more miles per week affects the cycle.

Myth: Irregular periods are normal for teenage girls.
Fact: Most teens have regular periods. If they're irregular for more than a few months, a hormonal disorder is likely.

For many women, the regularity of their cycle is reassuring, something that can be counted on in the midst of all in life that is unpredictable. When this regularity is lost, one more aspect of life seems to be slipping beyond control. This is particularly true for women whose cycles are troublesome; however, many women with smooth cycles like the monthly reassurance that everything hormonal is working right. For them, regular periods are part of being a woman, however inconvenient.

Some women, on the other hand, decide that they would just as soon not bother with periods. There are safe ways to do this; for the first time in human history, menstruation is a choice. By taking birth control pills on a customized schedule, women can pretty much decide when, if at all, they want to have a period. It may well be that at some point in the future, women will have forgotten that periods were once a month, just as many have nearly forgotten that in the past pregnancies could not be planned. (How to be in control of when you menstruate is explained in chapter 4.)

Given that regular cycles are a sign of hormonal health, unpredictable ones can create considerable anxiety. For years irregular periods have bedeviled women: When are they simply benign blips on the hormonal radar screen, and when do they indicate some deeper problem? Fortunately, research has given clear guidelines to help women determine if their cycles fit within normal. Oddly, considering that half of the human race menstruates, these guidelines are hard to find. This chapter will present simple criteria for checking your menstrual pattern, together with an explanation of what your hormones are up to over the course of each month.

The menstrual cycle does not exist for the purpose of having periods, but to make pregnancy possible. Menstruation is simply a way for the body to return to baseline when pregnancy has not occurred. Life would be simpler if hormones left everything in a steady state until pregnancy was desired, but that is not how human bodies work. On the other hand, the possibility of pregnancy each month does allow humans maximum flexibility to time having children, in contrast to lower mammals who are fertile only at particular times of the year.

WHAT IS INVOLVED IN A NORMAL CYCLE?

First, we need to define terms since they are used loosely in casual conversation. "Cycle" or "menstrual cycle" refers to the entire four-week (usually) duration from the beginning of one bleeding episode to the beginning of the next. "Period," "menstrual period," or "menstruation" refers to the time when bleeding is occurring. A cycle lasts about twenty-eight days, while a period lasts about five.

Though the most noticeable event of the cycle is bleeding from the vagina, the process actually involves the body at all levels. It begins in a brain structure called the hypothalamus, which also controls other cyclic body functions such as thirst, appetite, and body temperature. The hypothalamus sends chemical signals through tiny blood vessels to the pituitary, which is located just below it. The pituitary in turn re-leases the hormones that control the ovary (or testicles in a man), the adrenal, the thyroid, and lactation. Two pituitary hormones serve to orchestrate the function of the ovary during each cycle. First, follicle stimulating hormone (FSH) facilitates growth of the follicle—the structure that contains the egg cell. The other hormone, luteinizing hormone (LH), surges at mid-cycle to induce ovulation. After ovula-tion, the cells that surrounded the egg cell transform into a structure called the corpus luteum, which makes the large amount of proges-terone characteristic of the second half of the cycle. If ovulation does not occur, no corpus luteum forms and hardly any progesterone is made.

Though the hormones made by the ovary are invisible, their actions in the uterus produce a visible effect: the menstrual period. As estro-gen rises steadily in the first two weeks of the cycle, it causes the lining of the uterus to thicken; this is referred to as the proliferative phase. During the second two weeks of the cycle, high progesterone levels cause the endometrium to mature; this is referred to as the secretory phase. If pregnancy does not occur, estrogen and progesterone levels drop, causing the endometrium to shed. It is the blood and sloughed tissue that travel through the cervical opening into the vagina that form the menstrual flow.

Another pituitary hormone, prolactin, as its name suggests, pre-pares the breast for producing milk; high levels can suppress ovulation and menstruation. Breast feeding, however, is not completely reliable as contraception.

Irregular periods can be due to a disorder at any level of the system, from the hypothalamus to the vagina. With hypothalamic or pituitary causes, menstruation usually stops altogether and estrogen levels are low. When the problem is in the ovary, periods usually become infrequent, but when bleeding does occur, it is often heavy and prolonged. The most common form of ovarian dysfunction is polycystic ovary syndrome (PCOS), covered in detail in chapter 21. Some of the possible causes of irregular or absent periods are listed in the sidebar on page 50. In this book, I give particular attention to the common menstrual disorders for which women most frequently encounter difficulty getting diagnosis and treatment. Ironically, the unusual causes tend to receive the most medical interest. It is more difficult to find expert medical care for common disorders, such as polycystic ovary syndrome than for pituitary tumors, which are far rarer.

YOUR MENSTRUAL CYCLE: WHY IT FEELS THE WAY IT DOES

The easiest way to make sense of the changes that occur in your body during each cycle is to consider what happens week by week. Each week can feel slightly different. Keeping this scheme in mind will help you sort out the changes that occur over the month. (I use "month" here as a convenient way to refer to a cycle, even though most cycles are a few days shorter than a calendar month.)

By convention, the first day of menstruation is designated day one of a new cycle. This makes it easy to keep track of cycles, since the beginning of bleeding is impossible to miss. The days of bleeding mark the end of the old cycle and the beginning of a new one. The sidebar on page 51 gives the featured events of each week. The menstrual cycle is one of the most dynamic of biological processes—even within each week, hormones are changing.

You can refer back to this sidebar to refresh your memory when you are reading later chapters.

WHAT'S REGULAR?

The description I have just given describes the average cycle, but if you are one of the 10 percent of women whose cycle does not come every month, this scheme will not fit you exactly. Most of the variation occurs during the follicular phase (weeks one and two), which is often a few days shorter or longer than the nominal fourteen days in the generalized scheme I have given.

SOME CAUSES OF IRREGULAR OR ABSENT PERIODS

Tumors or other diseases of the hypothalamus or pituitary. Most common are those that make excess prolactin; unless very large, these are treatable with medication. If prolactin is under 30 or 35 ng/mL, a pituitary tumor is unlikely. Pituitary tumors do not fall into the category of hormonal vulnerability and so I don't discuss them further in this book. If you have pituitary disease, I strongly recommend that you seek care from an endocrinologist with special expertise in this area.

Hypothalamic amenorrhea. In this condition, the brain does not trigger cycles. It may be brought on by extreme exercise or dieting or from almost any debilitating illness.

Polycystic ovary syndrome (PCOS). This is the most common cause and is covered in detail in chapter 12.

Menopause, either premature or normal. Early menopause (before age forty) is often referred to as premature ovarian failure (POF).

Thinning of the lining of the uterus or blockage to flow are rare causes that can be detected by imaging procedures.

Even with regular cycles, there is some variation. Most of us vary the times when we eat, sleep, make love, and carry out other biological functions. Indeed life would be duller, and we would be much less creative, if we were exactly the same all the time. Our bodies are not like machines or computers. It is the same with menstruation. A meticulous study of healthy women who attended Northwestern University found that of 2,000 women, only one had her period exactly every twenty-eight days

A QUICK GUIDE TO THE MAIN EVENTS OF YOUR CYCLE

Week One: Recovery from the hormonal tumult of Week Four. The uterus sheds its lining, resulting in bleeding. Cramps may occur as the uterus expels the menstrual fluid. (When pain lasts throughout menstruation, endometriosis or another condition may be present.) Week One comes in like a lion and goes out like a lamb.

Week Two: Smooth sailing. For many women this is the easiest week. Though estrogen is rising, hormonally things feel relatively quiet. Weeks One and Two together are called the follicular or proliferative phase. These terms refer to what is happening in the ovary, where the follicle is developing, and the endometrium, which is thickening.

Ovulation: For reproduction, this is the main event. The egg, now mature, pops out of the ovary into the pelvis, where it will await possible fertilization. A small bit of fluid is released with the egg. Brief pain, mittelschmerz, may occur but is not a completely reliable sign of ovulation because other internal twinges can feel similar.

Week Three: Another transition week. Acne may be brewing under the skin, triggered by the dab of testosterone released at ovulation. Progesterone rises. Week three starts out smoothly, but by its end, PMS may be starting to rear its ugly head.

Week Four: This is the bad one. Some women breeze through it, but most have at least mild symptoms, and for the unlucky vulnerable ones, it is misery. Toward the end of this week, estrogen and progesterone levels fall, causing the endometrium to begin to shed.

In medical terminology week three and the first part of week four are referred to as the luteal or secretory phase. In the ovary, the corpus luteum has formed and is making progesterone. Under the influence of this hormone, the endometrium matures into the proliferative phase.

for two years. So if your cycle varies a bit from month to month, you are not really irregular.

Women sometimes think that to be considered regular, periods should come on the same day of the calendar each month. But months vary in length and, except for February, are all two or three days longer than an average cycle. As long as your period comes more or less monthly, it is regular. Some women's cycles are only twenty-four to twenty-six days; others have slightly longer ones, up to thirty, or even thirty-five, days. These are still normal patterns and indicate that everything is working right.

It is common for the average length of a woman's cycle, and of her period, to change slightly over time. In a sense, the ovary is a new gland every month because with each cycle a new follicle develops to make estrogen and progesterone. Hence, every cycle is slightly different. This variation is usually slight, however, because all the follicles in an individual's ovary start out with the same DNA and live in the same body. From time to time, most women will have a "bad" cycle, when PMS is worse and flow is heavier and more uncomfortable. Presumably conditions were a little different in the ovary that month. Or perhaps for unknown reasons the rest of her body was more vulnerable. An occasional uncomfortable cycle is not cause for anxiety. Though the treatments discussed in the following chapters can help, the discomfort is usually over before there is a chance to do anything about it. If difficult cycles are frequent, then you have PMS. Dealing with problem cycles is fully covered in the next three chapters.

WHAT'S IRREGULAR?

Though a few days' variation in cycles is perfectly normal, more than this may not be. Unfortunately, not all doctors pay much attention to menstrual patterns. Too often, women's questions about their cycles are brushed off casually by such remarks as, "It's normal for you." Obviously cycles that are really irregular are not normal and need to be diagnosed and treated.

To help you decide whether your cycle is really "normal for you" I've provided guidelines in the sidebar on page 53. When you compare your cycle to these yardsticks, keep in mind that an occasional cycle that falls outside these guidelines is generally nothing to worry about. The one exception is heavy bleeding, which may be due to miscarriage or other potentially serious condition. *If you are bleeding heavily, call your doctor right away!*

Evaluation for abnormal cycles should include pelvic examination, hormone testing—at the very least, prolactin, FSH, and testosterone—and sometimes a pelvic sonogram. You may have to be somewhat assertive to get the testing done. Working out the cause of menstrual problems can be rather complicated, and many nonspecialist physicians do not feel entirely comfortable doing so. This itself is understandable; no physician, or other mortal, knows everything. However, it's your body, and you are entitled to know what's happening in it. Don't hesitate to obtain a second opinion if you do not receive a clear diagnosis.

If you have had a thorough workup and everything is normal, then your pattern really may be normal for you. Some women just have more variable cycles; there is nothing wrong with this in itself. All too often, unfortunately, a hormonal disorder is present but is overlooked. This happens frequently with polycystic ovary syndrome PCOS. Clues to this are acne, unwanted hair, hair loss, and weight difficulties. If you have any of these in addition to irregular periods, you should check chapter 12.

SIGNS OF ABNORMAL CYCLES

If your *usual* pattern meets one or more of the following criteria, medical evaluation is indicated:

Periods are less than twenty-four days apart.
Periods are more than five or six weeks apart.
Bleeding lasts more than a week.
Bleeding is very heavy, for example, you need to use more than five to seven pads or tampons after day one or need both a pad and a tampon at the same time.
Cramps persist past the second day of bleeding or limit your activity.

STRESS AND PERIODS

Contrary to folk wisdom, only extreme stress will stop periods. Careful studies have shown that the ordinary pressures of life, such as difficult job demands, or even a change of environment, such as going away to college or traveling abroad, do not affect the cycle. On the other hand, women in truly terrible situations, for example U.S. Army nurses who were prisoners of war during World War II, are likely to stop menstruating.

In my experience, it is rare for hormone problems such as irregular periods or hair loss to be due only to stress. Explaining symptoms away as stress is basically a medical cop out. Almost everyone is under some stress, but most do not get amenorrhea, or hair loss, or any of the other symptoms commonly dismissed in this way. Of course, stress is unpleasant and can contribute to certain health problems. The symptoms that stress can cause are quite specific and familiar to most of us; they include shortness of breath, panic, sleeplessness, headaches, vomiting, diarrhea, and/or weight loss or gain. That some symptoms can result from stress does not mean that any can. If I sound emphatic about this, it is because literally every day in my practice I see women who were told their problems were due to stress when actually the cause was hormones. The *real* stress when this happens is frustration at not getting an explanation and precious time lost because the real cause was ignored.

NUTRITION, EXERCISE, AND PERIODS

Most people know that a high-level of physical exercise or excessive weight loss can cause periods to stop. Amenorrhea in this situation is thought to be a primitive mechanism for preventing pregnancy when the body cannot properly nourish the developing child. In men, too, reproductive function may be suppressed with excessive weight loss or extreme exercise.

Dieting makes periods stop only if it is extreme. Unless you are below the ideal weight range for your height, being thin is unlikely to cause any menstrual change. Nor will modest weight loss of even thirty pounds or less—unless you were thin to begin with.

A few women who are naturally very slender may menstruate less than monthly. This is not necessarily a sign of an eating disorder; some people naturally eat very little. Estrogen levels are related to weight, so very slender women tend to have low levels, while overweight women tend to have high ones. As we'll see in the next section, this is important because estrogen levels determine the health consequences of not menstruating.

It takes a lot of exercise to make periods stop. Marathon training may do it, but sports at high school or college level rarely do. Training for sports that require thinness can result in missed periods; those that result in bulking up do not. Ballet on a professional level is particularly hard on hormones. Ballerinas are often amenorrheic because they must train to an extreme degree and are under constant pressure to be thinner. Casual ballet for recreation or aerobics will not affect the cycle.

Being too heavy can also stop periods, usually as part of polycystic ovary syndrome, as discussed in chapter 4.

SO WHAT IF I DON'T GET MY PERIOD?

Irregular periods are important for three reasons. First, they may indicate a significant underlying disorder; some of these were listed in an earlier sidebar on page 50. Additionally, amenorrhea indicates low levels of estrogen or progesterone, either of which may have consequences. (The one exception is use of low-dose birth control pills, which sometimes make periods so light as to be invisible; this is harmless.) Finally, many—though certainly not all—women find it disconcerting to have no idea when their period will come. Restoring regularity with an oral contraceptive or monthly progesterone makes life just a little more predictable.

Deficiencies of estrogen and progesterone have different potential health risks. When estrogen levels are low, as they are with hypothalamic amenorrhea or early menopause, the possible ill effects are similar to those of menopause: hot flashes (sometimes), vaginal dryness, bone calcium loss, and a risk of early heart disease. Bone loss is of particular concern because women with low estrogen levels are usually thin anyway, which means that their bones may be somewhat delicate.

Treatment of low estrogen levels is actually fairly simple. Oral contraceptives have generous amounts of estrogen and are usually the best treatment. You'll need to use them in a way that provides estrogen all the time, rather than the usual three weeks on, one week off schedule. This can be done either by taking an OC on an extended schedule or by using some other form of estrogen during the fourth week. For younger women with low estrogen levels, it is actually safer to be on estrogen than not. The well-publicized risks of estrogen do not apply to women under fifty. Calcium and vitamin D supplementation is particularly important if you have low estrogen levels.

With anovulation, progesterone is not made. A typical pattern is for periods to be infrequent but heavy and prolonged when they do come. This is common with PCOS. With this condition, there is usually plenty of estrogen, so there are no hot flashes or dryness and bones are not affected. Instead there is an increased risk of cancer of the lining of the uterus (endometrium). Progesterone has a powerful protective effect against this form of cancer, but this protection is lost with anovulation. The simple solution is to take a form of progesterone regularly. OCs protect against endometrial cancer, as does progesterone itself in oral form. (Progesterone therapy is covered in chapter 26. For anovulation a good regimen is Prometrium, which is natural progesterone, taken for at least twelve days every month in a dose of 100 mg in the morning and 200 mg at bedtime. The synthetic Provera is an alternative in a dose of 5 mg daily, also for at least twelve days every month. Other variations are possible. Unlike the pill, progesterone does not provide contraception—which makes this a good place for a reminder that even women with infrequent periods ovulate occasionally, so contraception is still necessary.

WHAT TO DO ABOUT HEAVY BLEEDING

Some women tend to have heavier periods than others. If your period has always been heavy but only for the first day or two, has not gotten worse, and does not leave you anemic, it may be okay. However, if it has gotten heavier over time, a workup is indicated.

The medical term for excessively heavy bleeding or bleeding at the wrong time of the cycle is dysfunctional uterine bleeding (DUB). This rather vague term is left over from an earlier era when the causes were not well understood. With current diagnostic technology, it is nearly always possible to find the cause. Most common are lack of ovulation (anovulation) and fibroids. Anovulation is usually due to PCOS (see chapter 21), although it can occur as a normal variant in the early teens or in perimenopause. In general, the treatment for anovulation is either oral contraceptives or monthly progesterone.

It is common to have light spotting while on birth control pills, especially in the first month or two. This is innocuous and generally settles down, though if it continues for more than two consecutive cycles, changing pills may be appropriate. The lowest dose pills, such as Alesse, Loestrin 1/20, and Estrostep, are more likely to produce spotting. Demulen 1/35, once but no longer the first choice for women with hormonal hair and skin problems, also has a high breakthrough rate.

Other causes of DUB include endometrial polyps, which are benign growths, and excessive thickening of the endometrium, a condition called hyperplasia. Diagnosis can be made by ultrasound and an endometrial biopsy. The latter is an office procedure—somewhat like a pap smear—in which a small plastic device is used to take a sampling of the endometrium. It is slightly painful but is over in a minute or two. Taking an NSAID such as ibuprophen two hours before can reduce the pain. Because a widened endometrium on ultrasound always raises concern about cancer, endometrial biopsy is essential when ultrasound shows a lining thicker than 4 or 5 millimeters for a peri- or postmenopausal woman. During the menstrual years, the lining is normally somewhat thicker. Endometrial disorders can sometimes be cured by a course of a progestin. When abnormality persists after a course of progestin, the next step is hysteroscopy, which involves looking inside the uterus with a special instrument, or D&C (Dialation and Curettage) in which the lining is scooped out.

Fibroids, more correctly referred to as uterine myomata, are basically areas of overgrowth of uterine muscle. Most fibroids are innocuous. Up to half of all women have them; often they are found by chance when a pelvic ultrasound is performed. If fibroids are asymptomatic, they are usually best left alone. They can, however, be responsible for three kinds of problems. When located at the inner wall of the uterus, they can cause increased menstrual blood loss; periods come on schedule and last the normal number of days but are very heavy. OCs or NSAIDs may reduce the bleeding somewhat. Very large or numerous fibroids can cause abdominal discomfort or even bladder and bowel problems. They can also interfere with fertility by distorting the shape of the uterus.

The main medical treatment of fibroids is a drug called leuprolide (Lupron), which turns off the ovary so that estrogen levels plummet to menopausal levels. As you might expect, this can cause all the discomforts of menopause and so is not suitable for long term use. Once the leuprolide is stopped, the fibroids grow back to their previous sizes. The main use for this treatment is to get the uterus to a more normal shape to make pregnancy possible.

Fibroids can be treated surgically by several procedures, depending upon how large they are. Smaller ones can be removed through the laparoscope or hysteroscope. A new approach is embolization, a procedure performed by interventional radiologists in which tiny beads are sent into the arteries to stop blood flow to the fibroids. Though embolization is an easier procedure than surgery, there is some pain afterward, and the lumps can grow back. This way of getting rid of fibroids is promising but too new for any final assessment to be made.

When childbearing is no longer an issue, hysterectomy, though a bigger procedure, prevents any further problems with the uterus. When fibroids are extensive and have caused substantial uterine enlargement, this may be the only solution. Though hysterectomy was done far too often in the past, unnecessary ones are rare now, in my experience. After hysterectomy, most women are glad that they decided to have the surgery. Nonetheless, any major operation should only be considered in comparison to alternatives.

A final caution: Abnormal vaginal bleeding is only infrequently due to cancer, but it is obviously important to be sure the cause is benign. For this reason, any unusual bleeding needs proper evaluation by a gynecologist. Spotting is rarely significant, but when in doubt, it is always better to call.

4.

Birth Control for the Hormonally Vulnerable: Finding a Method That Respects Your Body's Sensitivities

Although the idea of contraception is not new, effective methods are. Earlier methods now seem rather fanciful, since they were not based on knowledge of how fertilization takes place. In ancient China, for example, women not wishing pregnancy would ingest ashes and jump up and down. China's population size tells us all we need to know about the effectiveness of this method. We now take it for granted that pregnancy will be a planned life event. The improvements in women's lives of the past 100 years would have been impossible without the ability to control the biology of reproduction. Yet, despite the immense advances in contraceptive technology, a method that is perfect for all women at all times of their lives has yet to be invented. If you are hormonally vulnerable, it may take special effort for you to find an effective method that does not cause bothersome side effects. Straight talk on the differences between methods is needed but is hard to find, in part, because much of what doctors know does not find its way into print. In this chapter, I'll share with you some of the inside information that hormonal contraception experts tend to keep among themselves.

CONDOMS AND DIAPHRAGMS: THEY WORK, BUT . . .

These are called barrier methods for the obvious reason that they place a physical and, usually, chemical barrier between the man's sperm and the woman's ovum. They have been around for a long time and are still widely used. The diaphragm has the advantage of being controlled by the woman, but some find it awkward to insert and the hard ring at its edge increases the trauma of intercourse. This is particularly true for younger women whose pelvic tissues have not become accustomed to penetration. Because the bladder is directly in front of the vagina and is a very delicate organ, it is particularly vulnerable to the repeated jolts from a diaphragm. A frequent result is bladder infection, which is easily cured but quite painful in the meantime. Because of these problems, plus a degree of messiness, diaphragms are not often used today. A more comfortable alternative to a diaphragm is the contraceptive sponge.

Condoms have the advantages of being easily available, inexpensive, and relatively reliable. Their biggest advantage is that they afford good, but not absolute, protection against STDs. Efficacy for both contraception and STD protection are greater with lubricated condoms with spermicide. Needless to say, condoms must be used in order to be effective. Sex is not always planned, and so sometimes no condom is available when unexpectedly needed. The best answer is to plan ahead. The second best is to use the morning after pill, as discussed below.

A condom problem that is not often discussed is irritation of the vaginal tissues by the latex of the condom. This happens less with lubricated forms, but it can still occur. It is more common in perimenopause, when natural lubrication tends to decrease. Use of additional sexual lubricant with spermicide (nonoxynol-9) may help but is not always adequate. In this situation, a gynecologic exam to detect infection or other factor is a good idea. Another method may need to be chosen; if so, it is vital that you know your partner's STD status. In a longstanding relationship, this is usually not a problem, but with a new partner, absolute honesty about such things cannot be assumed. Compounding the uncertainty is the fact that men may be infected with chlamydia, herpes, or HPV (the virus of venereal warts and cervical cancer) without being aware that they are. The only safe course is to insist on condom use when in doubt.

There are other problems with condoms. They interrupt lovemaking. Some men dislike putting them on and may lose their erection when doing so, although they may not admit that this is why they resist using them. As with vaginal irritation, this is more likely to occur in the forties than earlier years.

I do not intend to disparage condom use; the method works fine for many couples. But it is only fair to acknowledge problems that the family planning establishment, in its commendable zeal to reduce STD transmission, tends to underplay.

NATURAL FAMILY PLANNING AND "BEING CAREFUL"

Here's something all sexually active women should know: the man's sperm can live in a woman for about a week. This means that unprotected intercourse even a week before ovulation has some chance of resulting in a pregnancy. The woman's egg, however, can only be fertilized within forty-eight hours of being released. This means that sex is again safe after this interval. There's a big catch, though: The time of ovulation is difficult to predict accurately. This is particularly true if your periods are irregular and/or you have a hormone condition affecting your ovaries. Natural birth control is not a good option for women who absolutely want to avoid pregnancy.

"Being careful" refers to early withdrawal by the man before ejaculation. The problem with this method is that the man may not pull out in time, and, in any case, sperm may come out of the penis before ejaculation.

Some women with irregular periods assume that they cannot become pregnant. This is not necessarily so. Many women with irregular periods ovulate sometimes. Since there is no perceptible warning that will alert you that ovulation is imminent, it's not a good idea to take a chance.

HORMONAL CONTRACEPTION

More than 80 percent of American women use oral contraceptives at one or another time during their lives. Though some remain leery of them, their overall safety is excellent. In fact, overall mortality rates for women on the pill are *lower* than for those not taking it. I'll cover side effects and safety issues later in this chapter.

The situation with the pill has improved considerably in recent years. When I last wrote about this subject, I gave fairly elaborate advice about choosing a pill because each pill available had significant disadvantages. This made it somewhat difficult for hormonally sensitive women to find a pill that agreed with them. Now, there are several new OCs that are excellent for nearly all women. Still, since you have to choose, you will want to make the best choice, even if the differences are smaller than previously. And, if you are hormonally vulnerable, differences that are minor for other women may not be so minor for you.

WHY DO SO MANY WOMEN WORRY ABOUT OC SAFETY?

Although most women use an OC at one time or another in their lives, many still worry that pill use may harm them. It is natural to be concerned about anything that affects such basic body processes as menstruation and fertility. Nonetheless, based on the more than 25,000 studies published about the pill, it is clear that no matter how long a woman takes OCs, they have no permanent effects on the cycle or on fertility.

You may be wondering why there is so much concern. I think this has to do with the previous history of the pill. When first introduced, the main concern was to be absolutely sure that it would prevent pregnancy. As a result, the doses of hormones in the old pills were extremely high—two to three times the amounts in current low-dose OCs. Not surprisingly, there were many side effects, such as nausea and sore breasts. Before long, there were reports of more serious dangers, such as blood clots forming in the legs and traveling to the lungs. Soon after, reports came out linking pill use to heart attacks. Given that these problems are almost unheard of in young women, it was clear that something was going on.

Subsequent research has clarified these safety issues. First, by getting the estrogen dose down to a fraction of that which was in the early OCs, the risk of blood clots has dropped to extremely low levels. Second, it was recognized later that the heart attack risk was only in women who smoke. Hard as it is to believe now, the severe adverse effects of smoking on health were only beginning to be recognized at that time, and so the early studies did not consider smoking as a risk factor. *Current guidelines are that women who are more than thirty-five and smoke should not use the pill, and even for those who are more than thirty there is extra risk.* This issue is usually stated backward as an OC risk. Actually, the risk factor is smoking, which is made worse by the pill.

The most important advance in birth control pills has been downscaling the hormone doses. This has greatly reduced the chance of side effects, both those that are serious and those that are simply uncomfortable. Yet for some women, anxiety still lingers. Rumors don't help. Recently I had a call from a patient who'd been told by classmates that taking the pill would reduce her chances of being able to become pregnant. They were not correctly informed but did not hesitate to pass on their misinformation. Though gossip is as old as humanity, technology has made its spread far more efficient; Internet chat rooms allow rumor mongers to now reach thousands in seconds. The moral is simple: Get sound information for your health decisions, including contraception.

WHAT'S IN THE PILL AND HOW IT WORKS

Except for the rarely used "minipill," all OCs contain two hormones: estrogen and a progestin. Both are chemically modified to make them easily absorbed and able to last long enough in the blood to provide reliable contraception. Progestins are effective as contraceptives because they suppress ovulation, but when used by themselves, they tend to cause unpredictable spotting, a quite tiresome side effect. By accident, it was found that adding estrogen in a proper schedule could produce regular and predictable cyclic bleeding. So the combination pill was born. The addition of estrogen also increases contraceptive effectiveness and permits lowering the dose of progestin, important because some side effects are due to the latter hormone.

All currently used OCs contain the same estrogen, ethinyl estradiol, but they vary in the amount they contain. Form and amount of progestin they contain also differ from pill to pill.

The following sidebar summarizes the two hormones in the pill and explains what they do.

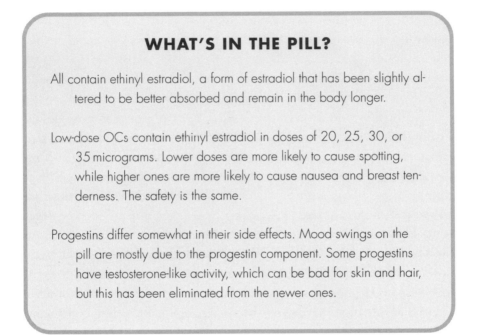

WHAT'S IN THE PILL?

All contain ethinyl estradiol, a form of estradiol that has been slightly altered to be better absorbed and remain in the body longer.

Low-dose OCs contain ethinyl estradiol in doses of 20, 25, 30, or 35 micrograms. Lower doses are more likely to cause spotting, while higher ones are more likely to cause nausea and breast tenderness. The safety is the same.

Progestins differ somewhat in their side effects. Mood swings on the pill are mostly due to the progestin component. Some progestins have testosterone-like activity, which can be bad for skin and hair, but this has been eliminated from the newer ones.

THE OC POPULATION EXPLOSION

Soon we may need birth control for birth control pills; there are now so many that it is hard to keep track of all of them. To keep things simple, I discuss only those I consider the best—or those that I suggest avoiding. Many others work perfectly well for contraception but have no particular advantages, so I do not discuss them here. If your pill is not mentioned in this chapter but has not caused you problems, there is no need for you to change.

In recent years, in part due to the influence of health insurance, generic OCs have become far more widely used than before. These are made by two companies, both of which have excellent quality control, so you can be just as confident with generic as with brand-name OCs.

The only problem with generics is that they have different names from their branded equivalents. In what follows, I generally use brand names since they are most familiar, though I also mention commonly used generics. My use of brand names is for simplicity, not an endorsement of a particular manufacturer. With so many variant names, it would be tedious if I listed all of them. If you are not sure whether your OC prescription was filled correctly, it's best to check with your pharmacist.

HOW TO PICK THE RIGHT PILL FOR YOUR PERSONAL HORMONAL BALANCE

I've already pointed out that the pill contains both estrogen and a progestin. Picking the right pill basically means picking the right form of each of these hormones for your body.

The Estrogen Choice Here the issue is not which estrogen—all current pills contain the same one, ethinyl estradiol—but how much. Doses are 20, 25, 30, and 35 micrograms. It would seem logical that the lowest dose would be safest but, surprisingly, this is not the case. Studies have shown that the risk of blood clots, the most serious pill adverse effect, is not lower and may actually be slightly higher with the very lowest dose. The difference is quite small, however. It does mean that with the pill, less is not always best. Spotting is more likely on 20 microgram pills, with the exception of Mircette/Kariva.

You might want to consider a 20 microgram pill if you are vulnerable to estrogen side effects, such as breast soreness or morning nausea. In this case you may feel better on Mircette or its generic equivalent, Kariva, the only 20 microgram OC I recommend. I say more about them at the end of this chapter under "The Best Pills."

You may be wondering, *Why take more estrogen than the minimum?* This is a logical question. The 30 and 35 microgram pills do have some advantages that are important for many women. First, the best ones are less likely to cause spotting than most of the 20 microgram ones. Second, although never proven, it is possible that the 20 microgram versions have a slightly higher incidence of "contraceptive failure"—the medical euphemism for getting pregnant when you don't want to. This may be especially true if you occasionally forget a pill—who doesn't? More important, if you are taking the pill for therapeutic reasons, such as suppressing testosterone to control acne or hair loss, the 30 and 35 micrograms may work a little better. They are also generally better if you are taking the pill to prevent ovarian cysts or for cramps.

The Progestin Choice The pills differ in subtle ways. Originally, different progestins were developed for business reasons: Having a unique one allowed the pharmaceutical company to patent its OCs and promote them under a brand name. Although at first new progestins were developed solely for patent purposes, they turned out to have subtle differences in their effects on the body. Not all OC experts consider these differences to be large enough to matter. In my experience, they clearly do matter. One reason may be the high proportion of hormonally vulnerable women in my practice whose bodies are more fastidious about what hormonal medications they will accept. I do not dispute that many women do equally well on any pill, but I still think that since you have a choice, you might as well try to get the best match for your body.

Progestins differ in two important ways: androgenicity and mood effects. Androgenicity refers to testosterone-like action. More androgenic progestins can produce unfavorable cholesterol changes and possibly a greater tendency to acne, unwanted hair, or scalp hair loss. Though some experts deny that such effects are significant, no one has yet come up with a convincing reason why progestin androgenicity would be good for anyone. Now most OCs prescribed are nonandrogenic, which is gratifying to those who, like myself, have been speaking out on this issue for many years. The newer, nonandrogenic OCs are listed under "The Best Pills" at the end of this chapter.

Most women feel fine on the pill, but a few do not. Overall, the incidence of mood changes with the pill is low, only about 2 percent; the trouble is, if you are one of those 2 percent, the pill may put a damper on your enjoyment of life. Since the pill contains versions of the same hormones that can trigger PMS, it is not surprising that it can induce similar emotional swings in some women. It is my experience that hormonally vulnerable women are the ones who are likely to feel depressed on an OC.

The most mood-friendly pills are Yasmin, Mircette, and Ovcon 35. If you are on a different pill and feel blue on it, try one of these as the next move. Some women, however, do not feel good on any OC; for them the only answer may be getting off the pill altogether.

The news about the pill and mood is not all bad. Many women find their moods are more stable on the pill, probably because it tends to even out hormonal fluctuations.

SOLVING PILL DIFFICULTIES

For most women, the pill makes life simpler. There's no need to worry about contraception at the time of sexual activity, and periods are predictable, light, and relatively comfortable. While the great majority of women feel fine on the pill, a few do have problems, and since this book is for women whose hormones complicate their lives, I need to say something about pill problems and their solutions.

Pill rumors Rumors are not harmless because they can trigger quite unnecessary anxieties. Before considering real pill problems, I need to dispel some of the common myths about OCs. Keep in mind that oral contraceptives have been in use for almost fifty years and that their effects have been studied in hundreds of thousands of women. We probably know more about the effects of OCs than any other medication. It can be clearly stated that the pill does not cause cancer. Breast cancer rates are definitely not increased, and the risks of ovarian and uterine cancer are *reduced* by half. Nor does the pill impair fertility. No matter how many years you take it, it will not lessen your chances of being able to become pregnant. It will not increase it either, so if you delay trying until your late thirties or forties, while you still may be able to become pregnant, the odds are not quite as good. But pill use does not affect this one way or the other.

Extra bleeding About 15 percent of women have spotting or light breakthrough in the first month or two on the pill. This is harmless and does not suggest that anything dangerous is happening internally. (If bleeding is more than light, however, you should check with your gynecologist, since there can be a variety of serious causes unrelated to the pill, such as ectopic pregnancy.) But spotting, even though harmless, rapidly gets on women's nerves. If you spot when you start on the pill, the first thing to do is wait because it usually stops after one or two cycles. If extra bleeding continues, then a change of pill is the next step. Even with a pill change, you may need to wait a cycle or two for the spotting to stop. If you need to change pills, there is no absolute way to predict which will better agree with you. Generally, it is better to switch to another that is also nonandrogenic. However, there is one exception: The pill that often controls bleeding when nothing else does is Nordette, one of the most androgenic. So if spotting does not stop after multiple pill changes, Nordette may be the answer for you. Even if you have an androgenic condition, Nordette will probably not make it worse, if you are on an antiandrogen such as spironolactone.

Migraine Studies show that migraine usually gets better on the pill, but sometimes gets worse. Since dips in estrogen are a powerful trigger for a migraine, a good choice is Mircette, which has the most even estrogen schedule. Another approach is to use an estrogen patch during the inactive week of the pill cycle. On the other hand, if you have one of certain rare forms of migraine in which there is weakness or paralysis during the aura, or an aura that lasts more than an hour, the pill is not safe for you. Migrane is covered in chapter 8.

Weight and the pill The most frequent question I am asked about the pill is, "Will it make me gain weight?" While the old high-dose pills may have had this extremely unpopular side effect, several studies indicate that modern ones such as Ortho-Cyclen, Ortho Evra (the patch), and Yasmin do not. Actually, Yasmin is associated with very slight weight loss of a pound or two in the first few months. It is far from being a diet pill, however, and will not solve weight problems. Basically, the pill is neutral as far as weight is concerned.

A few women notice an increase in breast size when they go on the pill. Although far less common than in past years, when estrogen doses were much higher, it can still happen. Unfortunately, it is usually just those women who do not want their breasts to get bigger who notice enlargement with the pill. This is because larger breasts are more responsive to estrogen. Usually breasts go back to their former size when the pill is discontinued. If you notice unwanted chest expansion on the pill, it is reasonable to switch to a 20 microgram pill such as Mircette (generic Kariva). Some very slender women also notice a slight increase in breast size. This is nothing to worry about unless the increase is asymmetrical, in which case you should get a breast exam to be sure the enlargement is not due to a tumor. Slight breast asymmetry is extremely common, however.

Weight and contraceptive effectiveness Recent research raises the possibility that OCs may be slightly less effective for women who are overweight. The cutoff weight is about 158 pounds at 5'2" and 169 pounds at 5'6". The cutoff for the Ortho Evra patch is slightly higher, about 198 pounds overall. There is no obvious solution for this problem. If you are over these weights, there is a very slightly greater risk of becoming pregnant, despite taking the pill—A second method can be used in addition, if it is essential to avoid pregnancy.

I do not think the risk of pregnancy is higher, however, for overweight women who have PCOS with irregular periods, so the pill is still part of treatment for this condition.

Sex drive and the pill Nonandrogenic OCs lower the active free form of testosterone by about 50 percent; this is usually advantageous because suppressing testosterone helps to keep skin and hair in good shape. Some women worry that the pill will decrease their sex drive, but this is actually quite unusual. The pill does not prevent pregnancy by making women uninterested. Because most women need only a tiny amount of testosterone to feel sexy, even if the pill lowers it, there is still enough left to enjoy the reason you started the pill in the first place. If you are one of the few whose sexual interest is suppressed by the pill, stopping it and using an alternative method is the simplest solution. Before you do this, be sure the problem is really the pill and not something else in your relationship.

Melasma Also referred to as chloasma, this refers to an increase in facial pigmentation caused by estrogen. It is common in pregnancy and can occur with the pill. Melasma is not necessarily unattractive, but some women find this change in their skin quite distressing, especially if the extra pigmentation is blotchy. Reducing the pill to a lower estrogen dose is a step in the right direction but does not usually completely solve the problem. Melasma usually reverses if the pill is stopped, though it can be expected to recur with pregnancy.

Use of so-called bleaching creams can help melasma. Most effective is probably EpiQuin Micro, but there are a variety of others, all containing hydroquinone. If you have any concern about increased facial pigmentation, you should be scrupulous about applying sun block (SPF 50) whenever you go out in the sun. This includes walking to work or hunting down your car in a parking lot, not just being at the beach.

Blood clots The medical terms for this are deep venous thrombosis (DVT), which refers to blood clots forming in veins deep in the leg, and venous thromboembolism (VTE), which refers to the clots breaking off and traveling to the lungs where they can interfere with oxygenation of the blood. VTE, the most serious pill problem, is fortunately extremely rare. If clots are going to occur, they usually do so in the first few months of OC use. Marked obesity is a risk factor, as weight tends to interfere with the return of blood from the legs. (As already noted, obesity may lessen the reliability of the pill for birth control.)

Symptoms of DVTs are swelling, redness, and pain in the lower leg, usually just on one side. If you develop such symptoms, you should have medical evaluation immediately. Some women worry that leg cramps may be due to DVTs. However, occasional leg pain is universal—even a very thin person's legs absorb a lot of mechanical stress. Achy legs without any swelling or tenderness do not suggest clots. Leg cramps are not a reason to stop the pill. However, if you are in doubt, you should call your doctor.

THE MORNING AFTER PILL

Sometimes it happens, and you weren't ready. Or the condom broke. Or you realized that you forgot to start your new pill pack. There are many reasons that women have sex, then realize that they weren't adequately protected. If this happens to you, postcoital contraception, more commonly termed *the morning after pill,* will reduce your chance of becoming pregnant by about half. It's best to take the morning after pill as soon as you realize that you need it. The standard guideline is to take it within three days of intercourse, but it may be effective up to five days after. The main side effect is nausea and vomiting.

Unfortunately, you need a prescription for the morning after pill, which may be hard to get at short notice, especially on a Sunday. I suggest you call your doctor early and have it phoned in. The reason a prescription is required is not medical but political. Although the FDA's Advisory Committee recommended over-the-counter availability, the agency deferred making the decision to do so. Unfortunately, governments still try to control women's bodies.

The brand name of the morning after pill is Plan B. Nausea and vomiting are possible side effects. If you vomit, the pill may not have been fully absorbed, and you may need another dose—you should call your doctor if this happens.

If you had intercourse without adequate protection and your period does not come when it should or is very light, you need to do a pregnancy test. The one called hCG quantitative is more sensitive in very early pregnancy than the home tests are.

The morning after pill is not suitable for use as a routine contraceptive because of side effects and because it is not 100 percent protective. So if you do need it, be glad it is available but take the experience as a wake-up call to start using an effective method.

There is a website with advice about emergency contraception: www.not-2-late.com. This is a good place to get updated information.

NOW YOU CAN DECIDE WHEN—OR EVEN WHETHER—TO HAVE A PERIOD

When the pill was invented in the 1950s, it was assumed without much thought that it had to be set up so women had their periods every twenty-eight days. However, when a woman is on the pill, it is the pill, not her ovaries, that decides when her period will come. Uterine bleeding occurs whenever levels of estrogen and progesterone drop, as happens with each cycle when the active pills are finished. Most OCs have twenty-one days of active pills; the period starts a couple of days after the last active pill. While a minimum of twenty-one days is needed for reliable contraception, active pills can be taken for much longer. Usually there is no bleeding until the pill is stopped. This means that if you continue the active pills instead of switching to the inactive ones, you can delay your period for as long as you want. This has long been popular with women doctors during training, so that periods will not come during rotations with arduous on-call schedules.

When I present this option to a patient, there are one of two reactions. Either she breaks out in a smile and says, "You mean I don't have to have periods? That sounds great." Or there is a look of concern and something like, "I don't think I'd be comfortable with that." The latter response is not surprising, considering that only for the last few decades of human history has it been possible for a woman to decide for herself when to have a period. Some are understandably concerned that having periods less than monthly will damage the delicate body mechanism that controls the cycle. Fortunately, this never happens. The body will not forget how to have a cycle, no matter how long it goes without one. Yet, there is no reason to use the pill on an extended schedule if you don't want to. In this era when a woman can choose how often to have a period, every twenty-eight days is still a reasonable option.

Only one oral contraceptive is set up for other than once a month bleeding. This is Seasonale, which, unfortunately, is somewhat androgenic. This makes it not a good choice for treatment of testosterone-related skin and hair problems. A major reason for using the pill on an extended schedule is treatment of hair loss, as explained in chapter 4. If you have alopecia or any other androgenic condition, it's better to use a nonandrogenic OC, such as Yasmin, Desogen, Ortho-Cyclen, or

HOW TO HAVE YOUR PERIOD
WHEN *YOU* DECIDE

Any standard OC is fine. (Of the current pills, only Mircette/Kariva is not suitable.)

For reliable contraception you must take at least twenty-one days of active pills in a row. You can take actives for more than twenty-one days, but not fewer.

To bring on your period, you need to stop the active pills for several days. Usually three or four days off will bring on a period, which may be light. To maintain contraception, don't take off more than seven days at a time.

Going many weeks without a period is safe, but it makes spotting more likely.

A regimen that works well for many women is twelve consecutive weeks of active pill taking (which requires four packs), then four to seven days off. If you take off less than seven days, your start day for each pack will change.

Check your pill pack carefully. The pills for the first three weeks pills are active while those for the last week are inactive. The inactive pills are always a different color, but this color is not uniform between brands. If you are in doubt, ask your doctor, nurse, or pharmacist. You will not be safe from pregnancy if you start the pack backward with the inactive pills.

Tri-Cyclen without taking the inactive last seven pills. How to do this is explained in the sidebar above.

The main reason women extend their pill cycles is the convenience of not having monthly bleeding. Some women do it only occasionally to avoid having their period on their honeymoon, vacation, or other special occasion. However, it can also benefit any condition that is helped by preventing dips in estrogen, including hormonal hair loss, migraine, and some kinds of female pain.

Using the pill on an extended schedule actually makes it even more effective for contraception. The downsides are few. Although periods are prevented, there is a greater chance of spotting than with standard pill schedules. This is harmless, but annoying. If you plan pregnancy soon, it may take slightly longer for periods to come back after you stop the pill. There is a consensus among OC experts that continuous pill use is as safe as the standard way. There has been some backlash; a few laypeople, none of whom is an expert on OCs, have raised an alarm that it will somehow harm a woman's body to not menstruate every month. While infrequent periods—when not on the pill—may be a warning sign of an underlying hormonal disorder, infrequent periods on the pill are harmless. When the pill is used in this way, the lining of the uterus, the endomctrium, becomes very thin. It is not that the periods do not get out of the body, but that they do not form in the first place. The endometrium rapidly returns to its normal state once the pill is discontinued.

THE PILL WITHOUT A PILL: HORMONAL CONTRACEPTION WITH THE PATCH, VAGINAL RING, OR IUD

The pill isn't the only form of hormonal contraception. Other types include patches, rings, shots, and the new intrauterine systems (IUS), which contain a form of progesterone. I'll take up the IUS shortly; the others are basically similar to the pill in that they contain forms of the two female hormones, estrogen and progesterone. The only difference is how you use them. Their main advantage is that you do not have to remember to take a pill every day.

The patch Ortho Evra has essentially the same hormones as Ortho Cyclen and Ortho Tri-Cyclen. Instead of taking a pill, you put on a patch and change it once a week. At the end of the third week, you take the patch off and wait a week before starting the next one. Your period will come during this no-patch week. It's important not to forget to start the new patch on time in order to be protected. Some women like the patch because it spares them a nagging anxiety that they will forget a pill and become pregnant. If you like the convenience, the patch is a good method, but if you prefer what is more familiar, the pill is just as good.

Side effects with the patch are similar to the pill. One difference is slightly more breast tenderness during the first two or three months. For most women, this is mild, but if you tend to have problems with painful breasts, I would not recommend the patch for you.

The vaginal ring, NuvaRing, contains hormones similar to those in Desogen and Mircette. It is placed high in the vagina for three weeks—which correspond to the three active weeks of the pill or patch. Then it is removed for a week—when menstruation occurs—and a new one is put in after seven days. Insertion is easy, but does require using your fingers to push it all the way up to your cervix. The NuvaRing has not been extremely popular in the United States. Some women are happy with it, but as with the patch, there is no advantage if you find the idea too odd.

Both the patch and the ring can be used continuously, just as the pill can. You either keep putting a new patch on every week until you are ready to have a period, or, with the ring, insert a new one every four weeks until you decide it's time for your period.

Lunelle is a monthly injectable contraceptive that was introduced in the United States a few years ago, then withdrawn. It is not clear when, if ever, it will be available again. It does not have the problems of Depo-Provera (see the next section) because it contains estrogen as well as progestin. It does not have any particular advantage over other methods, so I don't think its withdrawal is a great loss.

IUDS

The IUD became popular when first introduced, but use plummeted when one such device, the Dalkon Shield, was found to predispose women to infection and possibly uterine injury. This caused a backlash that tarred all IUDs, even those that were safe. Currently available IUDs are much smaller than the Dalkon Shield and rarely cause problems. (Even now controversy remains about the Dalkon Shield; what is important is that contemporary IUDs do not have the risks associated with it.) IUDs containing copper have been used for decades with good results. The newest ones, now called intrauterine "systems," rather than devices, contain a form of progesterone and work by a different mechanism. IUDs alter conditions in the uterus so that the sperm cannot reach the egg to fertilize it. Reliability is high. Merina contains the progestin levonorgestrel. I do not usually recommend OCs with levonorgestrel because it has some testosterone-like activity, but I do not feel this way about Merina because the progestin works directly on the uterine lining; only insignificant amounts find their way into the bloodstream.

The advantage of Merina is that you can have it inserted, then forget about it. Needless to say, it does not provide STD protection. Hormonal conditions that the pill can help, such as alopecia, acne, or PCOS, will not benefit from Merina; it is a contraceptive, nothing else. It does protect the endometrium against cancer if a woman is anovulatory, so it is an alternative to the pill or oral progesterone for this purpose.

Merina is a good alternative for women whose hormonal vulnerability makes the pill intolerable or for those who are sensitive to the latex in condoms. Because the hormone it contains is essentially unabsorbed, it will not set off sensitivities. It can be used even by women who have clotting problems, complex migraine, or other reasons to absolutely avoid the pill, patch, or ring.

THE CONTRACEPTIVE TO AVOID: DEPO-PROVERA

This one sounds great: You get a shot every three months, and you have 100 percent reliable contraception. It does not sound so great when you talk to some women who have used it. Depo-Provera (depot medroxyprogesterone acetate, or depot-MPA) is the injectable form of the synthetic progestin, Provera, which is notorious for producing mood changes. I had one patient who hated it so much that after switching to natural progesterone, she told me, "I don't ever want to hear the word Provera again." It's one thing if you take Provera in pill form for hormone therapy (it does not work for contraception) because you can stop it any time and its effects will quickly wear off. But the injection takes more than three months to get out of your body, a long time to wait if it makes you feel depressed. In addition, Depo-Provera lowers your estrogen levels, which can result in vaginal dryness and even bone loss. Some women stop having periods on it, which is okay, but others have frequent, light spotting, which can be aggravating. In men it has been used to turn off sex drive, and it may have this effect on some women. It may even cause weight gain.

If you are asking, "Why would anyone take this?" then you have gotten my message. The only advantage of Depo-Provera is that once you've had the shot, you don't need to think about contraception again for three months. This makes sense only for women who absolutely cannot remember pills or patches and especially for women in third world countries, where difficult living conditions make pill use complicated. For women in these unfortunate circumstances, the side effects of Depo-Provera may be better than giving birth to more children than they can support.

THE WOMAN'S QUICK GUIDE TO THE BEST—AND WORST—HORMONAL CONTRACEPTIVES

All OCs *work* for prevention of pregnancy, which is after all, why most women take them. Because there are now so many available, choosing can be somewhat overwhelming. Usually women simply take what is prescribed for them, and most do fine. But if you are hormonally vulnerable, which pill you are on may spell the difference between feeling great with clear skin and full hair or being tearful and bloated all the time. Information about pill differences is extremely hard to find, so I've given you the full details here. I have not hesitated to give my personal opinions because these are based on my experience treating several thousand women with particularly delicate hormonal constitutions.

THE BEST PILLS

Yasmin is currently the most widely used OC in the United States and is definitely at the top of the list. It has no testosterone-like effect because its progestin is similar to spironolactone, a testosterone blocker that I discuss at length in chapter 20. Spotting is infrequent. Another advantage is a tendency to soothe PMS symptoms, which makes it the one to try first if you are hormonally vulnerable. Even on Yasmin a few feel more emotional; there is no perfect OC for all women.

Ortho-Cyclen and Ortho Tri-Cyclen Sprintec, MonoNessa, and Tri-Nessa are generic versions. Norgestimate, the progestin in these OCs, has no testosterone-like activity. Like other nonandrogenic pills, these lower the active form of testosterone by about 50 percent, which is why they help clear acne. I was the lead investigator for the original study of Ortho Tri-Cyclen as treatment for acne and can testify that most women are happy with it. Cycle control is good. The only difference between Cyclen and Tri-Cyclen is that the latter varies the progestin dose slightly during the cycle. I see no advantage to deliberately introducing hormone swings, and so I generally prefer Cyclen to Tri-Cyclen.

Ortho Tri-Cyclen Lo is Tri-Cyclen with a slightly lower estrogen dose. It is fine for contraception but possibly not quite as good if you are taking the pill for a therapeutic reason, such as acne or PCOS.

Desogen is also non-androgenic and a good overall pill. The differences from Cyclen and Tri-Cyclen are small.

Mircette is a unique OC because it has active estrogen for twenty-six days out of twenty-eight, rather than only twenty-one. The advantage is that hormone levels are more even throughout the month. This is particularly good for migraine and when taken in perimenopause to supplement estrogen. The estrogen dose is low—only 20 micrograms—but bleeding problems are less common than with other pills with similar estrogen doses.

THE MIDDLE PILLS

Ovcon 35 has the lowest amount of progestin. For women with mood changes on other pills, it is sometimes the only one tolerable. However, Yasmin is a better bet to try first.

Ortho-Novum 1/35, Ortho 7-7-7, with many generic versions, contain the progestin norethindrone. These have served many women well in the past but have no real advantages unless you can get them very cheaply.

Nordette has both virtues and vices. It is among the most androgenic of low-dose OCs but is the best for controlling bleeding. If your cycle has been regular on other OCs, there is no reason to consider Nordette. However, if you need an OC but spotted with every other you have tried, Nordette may be your answer.

Diane-35 contains a progestin called cyproterone acetate (CPA, Androcur), which is a testosterone blocker. It is not available in the United States but is widely used throughout the world, and many women obtain it from Canada. CPA is a very effective testosterone blocker, but the amount contained in Diane-35 is too small to have much effect. The risk of blood clots with Diane-35 may be slightly higher than most other OCs. I do not think it has any advantages over nonandrogenic pills available in the United States, such as Yasmin, Desogen, Ortho Cyclen, or Tri-Cyclen.

THE WORST PILLS

These all work for birth control, of course, and many women feel fine on them. But for the hormonally vulnerable, other options are better. Nonetheless, if you are on one of these pills and not having any problems, there is no urgent reason to switch.

Loestrin 1/20 was, until recently, marketed heavily for women in their forties. Spotting is frequent. The low estrogen dose—implied by the name—has no safety advantages. Its cousin, Loestrin 1.5/30, is not particularly low in dose and has too much mood-unfriendly progestin.

Alesse is a low-dose pill with the androgenic progestin, levonorgestrel. Spotting is common. Although it is often prescribed, I can think of no advantage whatsoever for this OC.

Lo/Ovral, Levlen, Tri-Levlen, Levlite, and innumerable generic versions all contain the same progestin levonorgestrel contained in Alesse. Except for Nordette, already mentioned for bleeding problems, there is no advantage to any of these pills.

PUTTING IT ALL TOGETHER: QUICK GUIDE TO CHOOSING THE PILL BEST FOR YOUR BODY

Contraception: They all work. Yasmin or Ortho-Cyclen would be my picks, with Desogen a close third.

Weight gain: Yasmin and Ortho Tri-Cyclen have not caused weight gain in controlled studies.

Mood swings: Three options here. Yasmin is the best to try first. If you don't like that, you could try the low estrogen Mircette or the low progestin Ovcon 35. If your problems are estrogen-related (breast tenderness or nausea), I suggest Mircette. If progestin-related (moodiness), I suggest Ovcon 35.

Spotting on the pill: If you've tried several pills but none kept your cycle regular, Nordette will probably control your spotting, though it has some testosterone-like activity.

PCOS: Any of the nonandrogenic pills—Yasmin, Ortho-Cyclen, or Desogen—are suitable.

Migraine: Mircette has active pills for twenty-six days, instead of only twenty-one. This means it avoids the sharp and prolonged estrogen drop that other pills produce. If Mircette does not work, then using a different pill on an extended schedule as explained earlier in this chapter is the next thing to try.

Breast tenderness: Mircette, because it has the lowest estrogen dose of the nonandrogenic pills.

Age forty or older: A host of very low-dose pills have been hawked for this age group. However, they are no safer and have no particular advantage for women over forty. Mircette is the best of the very low-dose pills. Yasmin, OrthoCyclen, and Desogen are just as good choices for most women.

Cost: Generics work just as well as brand-name pills, so don't hesitate to use one if the price is better.

5.

The Week from Hell: PMS and Other Hormonal Miseries

THE HORMONE PROBLEM MEN DREAD

Josie was a homemaker who came to see me because she had started having mood swings. "I used to be a little weepy for a day or two before my period, but it was no big deal. Now I often cry a lot for no reason, and, even worse, I'm a real witch at home. And not just for a couple of days, now it's the whole second half of the month. It doesn't make sense. We recently moved to a new house, which I love. My husband is good to me, and we have two wonderful children. I don't like feeling the way I do for those two weeks, and I'm starting to worry about how long my husband will put up with me. The children notice too—they've learned to stay away from me on those days."

What was happening to Josie is pretty typical of premenstrual syndrome—PMS. Sad and angry emotions run wild. Of course, mood swings can signal that there is something wrong in a woman's life. More often, though, life is fine, but hormones aren't. Antidepressants are heavily promoted for PMS, but there are also a variety of herbal and natural hormonal approaches that I'll explain fully in the next chapter.

Josie felt her PMS had reached the point where her life would be in crisis if she did not get immediate relief. For this reason, she opted, not without some reluctance, for an antidepressant rather than slower-acting herbs and supplements. The first medication she tried upset her stomach. Luckily, a second, similar medication did not cause side effects, and when she came back to see me a month later, Josie was actually smiling. "I think I'm on the right track. I feel like I used to, and my family says I'm back to my normal, easy-going self."

An after-note: A year later, her husband came to see me. He reported that he had started to have mood problems, in part related to difficulties with his business. He attempted a smile, "I've seen how much the medication helped Josie; I'm hoping it can do the same for me." Women get most of the bad press for mood swings, but men can have them too.

Though many doctors—and even some women lucky enough not to have it—have dismissed PMS as imaginary, it is all too real. It's true that studies haven't shown definite differences in hormone levels between women with PMS and those fortunate ones who stay on an even keel throughout the month. This doesn't mean, however, that hormones aren't at the root of PMS. Recent research has shown beyond any doubt that *PMS is due to hormonal vulnerability.* PMS-afflicted women have the same fluctuations in estrogen and progesterone that other women do; however, their brain chemistry is more sensitive to these shifts. These brain chemicals cannot be measured in blood tests. Animal research is no help here because, so far as we can tell, lab animals do not get PMS (though a horse breeder once told me that mares do). Fortunately, even though we cannot directly measure the disruptions in brain chemistry during PMS time, we do know ways to calm them. Careful recording of symptoms can provide the information needed to design a regimen to stabilize these neurochemical shifts.

You may have come across the term PMDD (premenstrual dysphoric disorder), the more extreme form of PMS. This term has a very elaborate, multipage definition in DSM-IV, the official manual of psychiatric diagnosis. I prefer the older and more familiar term PMS, for premenstrual syndrome, because it includes physical as well as mental symptoms. There is an unfortunate tendency in medicine to rename things that are not understood, hoping that having a new name will hide the lack of knowledge. Basically, it does not matter whether it's called PMS or PMDD; it's still miserable. More elaborate diagnostic criteria can make it harder to get treatment, as fewer women who really do have the syndrome meet the definition.

THE HISTORY OF PMS

Presumably PMS has been around as long as there have been women, which archaeologists estimate has been about 100,000 years. We don't know about women in ancient times, but more recent records suggest that some famous women in history had PMS. Queen Victoria was a notorious PMS sufferer, and at "that time of the month," could reduce her ministers, among whom were the most powerful men in the world, to abject terror.

Yet, it is only in the past fifty years that PMS has been clearly recognized as a common problem in otherwise quite normal women. The first reference in medical literature was a paper by Dr. R. T. Frank of New York, who termed it "premenstrual tension," a phrase still occasionally encountered. But it was the British physician Dr. Katharina Dalton who first brought PMS into widespread public awareness. Dr. Dalton published her first medical paper on the subject in 1953 and subsequently established a clinic for this condition at University College Hospital, London. Dalton was a charismatic figure who did much to publicize PMS, including using it as a defense in a famous murder trial. This legal use of PMS was not entirely novel, however, as there are several court cases from the nineteenth century that accepted "blocked" menstruation as exculpatory for women who had murdered children. The use of PMS as a legal defense has actually kept the syndrome from being taken seriously because it created a backlash. The public felt, quite reasonably, that hormones do not excuse murder. Although women with PMS feel out of control, this manifests as verbal outbursts, not physical violence. Nonetheless, the loss of control in PMS can be destructive to important relationships.

Excusing violent crimes on the basis of PMS suggests both recognition that some women seem to have diminished self-control at certain times of their cycle and perpetuation of ancient superstitions that misconstrue menstruation to be the elimination of poisons from the body. The presumption seems to be that if the menstrual blood does not flow out, it will travel up to the brain and cause a sort of temporary insanity. This is completely fallacious, of course. Yet, a primitive terror of menstrual blood persists, especially on the part of men, although I've even known nurses who become distressed at the sight of menstrual discharge. (Needless to say, these women had the good sense not to specialize in gynecology.) Taboos against menstruating women were once widespread and included beliefs that menstrual blood could destroy crops, dull mirrors, cause cows to abort, turn wine sour, and even put out fires.

Though women with PMS, as well as those of us in medicine who try to help them, owe a great debt to Dr. Dalton, her influence has not been entirely beneficial. It is vital to a woman's well-being that PMS be recognized as a very real entity, one that can be effectively treated. It is fair to expect men to make allowances for women at these times. However, the use of PMS as a defense in murder trials tends to discredit women as being unable to control themselves in the face of hormonal storms. It reinforces the myth that hormones render women unsuitable for positions of high responsibility. This attitude has gone underground but has not been eliminated. Objective research has shown that PMS, while trying, is not generally incapacitating. Queen Victoria suffered from PMS, yet was held in awe throughout the world during her long reign. In our own time, studies show that overall functioning is not much affected by the cycle. For example, it has been shown that schoolgirls' academic performance is not affected by the stage of the cycle. Nor have studies shown that women are any more likely to commit crimes while premenstrual.

It is important to be clear about this. *PMS does not make women less capable than men, nor does it cause academic or career failure or crime. What it does do is make life much harder for women and, it must be admitted, for those around them.* Women afflicted with PMS must expend greater energy to maintain emotional control and meet others' expectations when they have PMS. They can carry on effectively, though they often fear that their self-control will slip. Fortunately, social attitudes are improving. Menstruation and PMS have mostly lost their stigma; most women talk about their periods without embarrassment. True, there are still PMS jokes, but they at least show that the topic is no longer taboo.

Ironically, PMS is better recognized in popular culture than within the medical profession; it is still an uphill struggle for affected women to get themselves taken seriously. I've lectured to doctors about PMS for many years and have gotten used to it receiving much less interest than the "real" diseases I also lecture about. (Nurses usually show more interest, not only because most are women, but also because they tend to be attentive to quality-of-life issues.) Behind the medical neglect is what I term "hormonal pessimism," the attitude on the part of many in health care that women can't do anything about their hormones except put up with them. This is the attitude, usually unconscious, that having a woman's body means not feeling well a lot of the time and that there is little that can be done about it—and, anyway, doctors have more important conditions to attend to.

I hear instances of this nearly every day. One woman I know, who lives in the United Kingdom and must get her health care from a system more concerned with reducing costs than with helping people, had periods that lasted ten days each month, of which the first two were accompanied by incapacitating pain. Her gynecologist, a woman, told her that her ten-day periods and severe monthly pain were normal for her. This was inexcusable. The solution was simple: Going on the right birth control pill solved both problems. Her doctor just did not want to bother.

This uncaring attitude is widespread. Consider this statement from the prestigious *Mayo Clinic Family Health Book* (David E. Larson, M.D., ed., William Morrow, 1996): "PMS can be hard to tolerate but, because it does not reflect any harmful underlying disease, it is not considered serious. There is no cure for it except menopause—although it usually disappears of its own accord before that." It's difficult to imagine a comment less helpful or more expressive of the condescending attitude held by so many in the health care establishment. Yes, PMS *is* less serious than cancer—but affected women still have a right to relief.

Odds are that if you are hormonally vulnerable, you have encountered this hormonal pessimism more than once. Though the women's movement has done much to reverse patronizing attitudes toward women, they survive in subtle form. The strong voices of women physicians have done much to increase recognition of the importance of quality-of-life problems. Yet, not all the doctors who disregard them are men.

I've summarized some of the ways doctors dismiss women's concerns in the following sidebar.

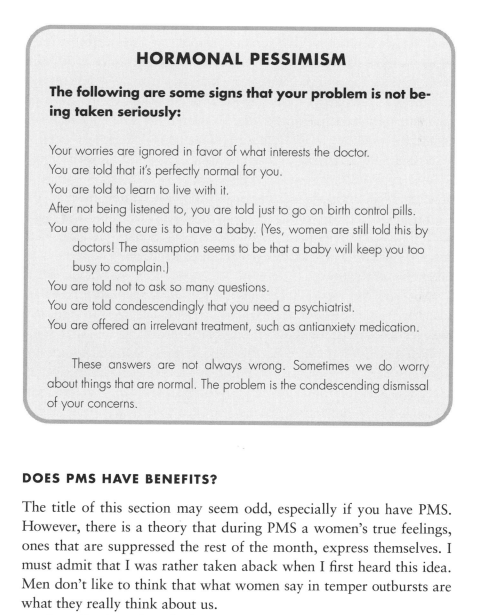

HORMONAL PESSIMISM

The following are some signs that your problem is not being taken seriously:

Your worries are ignored in favor of what interests the doctor.

You are told that it's perfectly normal for you.

You are told to learn to live with it.

After not being listened to, you are told just to go on birth control pills.

You are told the cure is to have a baby. (Yes, women are still told this by doctors! The assumption seems to be that a baby will keep you too busy to complain.)

You are told not to ask so many questions.

You are told condescendingly that you need a psychiatrist.

You are offered an irrelevant treatment, such as antianxiety medication.

These answers are not always wrong. Sometimes we do worry about things that are normal. The problem is the condescending dismissal of your concerns.

DOES PMS HAVE BENEFITS?

The title of this section may seem odd, especially if you have PMS. However, there is a theory that during PMS a women's true feelings, ones that are suppressed the rest of the month, express themselves. I must admit that I was rather taken aback when I first heard this idea. Men don't like to think that what women say in temper outbursts are what they really think about us.

On reflection, though this theory has a grain of truth, I do not think it is helpful. For one thing, the many patients I see for PMS do not tell me that they like the feelings they have premenstrually. They are usually baffled that, despite truly loving their children and husbands, they become infuriated with them during the premenstrual week. Indeed, this relationship damaging potential of PMS is what affected women most fear. We all have angry feelings toward those we love, yet we also know that just because of our love we often must suppress these feelings. PMS time may be an opportunity to be with these feelings for a while, but giving way to them can be disruptive and threaten a woman's most important relationships. If there are relationship problems, the time to discuss them is not when one feels out of control.

Significantly, PMS causes more problems at home than with friends or at work. With those with whom we are most intimate, our guard is down and our emotions, both positive and negative, flow more freely. As a result, it is those whom a woman most loves who are most likely to be the targets of her premenstrual loss of emotional control. Indeed, it is a sign that PMS is really getting out of hand when it starts to be taken out on coworkers.

Another PMS theory holds that the late luteal phase may be a particularly creative time for some women, perhaps because the hormonal changes are similar to those of very early pregnancy. Even if some women get their best ideas at this time, it may be a better time for thinking than doing because PMS diminishes patience and consumes energy. The notion that curing PMS deprives a woman of creativity is dubious, to say the least. I have never been told by a patient whose PMS I had helped that her inner life suffered as a result.

HELPING YOURSELF GET HELP

Experiencing PMS can feel like being trapped in a maze. So many things are happening that you feel helpless to escape. You can get back in control, however. The first step is paying attention to how you feel. Is the main problem mood swings or physical discomfort? Or do you have both? When during your cycle does each symptom occur? Though PMS is internal, in the sense that your hormones are the primary cause, external events often trigger or exacerbate symptoms. I often hear

EFFECTS OF PMS

Feelings

Anger

Irritability

Frustration

Dissatisfaction with yourself or others

Sadness

Crying for no reason

Fatigue

Sluggishness

Anxiety

Dizziness, light-headedness

Insomnia

Decreased sexual desire (sometimes increased)

Food cravings

Physical symptoms

Weight gain

Bloating

Edema (fluid retention)

Breast discomfort

Cramps

Pelvic fullness or aching

Discomfort with intercourse

Increase in hormonal skin problems (puffiness, oiliness, acne, unwanted hair, hair shedding)

Headache, including migraine

Diarrhea or, less commonly, constipation

women with PMS tell me, "I even cry at television commercials." While this may be an exaggeration, it is true that during PMS time, tears tend to flow at trivial matters. It's doubley annoying to know that they are trivial, yet be unable to control oneself. Certain kinds of stress may be harder to take at particular times of your cycle, especially embarrassment or frustration. Nor does PMS affect only the reproductive system; the gastrointestinal tract is affected as well. Foods that normally agree with you may make your insides uncomfortable. Energy and overall bodily comfort may be at their lowest at PMS time.

The sidebar on page 89 may help you sort out the specifics of your PMS. It may be helpful for you to copy this list, mark your specific problems on it, and bring it with you to your doctor.

Most of the symptoms I have listed in the sidebar are common; all women have most of them at one time or another. With PMS, however, symptoms are severe and recur with each cycle. You may be dry-eyed with the greatest of stresses during the first two weeks of your cycle but cry over the least little thing during week four. You may feel fit for three weeks, then out of shape during week four, when you become bloated, sluggish, and have diarrhea. Your dietary discipline may be good most of the month, but then you succumb to uncontrollable munchies as period time approaches.

WHEN DOES PMS HAPPEN?

The standard medical definition of PMS defines it as symptoms occurring only in the luteal phase—that is, the week or ten days before your period. Like many textbook definitions, this one does not always apply in real life. Many of the women I see for PMS problems do report that their symptoms are at their worst late in their cycles, but they can pop up at other times. This is because hormone shifts, though at their worst in the fourth week, can occur at other times during a cycle. To me the timing of symptoms is secondary. They are just as disturbing whenever they occur, and, if they are hormonally triggered, they can be treated in the same way.

A word of caution is needed here. Just as the symptoms in the list are common, they can be due to many conditions other than PMS. Emotional shifts such as sadness and tearfulness may indicate something wrong in your life that needs to be addressed or an underlying bio-chemical depression that is not primarily hormonal. Hormones, of course, can make any form of stress or depression worse. GI symptoms such as diarrhea can be due to irritable bowel syndrome (IBS) or to more serious conditions such as Crohn's disease. If you are fine all month except for PMS week, then symptoms are probably due to hormonal vulnerability, though it is always possible that something else is going on. If the symptoms have no clear relation to your cycle, it is more likely that another condition is contributing. For these reasons, an essential step in dealing with PMS is a medical and gynecological evaluation. Although only a few doctors take a special interest in PMS, most competent physicians can at least rule out other causes.

TOTAL PMS: WHEN HORMONES WON'T LEAVE YOU ALONE

Technically, PMS or PMDD can only be diagnosed when the mood swings and bodily discomforts are confined to the week or so before menstruation. I've already expressed my impatience with this sort of arbitrary, committee-decreed definition. The problem is that women's ovaries do not read the official definitions and don't confine their depredations to that premenstrual week. Unfortunately, there is no medical term for PMS-like problems that occur throughout the cycle, so I have coined the self-contradictory, but useful, term *Total PMS*. Since it does not fit the standard definition, Total PMS tends to be dismissed as depression or neuroticism. Doing so ignores the fact that the symptoms are exactly the same as premenstrual ones, except for when they occur.

Part of the problem is the way the menstrual cycle is taught in textbooks. They all have a diagram that makes the hormone changes look relatively smooth and predictable. What's left unsaid is that these diagrams oversimplify by leaving out the small, but still significant, estrogen fluctuations that occur from day to day and even hour to hour. These surges and drops don't get medical attention because they don't affect fertility. For hormonally vulnerable women, however, these swings can set off exactly the same miseries that would be called PMS, if they occurred during a different week. It's as if women are allowed hormone problems for only one week per cycle. Unfortunately, hormones hang around all month.

These hormonal undulations occur in cycles that are otherwise entirely normal. There is a dogma in endocrinology, which I must admit I too once believed, that if a woman is having regular cycles, her estrogen and progesterone levels must be okay. The question of course is, okay for what? Just because they function for ovulation does not mean they are functioning right for bodily comfort or emotional tranquility.

The lesson that ought to be taught, but isn't, is this: The only way to refine one's understanding of the menstrual cycle is to listen to women. Women doctors need to listen too because what the cycle feels like differs greatly among women. It's easy for women whose cycles are serene to assume that hormonally vulnerable women are simply complaining too much.

PREMENSTRUAL SYNDROME WITHOUT PERIODS?

A standard teaching is that women whose cycles are anovulatory (that is, who do not ovulate) do not suffer from cramps, mid-cycle pain, or PMS. Unfortunately, it doesn't always work out this way. Anovulatory cycles do have hormonal swings that can trigger all sorts of discomforts. Worse, they do not come in a predictable pattern. Many women who miss periods describe feeling as if they should get one but, since it does not come, they do not get the relief that menstruation usually brings. They feel premenstrual but cannot predict when this feeling will end.

I've heard this often enough that I've come to realize that premenstrual syndrome—despite its name—can exist without menstruation. Hormonally it seems to be a variant of Total PMS. Though progesterone is probably not involved, estrogen levels bounce up and down. If you are not having regular periods but do have PMS-like feelings on and off, don't let anyone convince you that they are imaginary. The treatments for PMS that I describe in the next chapter can still work.

A PMS NEAR-DISASTER

Thousands, perhaps millions, of American women's lives are almost destroyed by hormones. While they are basically healthy, they feel unwell so much of the time that life becomes a joyless process of struggling to cope. Often, they have to stop the activities they most enjoy because they just aren't up to them.

When I first saw Laura, she was one of these hormonal casualties. Years back she'd been a successful freelance writer, contributing many pieces to major women's magazines. She'd had a happy relationship with her husband from the beginning. Together they bought a house, and a couple of years later, she became pregnant and gave birth to a healthy baby girl. Then things quickly started to go wrong for her as a result of a severe postpartum depression. Much has been written about this problem, which can unexpectedly strike women who've never had mood problems in their lives. Sad to relate, Laura never bounced back, and six years later she continued to be severely depressed. She wondered why her husband, who stuck with her through these long, difficult years, continued to put up with her. The one area of happiness in her life was her daughter, Jennifer. The best parts of Laura's day were having breakfast with Jennifer and sending her off to school. While her daughter was at school and Laura was alone at home, she felt so tired and despondent she could barely move. Only the expectation of Jennifer's return in the afternoon got Laura through each day. Though Laura would have liked more children, she was warned not to get pregnant because of the risk of even more severe postpartum depression.

Several psychiatrists had done their best to help Laura, and for years she had been on multiple psych meds, which frequently had to be reshuffled to maintain the limited improvement they provided. Finally, just before she came to see me, her psychiatrist, probably frustrated that his treatments were not working, recommended electric shock therapy (ECT, electroconvulsive therapy). Though not quite as bad as it is portrayed in the movies, ECT is the absolute last resort. Laura refused to give up hope. Since her problems were set off by pregnancy and childbirth, she thought that the cause must be hormonal and hoped that there might be a hormonal solution. "I wanted to check this out before even considering electric shock, which terrifies me."

Laura had, in severe form, Total PMS. Mood swings and fatigue occurred throughout her cycle—which was ostensibly normal—not just during the last week. When I saw Laura, I agreed that hormones must be involved in this terrible change in her life. Yet her symptoms fit no established hormonal syndrome, and her extensive hormone tests, done by doctors she'd seen previously, were all normal. Of course normal lab tests are a familiar story for women who are hormonally vulnerable. Given that Laura was in her early forties, an age when estrogen levels start to decline slightly, and that her symptoms were quite compatible with this, I suggested that she start on an estrogen patch. (This was not a hard decision because the well-publicized risks of estrogen do not apply at her age.) I also made some adjustments in her thyroid treatment. The results were striking: Laura's depression started to lift, and for the first time in six years, joy came back into her life. Instead of worrying how she could get through each day, she started to think of resuming her writing career. She continued to use antidepressant medication because hormones may not have been the only factor adversely affecting her brain chemistry. But getting her hormone levels right was the critical step in her recovery.

I don't want to leave the impression that things were quite so simple. I did need to make some reductions in Laura's antidepressant medication, which was making her feel sluggish. And she had the challenging task of regaining self-confidence after the six long years during which hormones had put her life on hold. That she was able to do so is a testament to the courage of this remarkable woman.

ESTROGEN INSTABILITY AS A CAUSE OF HORMONAL VULNERABILITY

Laura's story demonstrates that estrogen does not wait until the perimenopause years to become unstable. Not only do estrogen fluctuations increase with age, the body seems to also become less able to tolerate them. Someone who did not notice swings at twenty-five might find them mildly uncomfortable at thirty-five and be made totally miserable by them at forty-five.

With estrogen instability, what is abnormal is not the levels of estrogen but how suddenly they change. The treatment for estrogen instability is estrogen, paradoxical as it may seem. Supplying the body with a steady stream of estrogen dampens the fluctuations.

Total PMS is harder to recognize than the standard variety but, fortunately, the same treatments usually work. Because Total PMS tends to be worse than the standard variety, you may need to use more of the therapies I list in the next chapter and adhere especially closely to the lifestyle and nutrition guidelines. Prescription antidepressants are more likely to be needed, but they supplement, rather than replace, hormonal treatment and lifestyle measures.

MEN AND HORMONES

It may seem unfair that women's bodies are changing day to day while men's are apparently constant. Actually, men's testosterone levels fluctuate a great deal, and sperm counts are cyclical as well. What is different is that hormonal swings in men are more random. Men, like women, feel better at some times than others. Given the importance of testosterone for well-being, it is plausible that changes in this hormone affect how men feel. The difference is that in men, hormonal shifts don't fall into a regular pattern and, of course, don't have the external marker of menstruation.

Women get an unfair rap for their hormonal swings. It's true that these may make certain days more difficult. But men don't necessarily feel at their best every day, either. Chronically low testosterone levels definitely cause low energy and mood. Then, too, men tend to feel better on days when their sexual feelings are stronger. This might be that sexual thoughts themselves create well-being, or it might be that both are due to there being a little more testosterone. Though men don't have cycles like women, hormones still affect how we feel.

DOING SOMETHING ABOUT PMS

Because I am convinced that hormonal self-understanding is key to overcoming any form of hormonal vulnerability, I have described PMS in detail. Recognizing that your problems are shared by millions of other women is comforting, though it does not solve them. The next chapter explains how you can make your PMS go away.

6.

The Comprehensive Program
for Overcoming *Your* PMS

To start out, there are two very important things I need to tell you about treatment of PMS: First, PMS nearly always gets better. *No matter how much misery you experience every month, no matter how many ineffective treatments you have tried, no matter how many times you have felt hopeless, you can feel yourself again.* Second, the cure for PMS is usually not one big thing but a combination of seemingly little ones. For this reason, I will go into considerable detail about a wide variety of PMS remedies. Some may be right for you, while others won't be. I've used this menu approach so that you can see all the options and choose which are right for you.

What will work for you depends not only on your biology but also on your lifestyle and values. Some women, like Josie in the previous chapter, may opt for the relatively quick effect and predictability of antidepressants. Others may prefer to work with lifestyle change and natural remedies. For those who find them harmonious, spiritual practices can be very helpful with PMS and can be combined with other modalities. For others, like Laura, who had been prescribed virtually every antidepressant with only slight relief, adjusting hormones was the only recourse.

What I have found most effective for PMS is a four-pronged approach: lifestyle, nutrition, herbs and supplements, and prescription medication. No woman will need all the treatments I cover, nor is there a single treatment that will work for everyone who reads this book. Since there are many options, you may get the most out of this chapter by reading through it once quickly, then returning to those sections that relate to you. *The key to successful treatment is a plan that is customized for your specific PMS.*

OVERVIEW: THE FOUR WAYS TO ESCAPE PMS

Lifestyle: Your way of life does not cause PMS, but it contributes to it. If you are hormonally vulnerable, you may not get away with the poor lifestyle choices—such as erratic meals and sleep—that some of your friends do. A consistent routine helps pacify wild hormones.

Nutrition: Eating right is not just good for overall health, it avoids provoking your hormones. Skipping meals is a common way busy women make their own PMS worse. Though carbohydrates have been demonized as of late, they can be therapeutic for PMS—if consumed in a healthful way.

Herbs and supplements: Thousands are available, but only a few actually work for PMS. You need to know which ones are worth trying, or you'll just waste your time and money.

Prescription medications: Antidepressants can work for PMS, but they're only one option. Spironolactone prevents fluid retention and is hormone-soothing. Estrogen supplementation, even before menopause, may suppress disruptive hormone surges. Since some medications such as strong diuretics and progesterone, especially synthetic forms, can make matters worse, it's just as important to know what *not* to take.

THE FOUR-POINT COMPREHENSIVE PLAN
FOR PMS RECOVERY

The four-point plan that I detail in the pages that follow is not an inflexible set of restrictions but a menu of options to guide you in developing a plan that fits your needs. Most who follow this program find that they start to feel better quite quickly—usually within one or two cycles. However, complete recovery usually takes somewhat longer, in part because strange as it may seem, it can take a while to get used to living with *you* being in control, rather than your hormones. It also takes time to get over that nagging anxiety that PMS will strike again next month. Because treatment addresses multiple factors at once, you may not know which part of the treatment made the biggest difference. In my view, this matters less than actually getting better. Someday, we'll know all about how hormonal vulnerability produces PMS. In the meantime, fortunately, we do know how to alleviate it.

Though prescription medication is only one part of the plan, the first step is a thorough medical evaluation to be sure there are no significant underlying hormonal or other disorders present. This evaluation ideally includes a thorough discussion of your past health history, current lifestyle, and nutrition, as well as the specific symptoms you are having and what triggers them. Your life situation and relationships should also be taken into account. Most doctors are not familiar with the intricacies of PMS treatment. Ideally, you will find one who is. If not, however, you can still apply the remedies I describe. Only a few require prescriptions, and for these you can ask your gynecologist or primary care practitioner. Here, as in so many forms of hormonal vulnerability, you will need to be your own advocate. This chapter will prepare you to do so.

The next important step is setting aside *hormonal pessimism,* the belief that having a woman's body means not feeling well a lot of the time and that nothing can be done about it. Many doctors assume this unconsciously, and some women get exposed to this attitude so often that they come to accept it themselves. In fact, hormonal pessimism is a fallacy and a dangerous one, since it may lead to unnecessarily accepting the status quo.

One frustrating aspect of PMS is how long it takes to see if a treatment is helping; the unit of time is not hours or days but an entire cycle. A headache remedy may work in half an hour, but it takes at least one cycle and sometimes several to see if a PMS treatment is helping. Because PMS is so variable, adjustments are often necessary to fine-tune your regimen as your body and hormones change. Here, as in so much of life, patience pays great benefits.

LIFESTYLE

Some of the most important steps in controlling PMS are simple, commonsense things that most of us need to be reminded about from time to time. In fact, some of the advice I give regarding lifestyle may sound like things your mother told you. Lifestyle advice used to come from mothers and grandmothers. Now, however, they are not always close at hand. Too, women's lives have changed so much in recent generations that what was good advice fifty years ago may be hard to apply now.

Self-awareness means being more conscious about how one's actions affect one's life on both a physical and spiritual level. My study of Eastern philosophies has convinced me that all of us have an instinctive knowledge of what is good for us, though this tends to be obscured by the stress and bustle of modern life. Cultivating this self-knowledge is desirable for everything, but especially when your mind and body give out confusing signals, as happens with PMS.

Eastern philosophies have much to teach us in the West because they have always given the highest priority to development of awareness of our true selves and its interaction with the universe. In Chinese philosophy this is referred to as knowledge of the Dao, or Way. The Way is many things: the road we travel in life, how we live, our ethics, the principles by which our bodies and the natural world operate, and, most of all, the wisdom to understand these things. When we do not feel well or are swept up in negative emotion, we can feel as if we are completely lost. Yet as the great Chinese philosopher Zhuangzi taught, although the Way may seem hidden, it is always there. By connecting with our innate knowledge of the Way, we can feel in harmony with life again. Cultivating this is particularly helpful with PMS, in which getting back a sense of control is so important. Some of the many practices your can use to cultivate self-knowledge, including prayer and meditation, are explained in chapter 28. You can find one that will fit your values and beliefs. Taking up one of these practices can augment the effectiveness of the other modes of treatment I describe.

If you have PMS, you may think that your hormones force you to be all too conscious of how you feel. You might think it would be better to be *less* aware. However, experiencing unpleasant feelings and sensations does not automatically mean recognizing what triggers them or what relieves them. A key part of lifestyle change is becoming conscious of behaviors that seem harmless but contribute to the instability of PMS.

Many pick up poor health behaviors in their teens and early twenties, only to discover sometime in their thirties that they can't get away with them anymore. Skipping meals, missing sleep, and taking in too much caffeine and alcohol are common examples. Smoking is particularly disruptive, not only to the lungs, but also to the nervous system. Cigarettes can seem cool when you are young but have decidedly uncool effects if you persist in using them. Bad habits such as these contribute to PMS, which is often a wake-up call that it's time to make changes in your life. Because bodies don't last forever, the sooner one learns to care for oneself, the better. Becoming more aware of how both internal and external factors affect your PMS helps you to adjust your lifestyle accordingly.

Here, then, are suggestions for lifestyle improvements as part of your comprehensive PMS recovery plan.

Consistency in timing of cyclic biological functions—such as sleeping, eating, working, and relaxing—helps mood and energy stay consistent. You may have tuned out your mother's admonitions to go to bed on time, not miss meals, not subsist on junk food, and so on. In adulthood, consistency becomes particularly difficult with the demands of school and work or career and family. The answer is not to stop doing what is important to you, but to impose as much order as you can on your routine.

The importance of sleep tends to be underestimated. In the heyday of the Freudian era, mood problems were diagnosed by interpreting dreams using rather fanciful theories. Now it seems what matters is not what happens in your dreams as simply having enough time to dream. A recent study found that the most important factors dragging down the mood of normal people were sleep deprivation and deadlines. (I am well aware of the unpleasant effects of both of these as I struggle to complete this book on time.)

Our culture tends to encourage resisting biological needs such as sleep because they seem to waste time that could be better spent in work or fun. Actually, the need for sleep interferes less if you have enough. This does not mean never staying up late, but it does mean trying to keep to a pattern as much as possible. Especially during PMS time, don't compromise on sleep if you can help it.

Most adults do not sleep as well as they would like. There is no single answer for this, especially since sleeping pills can be addictive. An essential lifestyle factor is to allow a period of calm before bedtime. This means not only no work from the office and no balancing the checkbook, but also no TV and no alarming newspaper articles. Ideally, the hour or two before bedtime—or as much time as you can free up—should be like a mini-vacation. A warm bath, chamomile tea, light reading, soft music—and sex—are all good ways to relax.

In addition to mental stress, physical pain is a common, though usually overlooked, factor in sleep disturbance. Aches you do not even notice during the day may become tormenting at night, when the brain becomes more sensitive to pain messages from the entire body. Slightly sore legs from a day on your feet, or stiff neck and shoulders from too many hours at the computer, are common enemies of sound sleep. When sleep is troubled by mild pain, NSAIDs, fully described in chapter 7, can make it more restful.

Timing of activities is always important, but especially so if you have PMS. Several of the most esteemed classics of Chinese philosophy, such as the *Tao Te Ching* and *I Ching*, pound home a simple message: The way to accomplish things is to learn to choose the optimal time to attempt them. Americans tend to want to be active all the time, but the ancient Chinese recognized that at times even the most ambitious person should withdraw from activity and await more favorable circumstances. Although Chinese philosophers did not mention PMS, their advice can be applied to it. Some women mark on their calendar or PDA when they expect to have PMS and try to avoid scheduling critical work activities as much as possible during these times. This may seem like giving in to PMS, and, in a way, it is. More important, it is respecting your body's needs. In chapter 3, I emphasized that normal cycles are not as regular as clockwork. Thus, PMS cannot be absolutely predicted. However, if you note the day PMS begins in your current cycle, you know that about four weeks later it may come back and can plan accordingly.

The problem is, of course, that few women are completely in control of their schedules. A century ago, well-off women could take to bed whenever they felt out of sorts. Few now have—or want—the luxury of turning menstruation into a holiday. Following the PMS recovery plan described in this chapter will result in your being much less limited by your hormones and far less bound by the calendar. Still, it is prudent to be as easy on yourself as you can during the most vulnerable days of your cycle.

Exercise Even twenty to thirty minutes of exercise is extremely effective in lifting mood. If you cannot exercise as well during the difficult times of your cycle, remember that some is better than none. Accept that your exercise tolerance will be a little less when you feel moody and bloated—this does not mean you are getting out of shape. An uncomfortable body cannot perform as much. Professional athletes have to push themselves through pain, but if you are exercising for health to do so is pointless.

For mood and mental well-being, thirty minutes of brisk walking or more intense activity such as cycling, jogging, or swimming three to five times a week will give considerable benefit. Exercising more, while it may be beneficial in other ways, will not necessarily further boost your mood. Overtraining can deplete energy and contribute to depression. Although exercise is one of the best ways to maintain mood, it is not a cure-all for mood swings or depression. If low mood persists, despite adequate exercise, you will need to use additional measures.

Stress reduction techniques Just as traditional societies recognized the need to attune human activity to natural rhythms, they also cultivated the natural healing abilities of both body and mind. In the past, self-cultivation practices were secret and taught only to a chosen few; fortunately they are now available for all who are willing to invest the slight time and effort needed to learn them. Everyone can benefit, but PMS sufferers especially so. Such practices include sitting meditation, yoga, tai chi, and regular prayer. All involve a lowering of activity level, which makes some people anxious at first, especially Type A personalities who are always on the go. By the standards of our fast-paced world, these practices seem to work gradually, but they do work. More detailed instructions can be found in chapter 28.

Even women with very positive outlooks find themselves surprised and disturbed by the negative thoughts provoked by hormones. For those not used to such thoughts, they can be alarming and guilt-provoking. There is a simple meditative practice that works well in this situation. Pick a powerful spiritual being with whom you feel a close connection and offer any negative emotion—such as anger, bitterness, self-blame for losing your temper—to her or him. The spiritual being might be Jehovah, Jesus, the Virgin Mary, the Buddha, Tara, the Great Goddess—even the ferocious Hindu goddess Kali, if you are in a particularly angry mood. What is important is that you feel this being's presence in your life. The basis of this practice is the desire of these beings to aid us; their spiritual power makes them able to take on our difficulties without the least strain. So next time you blow up at your children, apologize of course and make every effort not to do it again, but, instead of clinging to your anger and guilt, offer them to a higher power to dispose of. Negative emotions tend to be self-perpetuating, so letting go of them in this way greatly reduces their power over you. Note that letting go is a way to get quick relief; it is not a substitute for dealing with real problems.

Insight Sometimes the anger that comes out with PMS has a real basis. When you are calmer, ask yourself if your annoyance has a justifiable cause and what might be done to improve the relationship in which the anger has been festering. Or there may be an accumulation of frustrations, several of which need to be addressed. The problems may not be major, but just enough to push you over the edge when you are also coping with hormone shifts. Sometimes women are made to feel that being angry is their fault when it is actually quite justified. If your anger does have a real basis, you need to work on correcting the situation that is causing it. Hormones cause irritability, but not chronic anger.

Recognizing perfectionism and establishing priorities Many women feel that having PMS makes them failures. If you frequently feel angry at yourself for not doing everything right, then you are a perfectionist. I have become convinced that perfectionism is one of the most energy-sapping burdens that our culture inflicts on women. By perfectionism I don't mean high standards; rather, it is the feeling that *everything* one does, in every aspect of one's life, must be perfect. Women tend to be perfectionists about their bodies—can you think of anyone you know who is 100 percent satisfied with her shape and appearance? You may think the beautiful actresses and models on magazine covers are happy with how they look, but I assure you that they are among the most insecure. Housework is another area where much time and energy may be drained away in the drive for perfection. Having previously practiced pediatric endocrinology for many years, I am the last person to say that nurturing children is not important. Yet here, too, trying to get *everything* exactly right leads to frustration.

If, as you read this, you are thinking, "I'm not a perfectionist because I often fail to do things right," you have just confirmed beyond any doubt that you are. The true perfectionist never feels good about herself because she never meets her own standards.

Setting up standards you never meet does not encourage you to be a better person; on the contrary, it demoralizes you and saps your energy. An important part of overcoming PMS is setting priorities. All of us want to do more than we can. You'll get more out of life if you focus on the tasks that are truly important, and your family members will be happier, too.

Men can be perfectionists too, but women are more vulnerable because they are so often engaged in multitasking. Men tend to focus on one or a few important areas. At work they want to do well and advance. At home men want happy, healthy children, good meals, and good sex, but only a few pay much attention to the actual details of how these are brought about—except for the sex. To be sure, roles are changing, but for most the old division of labor still lingers. Men's priority setting tends to leave many things for the woman that won't get done unless she does them herself. The more tasks there are, the harder it is to do them all perfectly, and the greater the toll taken by perfectionism.

There are two things you can do about perfectionism. The first is to base your self-esteem on what is really important in each critical life area: the well-being of your family, the key courses if you are in school, those aspects of your work that are likely to be watched by supervisors, and recreation that actually gives you pleasure and satisfaction. Second, once you have started to let go of the need to do everything perfectly, get in the habit, before taking up a task, of asking yourself if it really needs to be done, and if it does, how well it has to be done. Some tedious tasks, such as paying bills on time, need to be done; others, such as cleaning the basement, can usually wait.

Moving beyond perfectionism involves a certain degree of pain because you have to accept not doing certain things as well as you would like to—and could if you had more time. However, careful goal selection pays off in feeling better and accomplishing more.

Lack of satisfaction Not all unhappiness is due to hormones, but hormones can make all unhappiness worse. If your relationship does not meet your needs, if your work is tedious or your boss oppressive, you are not going to feel good. Nearly all people have times in their lives when they feel trapped, imprisoned by obligations that they do not want but cannot escape. Energy can be completely consumed by the unsatisfying routine. Hormones can make you feel even more helpless. You probably know what you need to do: look for a new job, go back to school, find or end a relationship, set limits on family demands. Yet the energy needed to make these changes just isn't there. Treating hormones won't cure a life that leaves you unfulfilled. However, taking steps to correct hormonal vulnerability may be a prerequisite to recovering the energy and optimism you need to make changes in your life.

Goals are good but can be intimidating. It helps greatly to plan to do things in small steps. An ancient Chinese proverb reminds us that "a journey of a thousand miles begins with the ground under your feet." If you have gotten to the point of feeling unable to make life changes you know are necessary for happiness, an outside perspective is probably needed. Friends can help, but some may feel threatened by your proposed life changes and so may not give good advice. Or, with good intentions, they may just give blanket assurance that everything will be fine.

WHAT ABOUT PSYCHOTHERAPY FOR PMS?

Sometimes therapy is part of the treatment for PMS, not because the mood swings are all in your head, but to help overcome the demoralization that can result from years of struggling with hormonal vulnerability. I said *part* of the treatment because talk therapy will not change your hormones. Seeing a good therapist can help you find your way out if you feel trapped but is not a substitute for getting help for the underlying hormonal vulnerability.

Finding a good therapist is not always easy because style and competence vary greatly. It is particularly hard to find someone who can appreciate that your problems are as much organic as psychological. Studies show that if a therapist is going to be able to help, the client starts to feel better within the first few visits. My suggestion is not to succumb to the myth that psychotherapy is complex and esoteric. It is mostly common sense, and if your therapist seems lacking in that area, look for help elsewhere. *If you feel the therapist does not understand you, is unsympathetic, or does not share your values, he or she probably is not the right one for you.* The psychotherapy literature is replete with discussions of "resistance," which refer to the client resisting the suggestions of the therapist. Though there can be reluctance to face painful truths, more often clients resist because they are getting bad advice. If seeing the therapist makes you feel worse, the relationship is not benefiting you, and you should look elsewhere. The human psyche is delicate and precious and should not be laid open to anyone who does not deserve your trust.

NUTRITION

Frequent meals One day while walking in Central Park, I spent some time watching squirrels. Since it is late fall, all were already quite plump while they scurried around seeking a last few acorns to munch before hibernating. Squirrels, bears, and many other mammals can store up food, then go months practically without eating. We humans, however, cannot; many of us cannot comfortably go more than two or three hours without eating. Like sleep, regular eating is a biological necessity against which many rebel. Some feel positively virtuous when they skip meals; it shows how serious they are about dieting or how devoted they are to their work.

It is important to realize that fasting can trigger the release of stress hormones, such as adrenaline. This hormone not only prepares the body for emergencies, but also makes you feel as if you've just experienced one. Skipping lunch can set off the same adrenalin surge as a near-miss car crash. Our primitive protective mechanisms react the same way to a mild blood sugar drop as they do to a life-threatening event. If you have PMS or any other form of hormonal vulnerability, you'll feel a lot calmer if you don't go more than two or three hours without eating. If you are thin or if you typically feel yourself hitting the wall at certain times of day—11:00 A.M. and 3:00 P.M. are common ones—you'll do much better if you eat a small snack during mid-morning and mid-afternoon. The best time is at least thirty minutes before your usual slump. Good choices are one or two crackers with cheese or peanut butter, raisins and nuts, or an apple. Since healthy snack foods are not always available, it is prudent to carry your own.

If this suggestion is generating anxieties of weight gain, let me clarify that the snack is not in addition to what you would eat at a regular meal but is subtracted from it. You don't eat more in the course of a day but spread it out into five instead of three feedings. Research shows that eating small amounts less frequently is easier on weight than the same amount divided into the usual three-meal-a-day schedule. If you've been raised to think snacks are self-indulgent, remember that this is therapy, not loss of self-control.

Vegetarian diets can be beneficial for women with PMS. Avoiding meat seems to have an overall calming effect, though this may in part be that those who choose to become vegetarian tend to do other things, such as meditation, to improve their serenity. I suspect a biological basis, however, because animal protein and fat are much harder to digest than those from vegetable or even dairy sources. When the body uses more energy to break down food, less is available for voluntary activity. Heavy or hard-to-digest meals introduce yet another sort of internal chemical fluctuation. If you have PMS, it's best to stick to foods you know from experience are friendly to your insides, especially during the premenstrual week.

Though I am a vegetarian myself, I am the first to admit that many people feel deprived on this sort of diet. If you feel unsatisfied on a vegetarian diet, health benefits can still be obtained from simply reducing red meat. Most women have some changes in intestinal function before and during menstruation, and so it is best to stick to easy-to-digest foods—which can include fish and chicken—and avoid high-fat meals.

If you are considering becoming vegetarian, it is best to do so gradually, to give your body time to adjust. There are several books on vegetarianism that describe how to do this. Nutrition is another area in which it is easy to be undone by perfectionism. To change from the standard American diet to an ideal one is very difficult. Keep in mind that any move in the right direction will be beneficial for you. Nutrition need not be perfect to be healthy.

Soy Despite recent alarmist claims, soy is one of the healthiest foods you can eat. It seems to have a soothing effect on hormones, as shown by the fact that it can reduce menopausal hot flashes. I do not recommend soy in pill or capsule form from health food stores because these lack adequate amounts of the healthy substances contained in tofu or fresh soy milk. One cup of tofu or two cups of fresh soy milk a day is sufficient to give you adequate amounts of isoflavonoids and soy protein.

Despite all the antisoy propaganda, evidence of harm is lacking. The main evidence for health benefit is the much lower incidence of breast and prostate cancer in Japan. Japanese are generally much calmer than Americans, too; while culture is undoubtedly a factor, diet probably is as well.

Carbohydrates The low-carb fad is based on sound principles but ignores the fact that low-carb eating is not the best way for everyone. Many women notice that they crave carbs during PMS time.

Because carbohydrates have a soothing effect on mood and anxiety, Dr. Katharina Dalton recommended that PMS sufferers consume some carb-containing food every three hours. This may be overdoing it, but the principle is sound. I've provided some guidelines in the following sidebar.

CARBOHYDRATE GUIDELINES FOR WOMEN WHO ARE AT THEIR NORMAL WEIGHTS

Eat less, more often. This avoids setting off hormonal alarm systems.

Unless you have a condition such as PCOS, in which carbs should be avoided, include a modest amount with each meal. Good choices include fruit or whole grain bread.

Allow yourself healthy comfort foods such as fruit.

Don't replace real meals with sweets. A small amount at the end of a meal is okay because absorption then is slower.

Try to avoid binging. If you are hungry and irritable because you skipped a meal, eat a modest amount, then give it time to make you feel better. The Buddha's advice to his monks and nuns is good for everyone: Stop eating six bites before you are full.

Try to minimize high-fat foods such as red meat and duck, as they increase GI symptoms and bloating.

Limit or, if possible, eliminate alcohol and caffeine. If you need coffee to get going in the morning, one cup is okay.

Comfort foods Not all foods that make you feel good are unhealthy. Hot soup and fresh fruits or juices are good choices. Some chocolate has health-promoting effects. Small amounts are mood-soothing, but chocolate is not a good idea unless you can stop before you overdo it. Cocoa is probably a better way to get the mood benefits because it is less likely to be taken in excess. Contrary to general belief, cocoa's caffeine content is negligible. Substances called flavonoids, which are naturally present in cocoa, act as antioxidants and have slight positive effects on cholesterol. They may be removed in processing, so it's hard to tell which forms of cocoa and chocolate have health benefits—and there's plenty of controversy here. Dove dark chocolate bars and Cocoa Via products are processed to retain the flavonoids. There may be others as well.

Water and salt During the second half of the cycle, fluid and salt balance can be disrupted by several hormones. A progesterone-related hormone, 17-hydroxyprogesterone, promotes loss of salt, which sounds good, except that this provokes release of another hormone, aldosterone, which takes over and causes retention of salt. The brain compounds your troubles by making you crave salt, just when you are most worried you'll swell up.

Good water intake helps, though it does not cure, PMS. If you are someone who just does not remember to drink water, measure out one and a half liters (or quarts) every morning and make sure you have finished it by the end of the day. With sodium, things are more individual. Depending on which hormones win out in their premenstrual struggle, aldosterone (which clings to salt) to 17-hydroxyprogesterone (which flushes it out), you may need to restrict salt or increase it. The choice is not actually difficult and does not require measuring your hormone or sodium levels. If during PMS week or the first days of your period you tend to feel light-headed, weak, or dizzy, the salt-losing hormones are in charge at this time, and your energy may be better if you salt your food lightly. Most women with this pattern of premenstrual salt loss are quite thin. On the other hand, if you are twenty-five or more pounds overweight, and certainly if you have high blood pressure, increasing salt is not usually a good idea.

If your premenstrual week brings on ankle swelling and a bloated sensation, then aldosterone is winning the contest and causing you to retain more salt than you need. In this instance, doing your best to limit salt will help. This is one of those medical recommendations that sounds easy to follow but in practice is not for two reasons. First, salt craving accompanies fluid retention, and, second, low-salt food can be hard to find. Not only fast food but also virtually all restaurant and prepared food is high in salt. Even some foods that are otherwise quite

healthy, such as soups, tend to be high in sodium. Only if you can prepare your own food can you be absolutely sure that the salt content is
low. Fruit and salad are low in salt, although dressing may be high, so
it should be used sparingly.

Though premenstrual fluid retention seems like a cruel trick of nature, there is a purpose to it. Remember that the hormonal events of
weeks three and four of your cycle are designed to prepare your body
for pregnancy. Retention of water and salt is necessary for the increase
in blood volume needed to nurture a developing fetus. Unfortunately,
this happens whether you intend pregnancy that cycle or not.

Some women retain so much fluid premenstrually that they have a
disorder called idiopathic cyclic edema. (Calling a condition "idiopathic" is simply an elegant way to admit that the cause is unknown.
Edema is retained fluid in tissues.) In this condition, fluid retention can
be so extreme that clothes and shoes do not fit. Idiopathic edema is a
form of hormonal vulnerability in which the normal salt-retaining tendency of the luteal phase is greatly exaggerated. There is a temptation
to treat it with strong diuretics (water pills), such as hydrochlorothi-
azidc (Diuril and Dyazide, among others) or, even worse, furosemide
(Lasix). These provide quick initial relief—until the body realizes that
it is being tricked and redoubles its fluid-retaining efforts as the diuretic wears off. The result is an extremely uncomfortable seesawing
between fluid overload and dehydration. For this reason, strong diuretics should be avoided for treatment of premenstrual edema. While
resisting salt is the best thing, it does not always work by itself. The
only really suitable diuretic is spironolactone, which has a gentle diuretic effect without the rebound. It has other benefits for PMS too, as
discussed below with prescription medications.

SUPPLEMENTS

Many women with PMS want to try natural approaches, reasoning
that the menstrual cycle itself is a natural process. There is much sense
in this, and that is why I emphasize lifestyle and nutritional approaches in this chapter. Of late, the unrestricted availability of botanical supplements and vitamins has become too much of a good thing;
so many are available that choosing effective ones becomes a daunting

task. To help you make choices, I emphasize those few for which I've found evidence that they really work. There are surprisingly few well-conducted scientific studies of herbs. I've relied on these whenever possible, supplemented by my experience and the experience of other practitioners whom I respect. Gradually, scientifically sound studies of herbs and vitamins are accumulating. Eventually, the varieties sold should shrink down to a much smaller number that are actually effective. We are not at this point yet unfortunately.

Herbal medication is definitely an area where the consumer must beware. Sales personnel in health food stores are not reliable sources of advice. They are simply trained to sell. GNC, for example, has a sophisticated computer system advising its sales staff on what marketing messages are most effective at the moment. Be wary also of preparations that contain several ingredients. While they seem to be giving you more for your money, actually they give you less. Capsules can only hold so much; the more ingredients they contain, the less you get of each.

VITAMINS AND MINERALS

Multiple vitamins I recommend that all women take a standard women's multiple vitamin with iron. Mainstream brands such as One A Day Within or Centrum or generics are just as good as more expensive ones. All manufacturers buy their raw vitamins from the same group of suppliers. If you are considering buying special vitamin preparations that are supposedly good for specific conditions, check the ingredients list first. Often you'll discover that their ingredients were already present in your multiple anyway. While your multiple should include a maintenance dose of iron, higher therapeutic doses should be avoided unless tests have shown you to be iron deficient.

The medical establishment has traditionally been skeptical about the value of vitamin supplements, arguing that we all get enough in our food. Maybe so, but it's hard to be sure. The old calculations were based on the traditional high-meat American diet, which many people have moved away from. Nor were they designed for very active, but weight-conscious women. It seems to me that taking vitamins is an easy and cheap way to be confident that your nutrition is adequate. Certainly, if you have troublesome PMS, you want to be sure you are not subtly deficient in any vitamins.

VITAMINS AND MINERALS AS THERAPY FOR PMS

Pyridoxine (B$_6$) 100 mg per day. Dr. Katharina Dalton was skeptical of the value of pyridoxine and warned, correctly, that high doses can cause nerve damage. It is still worth a try; however, you must be sure you are not getting more than 100 mg per day from all sources, not just your B$_6$ capsules.

Vitamin E PMS dose: 600 to 800 units per day. Here it's important to read the fine print on the label. The most natural form is mixed tocopherols in the d form, not the d, l form, which is synthetic. It has been thought that vitamin E might be protective against heart disease. Recent studies have failed to confirm this, and one has suggested that more than the usual recommended preventive dose of 400 U per day may actually increase risk very slightly. This study is not consistent with others, however, and so it has been greeted with some skepticism. It's frustrating that research leaves us uncertain about important questions. My suggestion, given the uncertainty, is to continue to use vitamin E only if it makes a definite and significant difference in your PMS.

Calcium (Ca) 1000 to 1500 mg per day has been reported to help, possibly by its stabilizing effect on nerve cells. The citrate is probably best. Use one that includes vitamin D—you need 600 to 800 units per day, but standard multivitamins contain only 400. Although calcium has been recommended as a definitive treatment for PMS, it is not. The problem is failure to make a distinction between mild premenstrual symptoms, which most women have to some degree, and true hormonal vulnerability, in which PMS is highly disruptive. Calcium does help a little, and all women should take it anyway, but calcium is not by itself a complete treatment for major or Total PMS.

Magnesium (Mg) has also been reported to stabilize PMS and probably does. The usual dose is 200 mg orally of Mg citrate. It is also available in combination with calcium. Magnesium improves GI motility, which makes it worth trying if you tend toward bloating or constipation. In larger amounts, it acts as a powerful laxative. If magnesium gives you diarrhea, you should lower the dose until this problem is resolved. It is prudent to first try it when access to a bathroom won't be a problem.

BOTANICALS

Although it is commonly assumed that all natural products are safe, this is far from the case. Because information about safety of herbal medications is extremely limited. I recommend a conservative approach to botanical treatments at this time. An Internet search for reports of ill effects is probably a good idea before starting or continuing use of herbs.

Vitex (chaste tree or chaste berry) has been demonstrated to be effective in several well-designed studies. It evens mood and is one of the best treatments for breast pain. The dose used in the studies, which were done in Germany, was 20 mg of native extract once a day. The extracts available in North America do not seem to be as well standardized, and, therefore, doses are higher. Vitex is definitely among the first things to try for PMS, particularly if you have breast pain.

Evening primrose oil Early experience suggested a mood-soothing effect, but later studies have not confirmed any benefit.

Black cohosh There is evidence of some benefit for menopausal hot flashes, and so black cohosh may help PMS when estrogen instability is a factor, as it often is for women in their forties. Women below the age of forty or on birth control pills are less likely to have low estrogen.

Dong quai Used by hundreds of millions of Chinese women as a female tonic, usually as an ingredient in soup. It is taken for general well-being, rather than for specific symptoms. The name in Chinese is a pun on "time to come back." In traditional China, husbands might be away from their families for years at a time. Chinese women believed that eating dong quai soup would bring them home sooner. This idea is engaging but makes it hard to know whether the supposed benefits of dong quai are real or merely folklore. Scientific studies have not demonstrated benefit, and safety is uncertain.

L-phenylalanine (The l, not the d, l form should be selected.) Dose is 1000 mg in morning and 500 mg at night. This is a precursor of several brain neurotransmitters. There is not much published research, but a nurse midwife I worked with has found it helpful for some of her patients with PMS.

L-tryptophan was once widely used to help sleep, but deaths occurred due to toxic contaminants in some preparations. Supposedly the problem was solved, but I think it best not to take a chance.

Eleutherococcus (Siberian ginseng) This is not actually related to Asian ginseng except that both have a rather exotic taste and odor. It is said to be an adaptogen—that is, to improve a person's ability to deal with intense stress. The Russian cosmonauts apparently used it. It is worth a try if you have any degree of chronic fatigue, but, like most herbs, it works gradually.

American (Wisconsin) ginseng In traditional Asian medicine, ginseng strengthens yang and is therefore mainly for men. I'm not sure whether this represents wisdom or just sexism. There is, however, universal agreement that Wisconsin ginseng is suitable for both women and men. I like the tea bags made by Ten Ren Tea Company, which has stores in most Chinatowns. The Ginsana brand also has a good reputation. Raw root is available in many Chinese grocery stores, but English language instructions for preparation do not seem to exist. I suggest that you avoid the extremely expensive forms sold in Chinese herbal stores, unless you are a ginseng expert.

Immune system enhancers Some herbs, such as echinacea and pau d'arco have been recommended to boost immune functioning. My experience is that echinacea can work to stave off colds, although formal studies have been inconsistent. There is less information about pau d'arco. There is no reason to think that PMS has anything to do with immune deficiency, and so tinkering with the immune system does not seem prudent. Chronic fatigue is often attributed to immune problems but is more often due to the interaction of hormonal vulnerability with a high level of external demands.

Hypericum (St. John's Wort) This is widely used for mood problems. A recent, seemingly well-designed study showed efficacy for mild depression. Other studies have failed to show benefits for major depression. Improvement of mood is gradual, but safety has not been adequately studied. Side effects and drug interactions can occur with hypericum. It is not clear that hypericum is any safer than prescription antidepressants, and its effectiveness is less consistent. One problem may be variation between preparations.

Choosing which herbs and supplements to take The best evidence is probably for Vitex and calcium. Magnesium, natural vitamin E, and black cohosh also have some support. I suggest trying only a few alternative remedies at one time. It is easy to go into a health food store intending to buy one preparation and go out with a full shopping bag. This is costly and, if you feel better, you won't know which product helped you. There's also little information about interactions between supplements.

Safety of supplements Not all botanicals and vitamin preparations are safe. Some plants are poisonous and even herbs that are safe in themselves may be adulterated with pesticides and other toxins. Not long ago a Chinese herbal preparation that seemed to be effective against prostate cancer was found to be contaminated with rat poison. The State of California analyzed a large number of Chinese patent medicines and found that about a third contained poisonous heavy metals such as arsenic, mercury, and lead. Indian Ayurvedic preparations also may contain mercury or other toxic metals. It is lamentable that purity problems prevent us from getting the benefits of the Chinese and Indian traditions of botanical medicine.

Vitamins A, D, B_6, and possibly E are proven toxic in large amounts.

Despite the popularization of high-dose C by Linus Pauling, one of the great scientific geniuses of the past century, research has failed to confirm any benefit, and a recent study suggests that large doses may be harmful. The safety of taking other vitamins in high doses is generally uncertain because only recently have they come available in unlimited amounts; previously, vitamins were only obtainable in foods. It is chemical technology that has made them available as pills and capsules.

My suggestion is to use vitamins and supplements that have been around for at least a few years and resist the hyped-up claims for new supplements until they have been tested over time. It is prudent to first research a product online to see if there are reports of safety concerns. Although alternative medicine has much to offer, you need to exercise the same cautions you would about anything else you put in your body.

MORE ALTERNATIVE APPROACHES

Acupuncture can be worth a try, but it is time-consuming and expensive. I've had mixed reports from my patients who have tried it. Some have benefited, while others told me it made no difference. One problem is that acupuncture treatments are not standardized, so the same condition may be treated in quite different ways.

Acupuncturists, as well as herbalists, tend to say they have success with any condition they are asked about. No treatment works for everything, and so such claims should be interpreted with caution.

Be sure to pick a practitioner who is state licensed and uses disposable needles. There have been reports of needles being inserted too far into the chest wall, causing a dangerous condition called pneumothorax in which the lung becomes compressed, and surgery is necessary. Accordingly, common sense suggests that needle insertion into the chest wall be avoided.

Massage Massage therapy enhances overall well-being, and so it is not surprising that studies have demonstrated that it helps PMS. The benefit is entirely dependent on the skill of the therapist and how well he or she can attune him or herself to you. If you find someone good, massage is an excellent treatment, with the main problem being cost.

If pain is part of your problem, massage directed at trigger points such as acupressure, tui-na, or amma often works very well and lasts longer than merely soothing massage such as deep tissue or Swedish.

Some bodywork techniques claim to transfer energy from the therapist to the client. In my experience, only a few truly talented practitioners are effective at this. I don't think energy healing cures diseases, but some find that it enhances well-being. If something safe makes you feel better, then scientific proof is beside the point.

Fasting and detoxification Fasting is one of many ancient practices that has enjoyed a revival. Most mystical traditions employ some form of food restriction as a practice for spiritual development. It is also a very old healing modality, particularly in Ayurveda (traditional Indian medicine). It's important to keep in mind that religious fasting practices are intended to develop the ability to resist the demands of the body and are, therefore, too rigorous to be used for healing. If you want to try fasting as a spiritual exercise, it is best done on a retreat or other setting in which external demands are minimal. If you cannot tolerate missing meals, fasting is likely to be an unnecessary strain on your metabolism and probably is not for you. A day or two of eating lightly, but frequently, is a good alternative.

While orthodox medicine does not support the idea that toxins accumulate and need to be removed from the body, fasting and related techniques have become increasingly popular. Although some people do get a mood elevating effect from fasting, this usually takes a minimum of several days. Fasting does not mean complete starvation. It is best to take small amounts of food, preferably with easily absorbable carbohydrates, such as fresh fruit juice.

The mild euphoria induced is probably part metabolic and part spiritual. The setting is very important. My own experience was a week in a Thai monastery where only a single daily meal was allowed, at about 6:00 A.M. Refraining from eating was easy, since no food was available. Late in the day we were allowed a very small snack under the pretext that it was medicine. One day this "medicine" was small bottles of orange drink. I noticed that even this trickle of carbohydrate almost immediately improved how I felt. Fasting was workable because the environment was free of demands; nearly all one's time was spent in solitary meditation in a hut. For me to fast during a busy day seeing patients—or even writing a book—would have been far more difficult. The same would, I think, be true for any other kind of work.

If fasting appeals to you, I suggest that you first try it during week one or two of your cycle, when your hormones are quiescent, and at a time when your stress level is low. If you feel worse instead of better, fasting is probably not for you. Slender women and those with hypoglycemia symptoms often do not tolerate fasting well. How your body responds to fasting depends on individual metabolism, but fasting advocates do not necessarily allow for this.

Detoxification is a part of all the traditional healing systems of which I am aware. They range from drinking mineral water thought to have healing properties to sweating, to laxatives of various kinds, or colonic irrigation, which seems to be growing in popularity. Although contemporary orthodox medicine rejects any sort of detoxification as unfounded, such measures have been a part of healing for millennia. There is no scientific proof of benefits, but there is no proof to the contrary either. Some do report feeling better with these practices. Certainly no one should feel that she needs to be detoxified to stay healthy, nor that any disease will be cured thereby. So if you use such procedures or want to try, do so in moderation, and don't forget common sense. If you don't feel well, stop.

PRESCRIPTION MEDICATIONS FOR PMS

Lifestyle, nutrition, and supplements can do a lot for PMS, but many women also need prescription medication for complete relief. In this section, I discuss what medications work for PMS and what side effects to watch for.

Spironolactone (Aldactone) This is probably the single best medication for PMS. It can help hormonally vulnerable women in several ways. First, it blocks aldosterone, the adrenal hormone that causes salt retention and raises blood pressure. As already mentioned, it is the only diuretic suitable for prevention of premenstrual fluid retention. Spiro also blocks testosterone and, therefore, can help with premenstrual acne. (How to use spiro to help skin and hair is discussed in detail in chapter 20.)

For many women, spiro smoothes out mood swings. No one is entirely sure how it does this. Indeed, this benefit was discovered quite by accident when women who were taking it for other reasons reported that their PMS was gone. This may be partly due to its prevention of fluid retention, but I suspect it also works by insulating the brain from progesterone swings. Whatever the reason, spiro often works for PMS.

If you have mild PMS, spiro may be the only medication you need, though it usually works out best if it is combined with a birth control pill. Lifestyle and nutrition will still be important. It's also important to maintain a good water intake when on spiro. If you have tried spiro and did not feel well on it, most likely your water intake was suboptimal. As with all medications, however, spiro is not for everybody, and some women do not like how they feel while taking it. Also, you should not take it unless you are using effective contraception because spiro may not be safe for a fetus.

If your PMS is severe or Total, spiro will probably not be sufficient by itself, though it may be an effective adjunct to other measures.

NSAIDs (nonsteroidal anti-inflammatory drugs) These include Motrin, Advil (ibuprofen), and Aleve (naproxen), which can be very effective for cramps and overall bodily discomfort. If taken from the start of your period, they can also cut down the amount of flow by as much as half. The next chapter details what you need to know to get effective relief from NSAIDs.

Diuretics ("water pills") As I explained above, these get rid of excess fluid, but at a price. By dehydrating you, they set off a new cycle of fluid retention. Spironolactone is the only suitable diuretic for premenstrual fluid retention. As already emphasized, stronger ones, such as furosemide (Lasix), should be avoided.

Progesterone As I mentioned earlier, the PMS pioneer Dr. Katharina Dalton, strongly advocated use of progesterone to treat PMS. Reportedly, upon meeting another doctor for the first time, her first question was, "Do you prescribe progesterone or not?" Dr. Dalton's theory was that in women with PMS, the progesterone rises after ovulation is too weak. This theory is misleading at best. Women who do not make progesterone during their cycles seem to have less PMS than those who ovulate regularly. (They still may have mood swings and bodily discomforts due to estrogen fluctuations.) Further evidence against this theory is the fact that for many women, taking progesterone, for example, as part of postmenopausal hormone therapy, brings on PMS-like symptoms. Although the synthetic forms such as Provera (MPA or medroxyprogesterone acetate) are much worse in this regard, natural progesterone can induce moodiness in some women.

Another problem with progesterone therapy is that treatment becomes very complicated. Dosing schedules can get extremely elaborate. Dr. Dalton felt that oral forms did not work and prescribed progesterone as vaginal suppositories to be inserted as often as six times a day. The base of which the suppositories are made tends to trickle out. Needless to say this is messy; it is hard to imagine carrying out such a treatment if you have anything else to do on those days. Progesterone cream for skin application is now widely promoted, but evidence of efficacy is lacking. Because absorption from creams is inconsistent, blood levels vary widely, introducing yet another hormonal swing—the last thing hormonally vulnerable women need.

I have not found progesterone a good answer for PMS. If absolutely nothing else works, however, it can be tried. Although large-scale clinical trials have not found progesterone effective for PMS, such studies do not exclude the possibility that a small subset might benefit. Progesterone is now available in a well-absorbed oral form, which was not available when Dr. Dalton was practicing.

Estrogen patches These are discussed in chapter 26 on treatment of perimenopause/menopause. For women having estrogen swings, supplementation can even out levels of this hormone. For this purpose, patches are much superior to estrogen pills.

Tranquilizers These include Valium (diazepam), Tranxene (chlorazepate), Xanax (alprazolam), and several others. Because these can be addictive, I don't recommend them unless anxiety is incapacitating. If you are this anxious, I suggest seeking the help of a psychiatrist so that you get the most skillful possible management of your medications.

Antidepressants Although Prozac and related drugs have been a great boon to millions of sufferers from depression, lurid press accounts have frightened many away from trying them. Contrary to this impression, serious problems have been quite rare.

One of the biggest problems with antidepressants is not medical but semantic. In medical use, the term "depression" does not mean quite the same thing it does in ordinary usage. Clinical depression is a *syndrome*—not one symptom but a collection of them. Sadness is only one manifestation among others, which can include fatigue, lack of energy, irritability, insomnia, change in appetite, a sense of being bogged down—or just feeling overall unenthusiastic and blah. Many who have the medical syndrome of depression do not feel particularly sad. Indeed, low energy or lack of enthusiasm seem to be more common than sadness.

What these symptoms have in common is low levels of serotonin in the brain. Antidepressants can help all of them because these medications raise serotonin levels back up to normal. For this reason, antidepressants are not just for depression. Many who benefit are not unhappy, just lacking in zip.

PMS can feel much like depression; what is distinctive about PMS is that it is triggered by hormones. PMS sufferers are usually aware, even on their worst days, that they have no reason to be depressed. Though tearful, they know that life is really fine—except for hormones. This depression is hard to bear, despite the knowledge that it will go away once hormones settle down. Confusion is also part of PMS because mood seems to have nothing to do with what is actually happening in one's life.

It is of course possible to have both PMS and generalized depression. This is doubly difficult because unhappy feelings get even worse as period time approaches. If you are unlucky enough to have this sort of double whammy mood problem, I suggest that you consult an appropriate physician and at least consider antidepressant medication.

Biochemically, the unpleasant mental state during PMS involves the same loss of serotonin that occurs with other kinds of depression.

This is not the whole story, however, because some of the signs of PMS, such as sudden tearfulness over trivial frustrations—or for no reason at all—are much more common in PMS than in clinical depression. PMS also is more likely to involve feeling unappreciated. There is a lot of variation in how people feel with these conditions; my point is the unhappy feelings with PMS are not quite the same as those with clinical depression.

Most currently used antidepressants boost brain serotonin levels by preventing serotonin from being taken back into cells too quickly, hence their name of selective serotonin reuptake inhibitors (SSRIs). SSRIs usually reduce irritability and stabilize mood in PMS. They also boost energy, often dramatically, and dispel the inertia that makes it so hard to get up the initiative to work at important projects. A big plus of antidepressants in the treatment of PMS is that they are relatively quick and can work before you have had time to make adjustments in your lifestyle.

Though you won't find PMS listed in any manual of emergency medicine, it can suddenly becomes a crisis. Sometimes, as for Josie, whose story opened the previous chapter, the day comes when a woman with PMS feels she just cannot stand it any longer. If you are at the end of your tether with PMS, antidepressants are usually the quickest way to get relief.

Most with PMS who take an SSRI feel better, but not all. A few report feeling "wired" or, less often, a sort of apathy. However, only a small minority have such unpleasant reactions. Far more often, women tell me that the SSRI has helped them to feel their normal selves again. Antidepressants do not change anyone's basic disposition; they do not cause euphoria or unnatural happiness. If something bad happens, people still feel normal sadness. What SSRIs do is take away the biochemical sadnesses that have nothing to do with what is happening in one's life.

Deciding about antidepressant medication Many women with PMS are naturally hesitant about taking an antidepressant and not all need one. The decision of whether to try an SSRI generally depends on which symptoms are bothersome and how bad they are. If you feel a little blue for a day or two, but otherwise can go about your life normally, you certainly do not need this kind of medication. Lifestyle adjustments and nutritional measures should be sufficient. But if PMS puts your life on hold every month or seems to threaten relationships or career, it is reasonable to consider trying an antidepressant. You can reassess your need for the medication once you are feeling yourself again. However, if you notice a big improvement, it is probably best to stay on the medication for some time—especially if you are in a situation in which a slump would have serious consequences. For example, if you are facing final exams or starting a new job, it is safest to postpone going off the medication.

Many fear that if they start to take an antidepressant, they will become dependent on it or be stuck having to take it for the rest of their lives. Such fears are understandable but unnecessary. SSRIs and related drugs are not addicting because they do not give a pleasurable high, but simply bring low mood back up to normal. Starting an antidepressant does not commit you to staying on it for any specific period of time. If the medication helps, you may want to keep taking it—but nothing compels you to do so.

Is an SSRI needed all month? SSRIs, and indeed all antidepressants, do not work instantly. In general it takes one to three weeks to notice a difference. An SSRI called Sarafem has been shown to relieve PMS when taken only during the second half of the cycle. (Sarafem is actually Prozac under a different name; the generic name of both is fluoxetine.) This may work if your PMS meets the official definition, which states that you can only have it during the week before your period. If your PMS does not have the good manners to save itself for your premenstrual week, you will probably get a better result from an SSRI if you take it every day. As I've been stressing, the key to overcoming PMS is eliminating fluctuations in your life as much as possible. If you take an SSRI only part of the month, you'll be adding yet another change to your cycle.

Antidepressant side effects Side effects can occur with SSRIs but are generally mild and tolerable. Stomach upset is most common but nearly always goes away within a week or two. More problematic is the restless or anxious feeling a few get from SSRIs. Usually, though,

SSRIs calm anxiety. The wound-up feeling may be due to the improvement in energy SSRIs usually engender. If you've had low energy for a long time, you may feel restless when it starts to come back. Once you get used to the extra energy, you'll be able to find ways to put it to good use.

It is only fair to admit outright that SSRIs sometimes cause weight gain. This is not necessarily a reason not to try them, but if you are concerned about your weight, it makes sense to keep track of whether the medication is causing it to creep up, so you can stop it if your weight starts to climb. Lexapro and Prozac seem least likely to produce weight gain, while Paxil is most likely.

Another unwanted effect of SSRIs is on sexuality. Though most women are unaffected, some do notice less interest and slower arousal. For some women, this does not matter, though others are understandably unhappy about it. Addition of Wellbutrin (bupropion) may help as may so-called PDE-5 inhibitors (a.k.a. Viagra and its relatives). How to get your sexy feelings back again is discussed in detail in chapter 14.

Lately, there has been a lot of publicity about antidepressants possibly increasing suicide risk. Actually, this has been known for decades. What the media accounts leave out is that the suicides are people who were severely depressed, not those with PMS. (If you do find yourself thinking of suicide for any reason, you should seek professional help immediately.)

Which SSRI to try? Obviously, if you are going to take an antidepressant, you must choose a specific one. There do seem to be differences; if you are hormonally vulnerable, the right choice may make the difference between feeling better or feeling worse. Using the following guidelines will improve the odds that the first one you try will be right for you. However, if the first one does not work out, it's definitely worth trying another. There's a limit, though; if you've tried several different ones without benefit or they made you feel worse, SSRIs are probably not the answer for you.

The oldest SSRI, Prozac (fluoxetine), works as well as any. It is now available in relatively inexpensive generic form, so if cost is a concern, this is probably the best one to try. Prozac is considered activating or stimulating, which is great if you are struggling with fatigue but may not be so great if you have problems with anxiety. For some, however, it does help anxiety. Paxil (paroxetine) seems to have a more calming effect but, as I have already warned, it has a definite tendency to cause weight gain. Though also available as a generic, it is more expensive than fluoxetine. Celexa (citalopram) has more side effects than some others, at least in my experience.

Lexapro (escitalopram), a relatively new SSRI, is basically an improved version of Celexa. Of all the SSRIs, so far in my experience, it has the best success rate and the least likelihood of making people feel worse. For these reasons, it is usually the best one to try first. Lexapro also has a big advantage for women: At least for the first six months, it does not cause weight gain. Although more expensive than fluoxetine (generic Prozac), it is less expensive than some of the other branded SSRIs.

Effexor (venlafaxine) belongs to a related group of antidepressants referred to as SNRIs (selective serotonin and norepinephrine reuptake inhibitors). In my experience, Effexor is more likely than the SSRIs to have side effects when first started; however, these usually wear off over a week or two. It may be particularly helpful for obsessive symptoms and concentration difficulties and also has been reported to reduce hot flashes.

Wellbutrin (bupropion) is an antidepressant that is in a family by itself. In my experience, it is one of those things people either love or hate. Some women get a great result from it; others report it makes their flesh crawl. It does have two big advantages: It can help restore sex drive, and it does not cause weight gain. Bupropion is also used to help smoking cessation; for this it is marketed under the name Zyban.

IF YOU'VE TRIED EVERYTHING, AND NOTHING HAS WORKED

There is a last resort treatment for PMS that *always* works, even when nothing else has. It's safe when done properly but is somewhat complicated. This treatment is leuprolide (Lupron), which essentially turns off the menstrual cycle by putting the pituitary into a prepubertal state. The ovary becomes quiescent and hormonal fluctuations cease. Estrogen and progesterone levels drop to the very low levels that are present before puberty or after menopause. Since PMS and all its symptoms are due to the hormonal fluctuations of the cycle, it is logical that stopping these changes will prevent the PMS, and it does.

If you are wondering why I have left leuprolide for last, the reason is that this form of treatment is quite elaborate. To begin with, leuprolide can only be taken by injection. Fortunately, these are only needed every one to three months, but they do hurt. Second, when estrogen levels are lowered, menopausal symptoms such as hot flashes, night sweats, and vaginal dryness usually occur. To prevent these symptoms, as well as other problems from estrogen deficiency, estrogen and progesterone must be added back. This may sound self-defeating—why take one medication to lower hormones and others to restore them? The rationale goes back to the principle that I have stressed all along: The problem with women's hormones is not the hormones themselves but their fluctuations. Lupron treatment abolishes the hormonal surges and slumps that perpetuate PMS.

If PMS makes you seriously ill every month, Lupron may be well worth the effort. One woman I treated this way suffered from unstoppable vomiting each month as her period approached. Standard stomach-settling medications had no effect. Virtually every month she became so dehydrated that she ended up in the hospital plugged into an IV. After going on Lupron, though she did still feel nauseous once in a while, the vomiting stopped, and she could live her life again.

Unfortunately, Lupron is very expensive. If you have life-stopping PMS, it is worth battling your insurance carrier to get it covered. Otherwise, the less radical treatments I've explained in this chapter should be sufficient.

SOME LAST WORDS OF ENCOURAGEMENT

Don't let the cultural cynicism about PMS discourage you. It may take time to find the right doctor and the right treatment program, but PMS virtually always gets better. The best single bit of advice I can give you is to not give up in your search for help. Just as the causes of PMS are multiple, so must the treatments be. The key to PMS is finding the right combination. If you persevere, you'll find relief. Remember, though, that your mind and body will change over time, and this may necessitate adjustments in your regimen to keep you feeling good.

PART III

When Hormones Hurt

Female Pain: Cramps, Endometriosis, Fibromyalgia, and More

THE NATURE OF PAIN

Pain arising from their reproductive organs is a fact of life for most women. The pain may be cramps, twinges at ovulation, or those sudden internal jabs that women feel, but no one seems able to explain. While menstrual cramps usually get better with age, other kinds of pelvic pain tend to get worse during the hormonal years. But just because nearly all women sometimes have pain associated with their reproductive systems, does not mean you have to learn to live with it.

One of the most unfair myths about women is that they have higher pain thresholds than men because they must endure labor and childbirth. Recent research, however, shows the contrary: Women on average have lower pain thresholds. Women have no choice but to learn to cope with pain—the structure of their reproductive systems causes them to experience it frequently. Yet, no matter how well you can cope, recurrent or chronic pain, even if very mild, is energy-sapping. It lowers mood, impairs concentration, and interferes with sleep. Sleep deprivation, in turn, makes pain hurt more. This vicious cycle: pain → poor sleep → more pain → worse sleep, and so on is a major factor in many of the pain syndromes, especially fibromyalgia, that more commonly afflict women.

THE INS AND OUTS OF PAIN:
WHY INTERNAL PAIN IS WORSE

Women often fail to receive sympathy for their pain, especially from doctors and sometimes even from nurses. One reason is hormonal pessimism: The assumption that if you are a woman, you are going to have frequent pain in your life and had better get used to it. But there is another reason that has to do with the difference between the pains that men commonly feel and those that women endure. When healthy men have pain, it is usually relatively external—muscles or bones in the case of injury and the occasional headache or sore throat. Although this sort of pain hurts, it's easy to tell where it is and, usually, what caused it. Though women can have musculoskeletal pain too, specifically female pain is internal, which is physically and psychologically quite different. Because our insides are served by a primitive branch of the nervous system, internal pain cannot be localized except in a vague way—to upper or lower abdomen, pelvic area, front or back. Of course, different kinds of pain can be distinguished to some degree. Certainly a stomachache and a menstrual cramp feel different. But for many internal pains, it's very difficult to tell exactly where they are coming from. They also have a different quality than muscle pain, duller but somehow more pervasive.

Internal pain is insidious, it lingers at the back of one's mind and is all the more unsettling because you cannot tell what's causing it. When one's insides do not feel right, a foreboding arises that something may be seriously amiss. For this reason, internal pain has an emotional, as well as physical, component. Men have internal pain also, but far less often, and when we do, it is usually due to a well-defined disease that can be objectively diagnosed and treated. With women, the border between normal cramps and pathological pain is indistinct. This can be tragic because pain that is harder to diagnose hurts just as much. High-tech imaging studies often do not help because quite severe pain can come from normal structures, if they are hormonally vulnerable. Pain of this sort is too often dismissed as "all in the head" or "psychosomatic" because of failure to recognize that its source is not an injury in a specific area but an interaction between internal organs and hormones.

PAIN PROCESSING

Female pain occurs when estrogen and progesterone act upon the body structures that respond to them. Breasts, uterus, Fallopian tubes, and genitalia are, of course, exquisitely sensitive to these hormones. What tends to be overlooked, however, is the fact that nonreproductive tissues are also responsive to estrogen and progesterone. Skin, hair, muscle, the GI tract, the brain—all are affected. Intestines, for example, are hormonally vulnerable, as shown by the fact that most women tend toward diarrhea during their periods, and irritable bowel syndrome (IBS) is far more common in women. Hormones directly act not only on the organs where the pain occurs, but also affect the pain threshold. It has been clearly shown that this threshold is at its lowest during the week before menstruation—just when you don't want it to be.

High levels of hormones can trigger symptoms, but so can sudden drops. Despite the vital effects of hormone shifts on women's well-being, research on how hormones affect bodily sensation is surprisingly limited. Essential to my education in this area has been listening to women with hormonal problems describe how they feel. Medical journals will not publish this sort of information because they do not consider it scientifically objective.

Here's an example: Once, about a week after I gave a lecture about menopause to doctors, I received a telephone call from a woman who said, "You don't know who I am, but I want to thank you. I'd told my husband, who is a doctor, that it hurt to comb my hair. His answer was that I'm crazy. Now, because you mentioned this very thing in your lecture, he doesn't think I'm crazy anymore." Her husband was not unsympathetic; he'd just never been taught about the changes in sensation that are common with low estrogen levels.

Although mild, this sort of pain is unsettling because it feels so strange. There's no name for this combing-hair-pain syndrome, but there are general medical terms for abnormal sensation. Increased sensation is referred to as "hyperesthesia," while altered or abnormal sensation—things feeling weird or even creepy—is termed "dysesthe-sia." These strange-sounding words share the same root as "anesthe-sia," which means no sensation.

Though most of the time we do not feel pain, our bodies are actu-ally sending off uncomfortable nerve impulses constantly—clothes rub or press against skin, muscles are sore or stiff, our stomachs are too empty or our intestines too full, and so on. Normally, our spinal cords and brains filter out these signals so that we are not disturbed by trivial ones that do not really require our conscious attention. In a sense, these sensations are the spam of our nervous systems—we don't want them, and they serve no purpose but to annoy us. With hyperes-thesia or dysesthesia, this filtering mechanism has too low a threshold, and so discomfort or pain messages get through to consciousness too easily.

Hyperesthesia is the common factor in many female pain conditions, including daily headache (but not migraine), fibromyalgia, irritable bowel syndrome (IBS), and frequent urination. Because hyperesthesia is so common with menopause, it is clear that estrogen changes have pro-found effects on sensation. Hyperesthesia, then, can be a sign of hor-monal vulnerability.

Chronic fatigue is frequent with pain problems, but this connection was overlooked until recently. Pain, even if seemingly mild, results in sleep that is lighter and therefore not fully refreshing. Sleep depriva-tion, in turn, lowers the pain threshold. Before this vicious cycle was understood, there was no explanation for why the same person tended to have several seemingly unrelated forms of pain, as well as fatigue. A common response was to blame the patient and suggest, subtly or not so subtly, that the cause was neuroticism—a meaningless, as well as in-sulting, diagnosis.

Many female pain conditions are due in part to abnormal pain pro-cessing. Instead of being turned out, pain signals are amplified. It is not unlike being forced to listen to music you don't like. Played softly, it is mildly unpleasant; with the volume turned up, it is torture.

Hormone tests usually don't help because, once again, the problem is not the hormones themselves but how the body reacts to them: hor-monal vulnerability. Fortunately, if you have a female pain syndrome, there *are* effective approaches. I give the details later in this chapter.

A WORD OF CAUTION

Hormones can cause pain, but not all pain is hormonal. Any pain that is more than mild, or unexplained, needs medical evaluation. In this chapter, I focus on pain related to hormones because it is so often hard for women to get help for it. There are many other causes of pain that I do not have enough space to cover. In what follows, I am assuming that you have had a thorough workup for your pain and that nonhormonal causes have been ruled out. Pain problems are not for self-diagnosis. This chapter is intended to help the many women who, after serious causes have been ruled out, find that they are left without any treatment to control the pain. My view is that if you do have chronic pain, you have a right to relief.

WHAT WORKS FOR PAIN

Despite the ubiquity of pain, and the desire that we all have to avoid it, the medical profession has tended to undertreat it. So serious is this that the State of California has instituted a requirement that all physicians take a course in pain management. An old, and reprehensible, slogan in medicine is, "Pain never killed anybody." It's true that in certain serious illness, the urgency of other problems requires that pain relief be briefly deferred. This does not justify failing to treat pain, however.

With pain, like any other symptom, the best thing is to treat the cause. Difficulties arise in situations when there is no ready way to do this. With appendicitis, the offending organ can be removed without any loss of function. No one regrets having to do without their appendix. This is not the case, however, when the pain arises from the uterus, intestine, or other vital organs. In such cases, a way must be found to stop the pain without sacrificing a vital part of the body. There are many ways to do this, but they are conceptually more complicated than following the old surgical maxim, "When in doubt, take it out." I have no intent to belittle surgery here; it saved my life when I had a perforated appendix as a medical student. I simply want to explain why pain relief is sometimes more intricate than one would wish.

One bit of advice before I get down to specifics. If you have any of the pain syndromes I discuss, you probably have already tried several treatments, including some that I describe here. If so, you may have found that they did not work well enough. I suggest you be open to trying again because, in my experience, when these treatments fail, it is because they were not properly prescribed or because the directions were not clear. If you are troubled by chronic or recurrent pain, the odds are that one or more of the treatments in this chapter will work for you—but you need to be willing to give them a fair trial.

I've given an overview of treatment approaches in the sidebar on page 137. The remainder explains how they can be used for specific conditions.

MENSTRUAL CRAMPS AND WORSE: PELVIC PAIN

Like acne, menstrual cramps (dysmenorrhea) are too often met with dismissive comments like "You'll grow out of it." This is not much help while you are actually having cramps, especially if you've reached your thirties and are still waiting to grow out of them. Furthermore, more than very mild cramps past the early twenties are definitely not normal and an underlying cause should be sought, especially if they have been getting worse rather than better.

The myometrium, the muscle layer of the uterus, is smooth muscle akin to that in the GI tract; when smooth muscle contracts it tends to be uncomfortable, as with stomachaches or intestinal cramps. Uterine contractions are always painful. Weaker, but still painful, contractions occur with menstruation and, sometimes, with an intense orgasm. Contractions during menstruation serve to help stanch bleeding and expel the menstrual fluid. That these contractions perform a useful function does not make them any less painful. Both the contractions and the pain are due to the effects of a local hormone called prostaglandin F2-alpha that is made within the uterus. Severe cramps are due to too much PGF2-alpha being formed in response to progesterone. Cramps, then, are a form of hormonal vulnerability.

Bad cramps can be effectively treated with an NSAID (discussed below) or an oral contraceptive. NSAIDs work by preventing the formation of PGF2-alpha. Once this substance is formed, however,

APPROACHES TO PAIN

Eliminate the cause When the cause can be found and eliminated, pain is only a temporary problem. Pain due to infection in the bladder or tubes, for example, quickly goes away with antibiotics. For the more difficult forms of female pain, the cause is elusive, making direct treatment impossible.

Suppress inflammation This can be done with NSAIDS, such as ibuprofen (Advil, Motrin) and naproxen (Aleve or Anaprox). Glucocorticoids (cortisone-like medications such as prednisone, that inhibit inflammation) are usually not helpful for female pain syndromes.

Reduce or block hormonal pain triggers Oral contraceptives work in this way for mild pelvic pain. Other, less familiar, medications can lower estrogen or block its effects.

Dull the brain's pain awareness This is how opiates work. Unfortunately, in addition to being addicting, they dull the brain overall and so are mainly useful for severe but temporary pain.

Improve pain filtering in the central nervous system A variety of medications originally developed as antidepressants or anticonvulsants keep pain signals from reaching conscious awareness. Because they do not cause brain fog, they are suitable for long-term use.

Lifestyle Adequate sleep, recreation, regular meals, and exercise raise the pain threshold.

Physical methods These include massage and specific exercises. Biofeedback can help, too.

Spiritual practices Meditation can moderate the distress that pain engenders.

pain will take longer to go away. Hence, it is important to start the medication as soon as you notice any discomfort, rather than waiting to see how bad the cramps will be this cycle. If you do not start the medication quickly, it will still work, but will take longer. NSAIDs have another benefit: They make periods much lighter. Oral contraceptives seem to help cramps by making the uterine lining thinner so that much less PGF2-alpha is produced in it. This thinning makes periods lighter also. It can take more than one cycle for an OC to help your cramps, so don't give up on the pill if it does not help much the first month.

ENDOMETRIOSIS

After menstrual cramps, endometriosis is the commonest cause of pelvic pain. If you have endometriosis, early treatment is important to minimize the chance of it affecting your fertility. Endometriosis pain typically lasts throughout the days of menstrual bleeding, whereas ordinary cramps rarely last past day two of menstruation.

In endometriosis, tiny bits of endometrial tissue become lodged inside the pelvis. Endometriosis seems to be caused by menstrual flow going backward. Bits of the shed tissue then lodge inside the pelvis, where they cause pain by oozing during menstruation and by pressing on nerves. Hormonal vulnerability is involved also because the endometrium of women with endometriosis seems to be overly sensitive to estrogen. Occasionally, endometriosis tissue can lodge itself onto the intestinal wall, resulting in constipation and other symptoms. These extreme degrees of endometriosis are less common today because of much earlier diagnosis and better surgical methods. The most common effect besides pain is infertility, probably by distorting the shape of the tubes and surrounding tissues, making it harder for the egg and sperm to meet and for the fertilized egg to travel into the uterus in timely fashion.

Endometriosis is said to be getting more common. Pregnancy lessens the chance of this condition developing, and so the trend toward fewer and later pregnancies may account, at least in part, for this increased incidence. I suspect, however, that improved diagnosis is also a big factor. Though matters are far from perfect, the health care establishment is becoming more willing to take women seriously when they complain about pain.

If you have pain throughout your period, you probably should be checked for endometriosis, especially if standard measures such as OCs or NSAIDs do not relieve the pain. The only really effective way to check for endometriosis is to have a skilled gynecologist use a laparoscope to look inside, directly at your uterus, ovaries, and surrounding pelvic tissues. This procedure does require general anesthesia, but usually can be done on an outpatient basis. Ultrasound should always be done for pelvic pain, but is not adequate to diagnose endometriosis because the bits of abnormal tissue are usually too small to show up. When endometriosis is found with laparoscopy, it can be vaporized by laser during the same procedure.

Progesterone-like medications have been used for endometriosis when NSAIDs and oral contraceptives do not give adequate relief. The most effective of these, danazol (Danocrine), has significant testosterone-like activity and so can cause increased hair growth and scalp hair loss. For this reason, it is rarely used now, and I do not recommend it. High doses of the synthetic progestin Provera may help, but can cause depression. My own view is that if you have definite endometriosis, laser or other surgical treatment are both more effective and less likely to have adverse effects than these hormonal treatments. For intractable endometriosis pain, hysterectomy with removal of the ovaries is almost always curative, but is obviously the last resort.

FIBROIDS (UTERINE LEIOMYOMATA OR LEIOMYOMAS)

Fibroids are local overgrowths of uterine muscle; they are extremely common in the hormonal years. Very large fibroids can make a woman feel as if she is four months pregnant because the uterus gets just as big. Although they do not cause pain directly, fibroids can make the abdomen protrude uncomfortably and can press on the bladder, causing frequent urination. Less often they can encroach on the rectum or other structures. Fibroids are easily diagnosed by ultrasound. Treatment for fibroids is covered in chapter 3.

ADHESIONS

To put it starkly, adhesions are areas where a person's insides are stuck together. They result from irritation and inflammation inside the pelvis, as may be caused by prior surgery, an infection in the tubes, or a burst appendix or ovarian cyst. Extensive adhesions can cause pain. Diagnosis usually requires laparoscopy. Because adhesions can be hard to find, the procedure should be done by a gynecologist who is experienced in treating this kind of condition. Surgery may consist simply of separating the stuck together areas ("lysis of adhesions"), or in extreme cases, hysterectomy.

The best thing for adhesions is to prevent them. A common preventable cause is infection in the tubes (PID or pelvic inflammatory disease), which is caused by STDs. This is one more reason to practice safer sex. Another preventive, for women who are considering pregnancy in the future, is to avoid any pelvic surgery that is not absolutely necessary. One example of surgery that is generally best avoided is ovarian wedge resection for PCOS. This issue is discussed in chapter 21.

OTHER INTERNAL PAINS

The peritoneum, the lining of the inside of the abdomen, is very delicate, and any fluid leaking onto it can result in pain. This happens commonly at ovulation but can also happen when an ovarian cyst—which you probably were not aware of—pops. Pain from fluid or blood leakage can last from about a half an hour to several hours. This is not something for self-diagnosis; significant abdominal or pelvic pain needs prompt medical evaluation.

Many women have sudden, sharp pains within the abdomen that strikes without warning but lasts only a few minutes. These are disconcerting to say the least. Tests are rarely helpful because the pain is usually gone before they can be done. Most likely they are due to brief spasms of the intestines. Though startling, this sort of pain does not by itself indicate serious underlying disease.

I've mainly covered pain that arises from the female organs. Internal pain can come from several other sources. Irritable bowel syndrome

(IBS) is quite common in women and manifests as pain with variable degrees of diarrhea and/or constipation. It can be exacerbated just before and during menses. Treatment for this has been improving. As I've emphasized, any persistent internal pain should prompt medical evaluation. Pain originating from the gastrointestinal system involves a quite different set of issues that space does not permit me to cover in this book.

BREAST PAIN

Breast tissue is very delicate, and, to aggravate matters, it is placed in an unprotected location in front of the body where it is susceptible to being bumped. Given this, it is hardly surprising that as many as 70 percent of women have some breast pain from time to time. In 10 percent, the pain is enough to sometimes limit activities. Both estrogen and progesterone stimulate the breast, though in different ways, and so both can contribute to mastalgia (the medical term for tender or sore breasts). Both large and small breasts can be affected, though they have somewhat different vulnerabilities. Large breasts put strain on supporting tissue and are more likely to be compressed by tight bras, especially with underwires. Smaller breasts have less fat tissue, leaving the delicate breast tissue less protected.

Breast pain is not a sign of cancer, nor of increased risk of cancer. However, pain does not rule out breast cancer either. If you find a lump, it should be checked out—whether it's painful or not. (Even if you don't have any lumps, don't forget that you should have regular mammograms and breast ultrasounds yearly after age forty. Breast self-exams are a good idea also.)

Mastalgia is yet another instance of hormonal vulnerability. Estrogen and progesterone levels are not elevated, rather the breast is hypersensitive to one or both. There are effective ways to desensitize sore breasts, but as with other forms of hormonal vulnerability, it takes some effort to find a physician who is knowledgeable about treatment. Before jumping to medical treatment, however, you should do something that may seem too obvious to mention: Be sure your bras fit you properly. A recent study found that the majority of women wear bras that are the wrong size for them. A bra that is too loose does not support adequately, while a tight one squeezes tender tissue. Metal underwires are particularly hard on breasts if they are tight.

Most bras are designed for shape, not comfort. The importance of bras is underscored by another study that showed that women who switched to sports bras had substantial reductions in breast soreness. The first step, if your breasts are sore, is to be sure your bra fits; and it's even better to wear a sports bra whenever possible.

Sexual partners responding to the erotic appeal of breasts may not realize how gently they should be handled. Men don't have breasts and so will not necessarily understand that overenthusiastic squeezing is not the best way to appreciate them.

The best single treatment for tender breasts is the herb vitex (chasteberry or chastetree), which has been proven in several excellent German studies to reduce pain. Vitamin E in a dose of 600 mg daily may help as well.

If these simple measures do not restore breast comfort, there is a medication that will: tamoxifen (Nolvadex) in a dose of 10 mg daily. Tamoxifen blocks the effect of estrogen on breast tissue and so relieves the pain. Its primary use is for treatment of estrogen receptor positive breast cancer. It does affect the uterus, however, and may cause erratic bleeding. Tamoxifen slightly increases the risk of uterine cancer in women who take it for several years. Progesterone can be protective; this issue should be discussed with the doctor who prescribes it for you. After a course of three to six months, the tamoxifen can be stopped; usually the pain will not return.

FIBROMYALGIA

Though this condition does not involve the reproductive organs, it is particularly common in hormonally vulnerable women. Fibromyalgia refers to generalized pain in the muscles. Unlike arthritis, it does not directly affect the joints but rather the muscle and fibrous tissue around them. The neck and the area between the shoulder blades are most commonly affected, but all muscles can be involved. Activities that require holding the body in a rigid posture and using the same muscles repetitively can produce this sort of pain. Those who spend hours every day in front of a computer—as I am while writing this book—are particularly vulnerable to this sort of generalized achiness. Muscles feel good when they can move fluidly; they protest when they are held too long in static positions. Evolution did not have computers in mind when it designed our bodies. Some women, however, have fibromyalgia without any clear relation to how they use their muscles.

Fibromyalgia is a pain-processing disorder. Muscles and joints depend on a night of sound sleep to heal from the stretching and pounding they absorb during the day. When sleep is not deep enough, this natural healing process is incomplete, leaving muscles and joints still sore the next day. This situation perpetuates itself because the next night the pain makes sleep shallower. And so on, until something is done to break the cycle.

Often fibromyalgia and chronic fatigue are two aspects of the same condition. Treatment should be directed at both aspects. Adequate therapy with NSAIDs is important. Because daily use can cause stomach irritation and even ulcers, this may be a situation in which celecoxib (Celebrex) should be considered. When fibromyalgia is not constant, it is still best to take the medication for several days after the pain becomes tolerable, because even slight pain may still be enough to interfere with sleep. As discussed below, certain antidepressants are effective in improving the ability of the spinal cord and brain to filter out pain signals. Amitriptyline (Elavil) in low doses of 10 to 50 mg at bedtime is particularly effective for fibromyalgia because it also helps sleep. With chronic pain, sleeping pills and opioids are best avoided or minimized as potentially addicting. However, the herb valerian, which has been used to help sleep since the days of ancient Egypt, is worth a try. Diphenhydramine (Benadryl and generics), a very sedating antihistamine available without prescription, works for some.

GETTING RELIEF FROM PAIN

NSAIDs are the most commonly used pain relievers. Most women have used over-the-counter forms such as Advil (ibuprofen, also available by prescription as Motrin) and Aleve (naproxen). NSAIDS are very effective for cramps and overall bodily discomfort. They also cut down the amount of menstrual flow by as much as half. This contributes a lot to making difficult periods easier.

Prostaglandin F2-alpha, already mentioned as the inciting chemical in menstrual cramps, is the trigger for pain in many other tissues, including muscles. NSAIDs stop production of PGF2-alpha, thereby preventing pain. Once this unpleasant chemical is formed, however, NSAIDs have much less effect. For this reason they work best if you take them early to prevent PGF2-alpha from building up in the first place. Fortunately the evil PGF2-alpha is rapidly eliminated; NSAIDs can still work after pain starts but relief takes longer. For the same reason, it is best to take them often enough so that they do not wear off. If you delay, the pain will return so that you must wait once again while the next dose starts to work.

Choosing the best NSAID depends on how long the pain is expected to last. Ibuprofen is eliminated from the body within two to four hours, so it is mainly good for brief pain, such as headaches. To keep active levels of ibuprofen in your blood, you need to pop them pretty often—at least every four hours. If your menstrual cramps last only a few hours, then ibuprofen will work fine. Women who are hormonally vulnerable, however, typically have cramps which last longer, often several days. To try to keep up with the optimum every four-hour schedule with ibuprofen is virtually impossible. Fortunately, there are several longer-acting alternatives. Naproxen is available without prescription as Aleve or with prescription as Anaprox. Generic forms, which are much cheaper, are just as good.

When I recommend naproxen in the form of Aleve for menstrual cramps, many women tell me that it didn't work when they tried it. I often hear the same about ibuprofen. The difference is that naproxen, if taken right, works really well, whereas ibuprofen often doesn't for just the reason I gave—it doesn't last long enough. The problem with nonprescription naproxen is simply the dose—the 220 mg in each tablet is not nearly enough. As a point of comparison, the standard strength of the prescription form is 550 mg. You can get the same relief with the nonprescription form by taking two and half tablets about every twelve hours. (You may need a pill cutter, available in most pharmacies, to split the tablets.) Naproxen should be continued twice a day until you are past the time of your cycle when you have cramps. Women with very mild cramps may get by taking it only once a day.

If naproxen doesn't do it for you, another NSAID, often prescribed by arthritis specialists and shown to be effective for menstrual pain as well is diclofenac (Voltaren). The dose is 50 mg three times a day.

NSAIDs, COX-2 inhibitors, and your stomach The main problem with NSAIDs is stomach irritation. The can lead to ulcers and even hemorrhage from the stomach. While this is rare in younger women, if you tend to have a queasy stomach or any signs of gastroesophageal reflux (GERD), frequent use of NSAIDs may make matters worse. For this reason, the pharmaceutical industry has developed a class of drugs called COX-2 inhibitors (so-called because they inhibit an enzyme called cyclooxygenase 2) that are easier on the stomach. This group unfortunately includes the now notorious Vioxx (rofecoxib), which increased the risk of heart attacks in elderly patients with arthritis. A similar risk was shown with another COX-2, Celebrex (celecoxib), but only at high doses in patients with advanced cancer, not at the 200 mg once-a-day dose used for menstrual cramps. Until we have more complete information, it is better to use naproxen—which may even reduce heart attack risk—unless you have stomach problems. An even more recent study shows increased risk with naproxen, although earlier studies have shown an aspirin-like protective effect against heart disease. The only honest way to sum up the present state of knowledge is that we do not know whether, or how much, these medications affect heart disease risk. For perspective, keep in mind that the studies were done in mostly older patients with arthritis or cancer. Most likely, there is no risk for younger women who take an NSAID or COX-2 for only a few days per month in normal doses.

Celecoxib is quite expensive, more than two dollars a pill. The dose for cramps is 200 mg twice a day on the first day and then once a day as long as cramps are likely.

I haven't mentioned aspirin or acetaminophen simply because they are not very effective, and if you have read this far, you have almost certainly tried them and found they didn't do the job.

Oral contraceptives OCs have been a mainstay of treatment of menstrual cramps for decades. They prevent the progesterone-induced thickening of the endometrium, which is where prostaglandins are produced. All seem to work equally well, though if the first one tried does not give adequate relief, trying another is reasonable. My experience suggests that the very lowest dose pills do not work as well for cramps, so I suggest first trying one that contains 30 or 35 micrograms of estrogen. (Pill choice is explained in detail in chapter 4)

Some women whose cramps are a manifestation of hormonal vulnerability find that OCs do not give adequate relief. For an unlucky few, the pill gives no relief at all. If this is your situation, addition of an NSAID to the pill is the next step. Endometriosis is a possibility to be considered when cycle pain does not respond to these treatments.

It is not unusual, when starting the pill, to have your first period be somewhat heavier than expected. This seems particularly common with PCOS. The cause is probably that the endometrium was thick when the pill was started, making the menstrual shed more uncomfortable—a thick endometrium churns out more pain-inducing prostaglandins. For subsequent cycles, the OC keeps the endometrium thin so that periods become much easier.

For intractable pain related to estrogen stimulation of vulnerable tissues, leuprolide, already mentioned as the last resort for PMS treatment in chapter 7, may sometimes provide dramatic relief, though it is not always suitable for more than a few months. For this sort of treatment, you should be under the care of a gynecologist with special expertise in pain problems.

Opioids Uncommonly, cycle-related pain can be so severe that narcotic pain relievers are considered. When pain is chronic, these can create more problems than they solve. Opioids produce a groggy state that often makes normal activities impossible. Possible addiction is another concern. In general, it is better to find other ways of pain control.

Neuroactive drugs We think of pain as happening where it hurts. From another perspective, pain occurs in the spinal cord and brain because that is where we are conscious of it. As already explained, we never become aware of most potentially painful sensations because they are filtered out by switching circuits in our spinal cords and lower brains. With chronic pain, this filtering becomes less effective. Because the same kind of signal passes so often through the same neural circuits, they become like a well-traveled path that allows pain impulses to travel to the brain without impediment. Over time, pain becomes a larger and larger part of the person's life. Treatment must then be directed at multiple sources of pain.

Fortunately, there are a number of drugs that seem to work by helping the central nervous system to better filter out pain signals. They can be effective, even though all were originally developed for other brain disorders. One that is often effective in diminishing pain sensations is amitriptyline (Elavil), an older antidepressant. It is quite sedating, a disadvantage for an antidepressant, but a benefit if pain is interfering with sleep. Amitriptyline can have serious cardiac effects at very high doses; however, 25 to 50 mg at bedtime is safe. It absolutely must be kept out of reach of young children. Although the newer antidepressants, the SSRIs and SNRIs discussed in the preceding chapter work better for depression, I have been less impressed by their effect on chronic pain. A new one, duloxetine (Cymbalta), is effective for diabetic nerve pain and so is the best among the SSRIs as an alternative to amitriptyline.

I need to emphasize that the effectiveness of antidepressants does not imply that the pain is imaginary or "all in your head." The reason antidepressants work has to do with improving pain filtering. Depression is often a secondary factor in pain because pain that won't go away is depressing, to say the least. Depression, in turn, lowers the pain threshold. Both pain and lower mood interfere with sleep, and sleep deprivation makes pain and mood worse. This pain-insomnia-depression nexus needs to be interrupted in order for chronic pain to get better. Specific antidepressants such as amitriptyline and duloxetine can help interrupt this disastrous cycle.

If these do not work, certain anticonvulsants can also help chronic pain. Side effects and drug interactions can be significant with the class of drugs, so they are not the first things to try. If you need such measures for chronic pain, you should be under the care of a neurologist or pain specialist.

NATURAL PAIN RELIEF

Although herbs have been recommended for pelvic pain, in my experience they work mainly to ease mild forms. Exercise does help, however, at least with normal menstrual cramps. Meditation or yoga can be very useful. In my experience, the most effective form of meditation for pain control is vipassana, which I explain in the final chapter. This can change the way you experience pain by reducing the distress it causes. A high-tech version of meditation, termed biofeedback, helps too, but unlike meditation it requires special equipment. Pain centers can provide referral for instruction in this technique.

Massage or physical therapy can be very effective for chronic pelvic pain and for fibromyalgia. Ordinary massage, referred to as Swedish or deep-tissue massage, is soothing and can certainly make you feel better. The problem is that the relief is often quite brief, and few can afford—or make time for—a massage every few days. Far more effective are methods to stop the spasm that contributes greatly to many forms of pain. The medical term for this is trigger-point release. With pelvic pain, effective trigger-point release may involve pressure applied near the vulva. Though this is not sexual in nature, it is obviously a sensitive matter. Only a few physical therapists are skilled in such techniques, but if you can find someone who is and with whom you feel comfortable, this can be extremely effective. Some large medical centers have such therapists available, usually through the urology department. The traditional massage techniques that also apply pressure to release spasm include Shiatsu (Japanese) and tui-na and amma (Chinese). The latter is traditionally done by blind people. A skilled practitioner can sense the trouble areas and release them in half an hour or so. Unfortunately, I know of no specific way to find a skilled practitioner other than word of mouth or trial and error.

*   *   *

As with other conditions involving hormonal vulnerability, the quest to find help for chronic female pain can be a long one. As I have indicated in this chapter, however, many effective modalities are available and patience in fine-tuning your regimen will pay off.

8.

When Hormones Go to Your Head: Migraine and Other Headaches

Migraine is another one of those conditions that women figured out was hormonal before doctors did. Almost one in five women suffers from migraine. Headaches become a medical problem when they are very frequent or so severe as to require you to stop your normal activities. I begin this chapter with a patient's story that illustrates both the disruption that migraine can cause, and some of the ways treatment can bring it under control.

MIGRAINE AND THE EVENING NEWS

Valerie was a TV news producer who thrived on excitement and deadlines but felt her career was now threatened by headaches that were so severe she could not work. Unable to drive when an attack hit her, she would ride home in a taxi, hoping with every bump in the road that she would not throw up. Once home, she would lie down in her bedroom with the shades drawn. Val knew to expect a headache for the first three days of her period, but now she had them at other times as well, unpredictably.

We discussed the possible role of stress. "My work is very stressful, but if it weren't, I'd be bored and that would be even worse." Changing to a less demanding job, even if it meant fewer headaches, would not have been the right thing for her.

Because she would have to leave work suddenly in a job with unforgiving deadlines, Valerie was afraid that her career would be in jeopardy if she missed many more days of work. Although she was tough enough to travel to some of the world's worst trouble spots and to work without food or sleep, Val was tearful as she told her story.

Recent studies document that most people who have migraine never get effective treatment. For Val, pain remedies from the drugstore no longer worked, and she was afraid—rightly—to use the narcotic pain reliever she had been prescribed by another physician. We worked out a regimen involving three medications. She took one of these, amlodipine (Norvasc), every day; it prevented most of the attacks, but not the ones during her period. On those days she used an estrogen patch and, sometimes, naratriptan (Amerge), a drug that is particularly good for menstrual migraine. The third medication was for emergencies—sumatriptan (Imitrex) injections that she could give herself on the rare occasions when she was in the field and got a migraine, despite the amlodipine. She'd only needed it twice in the past six months but told me it was her security blanket—when she had it with her, she knew she'd be able to complete her assignment no matter what.

Although Val's treatment was much more elaborate than most migraine sufferers want—or need—it was worth it for her because it enabled her to stay with the job she loved. She no longer worried she'd be thought unreliable by her colleagues in the field.

We now know that menstrual migraine attacks are triggered by sudden drops in estrogen, which cause blood vessels to clamp down, followed by massive release of pain-inducing inflammatory chemicals. Women with menstrual migraine have brain blood vessels that are particularly vulnerable to drops in estrogen. Migraineurs may be sensitive in an artistic sense as well—it has long been observed that there is a link between migraine and creativity. This, however, is not much consolation when one is in the throes of an agonizing attack.

NOT ALL HEADACHES ARE MIGRAINE

All headaches hurt, but not all are migraine. It's important to know what kind of headaches you are having in order to fit the treatment to the cause. Though many think that migraine simply means a severe headache, the term refers to a particular kind of headache that is caused by stretching of the blood vessels around the brain. Migraine can range from mild to severe. Some, but not all, migraine is preceded by an aura—funny feelings, flashing lights, or other visual changes. These go away as the headache begins.

Because migraine is the most common type of severe headache, and the one most linked to hormones, I'll discuss it in detail. First, though, I'll briefly cover some of the other forms of headache that commonly occur in women.

TENSION HEADACHE

Nearly everyone gets tension or muscle-contraction headaches, at least occasionally. Pain results from spasm of the muscles at the sides of the head and back of the neck. Because these muscles must hold our heads up against gravity, they do not get much chance to rest during the day. As the name suggests, tension is a factor, but anything which strains these muscles—such as driving or working at a computer for long hours—can give rise to this kind of headache. The pain can be quite severe, probably because the pain nerves travel a short path from the sore muscles directly into the brain. Muscle-contraction headaches can be related to stress, but they do not necessarily occur on the most stressful days.

Getting upper body and head muscles in shape can reduce contraction headaches. Most exercise, however, emphasizes the lower body. Jogging and cycling won't help must but swimming can. Massage may give temporary relief. Meditation can definitely help. Of medical treatments, NSAIDs work the best. The specific medications for migraine that I discuss in the pages that follow will not help headaches that are due entirely to muscle spasm.

CHRONIC DAILY HEADACHE

Some unlucky people get headaches nearly every day. While migraine can be a factor in these chronic daily headaches, they are not the primary cause. Understandably, people suffering from these frequent headaches take pain relieving medications like acetaminophen or ibuprofen on a continuing basis, but this may perpetuate the problem by lowering the pain threshold. Tapering off the medication, usually with medical supervision, is the only way to stop the headaches.

I vividly recall Irene, a patient I saw for chronic daily headache. She was taking nonprescription pain meds several times a day, every day. I explained that overuse of these medications by lowering her pain threshold perpetuated her headaches and worked out a tapering schedule for her. When Irene returned two months later, she happily reported that her headaches were virtually gone. But she went on to say, "When you told me that the meds were causing the headaches, I went home and cried. It made no sense, and I didn't believe you. But I'd run out of options, so I tried it and to my surprise, it worked."

Irene's story illustrates an important truth about overcoming not only pain but also many other women's conditions as well—treatments have to be given a chance.

COMMON HEADACHE MISDIAGNOSES

While sinus problems are often blamed for headaches, most headaches—including those on the forehead—are not due to sinus problems. Recurrent headaches are not likely to be sinus-related because acute sinus infections are sudden and produce steady pain until cured with antibiotics. Also commonly overdiagnosed are temporomandibular joint (TMJ) disorders. Before concluding that your headaches are due to TMJ and agreeing to surgery or other expensive treatment for it, I suggest consultation with a neurologist who has no financial interest in your decision.

WHAT IS MIGRAINE?

Migraine is a unique form of headache that is due to blood vessel changes inside the head. For reasons we do not understand, these arteries first contract, then overexpand. The contraction phase can produce symptoms referred to as the aura that are due to inadequate blood flow to parts of the brain. Effects of the aura include visual changes, such as spots in front of the eyes or a decrease in visual fields—not being able to see from one side of the eyes. The aura may also produce strange thoughts and feelings that cannot be put into words but which warn of the headache to come. Most auras last a few minutes, but some are longer. In extreme cases, the aura may produce partial paralysis. In this severe form, and when the aura lasts more than an hour, neurological consultation is essential.

So-called "classical migraine" is preceded by an aura. Nonclassical migraine is not. These terms are actually a little misleading because the so-called nonclassical form is actually the most common.

As the blood vessels open up, the aura stops, and the pain begins. There seem to be two factors involved in the pain. When the walls of the arteries, which are made of smooth muscle, stretch, it hurts. To make matters worse, pain-producing inflammatory hormones ooze out of the blood vessels into the surrounding tissues.

A migraine is usually one-sided, at least at first. The pain of migraine is pounding because each heartbeat sends blood surging through the arteries, stretching them more. Light and sound are very bothersome. There may be nausea and even vomiting, which sometimes relieves the headache.

Downtime caused by migraine is considerable. While it is possible to work with a mild migraine, with a bad one, all you can do is go into a dark room and try to sleep. Sleep often relieves the headache, but at the cost of several hours lost from your day.

Most migraine has no ill effects on health, other than the recurrent disability produced by the pain. Rare forms of migraine can have complications, however. The danger is during the aura, when blood flow is decreased and permanent brain injury can occur. This occurs mainly with auras that last longer than one hour or have severe effects, such as partial paralysis. Oral contraceptives may increase stroke risk with these unusual forms of migraine and so are contraindicated. If you have more than mild symptoms during the aura or if your migraine has suddenly become more severe, you should have neurological evaluation. If in doubt, consultation is always the safest course.

HOW HORMONES TRIGGER MIGRAINE

At last, medicine has come to understand how women's hormones can trigger migraine. Because estrogen functions to help keep blood vessels open, a sharp drop in the level of this hormone can lead to arterial narrowing, which is the first event leading to a migraine. All women's estrogen plummets shortly before their periods, and some, as I have stressed, have additional, unscheduled estrogen plunges at other times during their cycles. Not all women get migraine, however, because not all have arteries that are vulnerable to these estrogen slumps. Menstrual migraine is a classic example of hormonal vulnerability in that hormones are normal, but the body's reaction is not. Typically, it starts just before or at the onset of menstrual bleeding because that is the time during the cycle when a woman's estrogen levels are at their lowest. It may seem strange that headaches and menstruation are triggered by the same hormone shifts, but remember that both have to do with blood circulation.

Not all hormonal migraine occur around menstruation. Some women get them at other phases of their cycles, probably because of the unscheduled estrogen swings with which hormonally vulnerable women are all too familiar.

There are other triggers for migraine besides hormones. Stress is one such trigger but, paradoxically, it is often when stress is relieved that the headache begins. Traditionally listed as a precipitant for migraine is the tyramine contained in certain foods, such as aged cheese and red wine. Wine can definitely trigger a headache, as can any form of alcohol. Cheese as a trigger seems much rarer.

GETTING RELIEF FROM MIGRAINE

There are two kinds of migraine treatment: Those that prevent them in the first place, and those that take them away after they have started. Many women with migraine need both. Hormonal treatment is mainly preventative; I'll start with this because it is usually both simple and effective. Then I'll discuss other medical approaches.

Treating the hormonal cause Menstrual migraine has a reputation among neurologists as being difficult to treat. Actually it can be easier to control than some other forms because the headaches are somewhat predictable. Keeping a simple calendar recording when during your cycle the headaches come will help determine the role of hormones in setting off the attacks.

The key to preventing menstrual migraine is stabilizing estrogen levels. There are several ways this can be done. One is to take an oral contraceptive. Sometimes this helps by itself, but for a few, taking the pill the standard way can make migraine worse because of the sharp fall in estrogen after the last active pill (day twenty-one of a cycle). One OC, Mircette (generic Kariva), has active estrogen for twenty-six days per cycle, instead of only twenty-one. This gives more stable levels and is the first choice OC if you have migraine. Another option is to take a standard OC on an extended schedule to avoid the monthly estrogen drop. How you can use OCs with an extended schedule is covered in detail in chapter 4. A third way is to take an OC according to the standard schedule and to use a 0.1 estradiol patch during the week of inactive pills. Climara is a convenient brand because each patch lasts a week—just the length of time you need it. If you do not want to take an OC or it would not be safe for you, you can use an estrogen patch at times of your cycle when estrogen levels tend to drop. One way is to put one on as soon as you feel any signal that your period is coming. The schedule must be individualized, so you really need a doctor who is willing to work with you on this. (Estrogen is contraindicated if you have the severe form of migraine discussed on pages 154 and 155.)

Stabilizing estrogen by one of the methods usually works very well. If it does not work for you or if it stops your menstrual headaches, but you still have them at other times, any of the preventive approaches I describe in a subsequent section can be used.

Medication to stop attacks A variety of new medications have been developed during the past decade to stop migraine. With mild migraine, many get adequate relief from acetaminophen (Tylenol and others) or NSAIDs, such as ibuprofen (Advil) or naproxen (Aleve), which were discussed in the previous chapter. If these work, there is no need for any other medication.

The new migraine medications belong to a family referred to as triptans; they work by reversing the blood vessel stretching that causes the pain. The first fully effective drug was sumatriptan (Imitrex). This is available in oral, injectable, and nasal spray forms. The nasal spray acts almost as quickly as the injection and faster than the tablets, but many dislike the taste. Some of the other newly introduced medications for stopping attacks are dihydroergotamine nasal spray (Migranal), zolmitriptan (Zomig), and rizatriptan (Maxalt), which are tablets. I have not been impressed that one is clearly better than the others, but some find that a particular one works better for them. Maxalt may start to work a little sooner with the first one. If the first one you try is not fully effective, it's worth trying one or two of the others to see if it does the job for you. With any triptan, it is important not to exceed recommended doses.

For migraine sufferers whose headaches usually last longer than a few hours, naratriptan (Amerge) often gives better control because it works for twelve hours, while the others last only three or four. If you have menstrual migraine that lasts for several days, the shorter acting triptans will not give adequate control. If estrogen stabilization has not worked for you, Amerge, in a dose of 2.5 mg every 12 hours usually does.

Side effects with triptans are all too common. Because these medications work by causing blood vessels to constrict, they also decrease blood flow throughout the body. This does not cause permanent problems, but some find the feeling they get from triptans extremely uncomfortable, though hard to describe in words. Those with severe migraine usually feel the pain relief is well worth the odd feelings, but those whose attacks are mild may not. For this reason, I suggest trying other measures, such as hormonal therapy or NSAIDs first.

WHY SOME NEUROLOGISTS CAN'T TREAT MIGRAINE

- Because the brain is the most complex organ in the body, neurology is a highly intricate field. Specialists in neurology, having mastered the extremely intricate workings of the brain, tend to be more interested in diagnosing obscure diseases than in treating common ones.

- Neurologists aren't taught about the menstrual cycle—even though the brain controls it—so they may not feel comfortable working with cycle-related headaches.

- Migraine treatment is as much art as science. Doctors and sufferers need to be patient enough to try different treatments until the best one is found. Often, neurologists aren't interested in this rather unglamorous task.

Neurologists are, however, best at ruling out other serious conditions that may be associated with migraine.

Preventive treatment for migraine Better than making a headache go away is not having it in the first place. If your migraine headaches are infrequent, there is no reason to take daily medication to prevent a headache every few months. But if you are one of the unlucky ones who gets them frequently, preventive treatment may make a big difference in your life. Not all doctors are familiar with preventive treatment for migraine. It is worth searching for a doctor who is; he or she might be a specialist in female hormone problems or a neurologist with a special interest in headache.

Typically, prophylactic treatment for migraine can achieve a 50 percent improvement: half as many headaches that are only half as painful when they do occur. Many get a good enough result that headaches no longer restrict their lives.

Three classes of medications are effective as migraine prophylaxis: beta blockers, calcium channel blockers, and certain anticonvulsants.

Beta blockers include propranolol (Inderal), atenolol (Tenormin), and nadolol (Corgard). I think the second two are slightly better in terms of effectiveness and side effects. Although there is some suspicion that beta blockers can exacerbate low mood and energy, this is uncommon, and many migraine sufferers do quite well with them. Contraindications to beta blockers include asthma and low blood sugar. Calcium channel blockers—such as verapamil (Calan SR) or amlodipine (Norvasc)—seem nearly free of side effects, but their effectiveness may be slightly less than the beta blockers. It is sometimes necessary to try several medications in these classes before you find one that works for you.

Of late, anticonvulsants are being used more frequently for migraine prevention. Those that can be effective include Topamax (topiramate) and Tegretol (carbamazepine). Although these can be extremely effective, they have more potential adverse effects than the other preventive treatments I've discussed. Also, anticonvulsants have many interactions with other drugs, so you need to be sure that anything else you take is compatible. None is safe during pregnancy. If nothing else works, these are a reasonable option but should be prescribed and monitored by physicians experienced in their use.

Coffee and migraine Many migraineurs discover that caffeine can delay or stop attacks. Unfortunately, the effect of caffeine quickly wears off, so that the headache often returns, unless you keep drinking more and more coffee. In fact, caffeine withdrawal can trigger migraine. As a result some heavy coffee drinkers get a migraine if they miss their usual caffeine fix. If you have migraine and are a heavy coffee drinker, caffeine may be perpetuating the problem; decreasing your intake may reduce the headaches. You'll need to taper slowly; I suggest decreasing by a half cup a week. The tapering should be part of an overall treatment plan to control your migraine. If you don't want to do without the smell and taste of coffee, as you taper, you can replace each cup of real coffee with a cup of decaf. Of course, you'll need to consider all sources of caffeine, not just coffee.

Natural treatments for migraine The herb feverfew has been used for migraine prevention. It is certainly worth a try before going on prescription medications. Sometimes it is used together with magnesium and the vitamin riboflavin. However, if your migraine has reached a crisis point, in which you frequently have to leave work or have difficulty managing your children, you may want to start with the prescription treatments. Later on, you can see if natural approaches will maintain the benefit.

Acupuncture is another avenue to look into. One reason I am not more enthusiastic about this technique is the inconvenience; frequent visits to a practitioner are required. But if other measures have not worked, acupuncture is definitely something to consider.

My personal experience suggests that meditation may be effective for migraine. As I discuss in the final chapter, I had migraine headaches since my early teens, but they stopped completely after I had been practicing meditation for a few years. Meditation, like most skills, takes sustained practice; the best time to start is not in the midst of an attack! I'm not sure that meditation will be sufficient by itself for bad hormonal migraine, but it offers a real chance of naturally lessening attacks. Since meditation has many other health benefits, if you are interested, I definitely recommend establishing a regular practice. I provide simple instructions for getting started in chapter 28.

SOME FINAL WORDS OF ENCOURAGEMENT

Research has identified an odd fact about migraine: Most sufferers don't even mention it to their doctors. Presumably, they assume that nothing can be done. I hope that this chapter has convinced you otherwise. If you suffer from migraine, it is definitely worth seeking help.

PART IV

Hormones Make Sex Possible—or Nearly Impossible

9.

Why Have So Many Women Stopped Enjoying Sex?

Women's sexuality has been with us since Adam and Eve. Why then are we hearing so much more about it as of late? Apart from the obvious reason that sex is a perennially exciting subject, sex is newsworthy now because for the first time in human history, medications are available to enhance the internal chemical reactions that underlie sexual pleasure. Men's sexuality got its turn first, when Viagra was introduced, accompanied by endless commentaries and jokes. Now it is women's turn: testosterone, first assumed to be exclusively a male hormone, turns out to be a pro-sex hormone for women also. Better still, testosterone does not change sexual feelings or interests in unwanted ways; it simply restores the ability to enjoy sex. Yet, testosterone is a mixed blessing because it has the potential to produce disturbing skin and hair changes in vulnerable women. This section will explain the revolution in sexual enhancement for women in a responsible fashion; both potential benefits and adverse effects will be disclosed so that you can make an informed decision regarding the use of testosterone.

Sex is hardly new as a human preoccupation. The first two classics of Western literature, the *Iliad* and the *Odyssey,* describe events set in motion by men's love for women: Paris's abduction of Helen and Odysseus's long voyage back to his wife Penelope. It's easy to forget that while the so-called sexual revolution of the sixties and seventies brought with it many changes in attitudes and behavior, it did not invent sex. What *is* new is open public discussion of sexuality in all its variations and convolutions. Whether or not people are having more sex is a moot point; they are certainly talking about it more. Previously, at least from a man's viewpoint, sex was simple: The penis was put into the vagina—although getting to that point, as now, often took considerable negotiation—then it was moved back and forth, there was an orgasm; all of this felt good. Pregnancy happened, or it didn't; this outcome was happy or not, depending on whether the woman was married to the man—among other factors. In our time, not only is discussion of sexuality more forthright, but also women now participate. This may be why women's sexual problems seem new—only recently have women been permitted to speak out concerning their sexual needs.

This greater openness is part of the enfranchisement of women's sexuality, a recent event in human history. The Victorian era had left as part of its legacy the idea that decent women did not enjoy sex, at least not too much and only if they were married to their partners. Even if seduced by the man, the woman was blamed because it was her moral responsibility to resist. A strong female sex drive could even be deemed a mental disorder. These repressive attitudes are now hard to comprehend. A common theory regarding the suppression of women's sexuality is that men felt threatened by strongly sexual women. No doubt there is some truth in this, though there is also an evolutionary explanation: If the wife has a low sex drive, it is less likely that her children will be fathered by a man other than her husband. With the availability of contraception, if a wife has sex with a man other than her husband, it is less likely to result in children carrying another man's DNA. In the modern era, fidelity is viewed less as a means to ensure perpetuation of the man's genes than as an essential prerequisite to an honest relationship. This shift toward openness in relationships brings recognition that a complete relationship involves sexual satisfaction for both partners. Being able to sexually satisfy a woman is now part of the masculine persona. This motivates men to polish their bedroom skills, but at the same time can make them insecure as to how they measure up against the competition. Women, too, worry about how good they are in bed. The sexual revolution has established a right to good sex, but also a nagging anxiety that what you are getting is not quite as good as you deserve.

At the risk of disappointing some readers, I regard the role of medicine not as making sex ecstatic but as ensuring that the pleasure apparatus stays in working order. The ecstasy is the responsibility of you and your partner. Some have criticized what they consider the "medicalization" of sexuality—implying that the medical establishment is somehow taking over sex. This seems nonsensical to me. Most people have perfectly good sex without the help of doctors. Yet, sex does depend on the body and brain; restoring these to normal when they are malfunctioning has been the province of medicine since the dawn of human culture. If your sex life is fine, then you do not need medical intervention. But if it is not working right, then the information in this section can help restore sex to its rightful place in your life. What this place is, of course, is up to you.

LOW SEX DRIVE: REPRESSION OR HORMONES?

Freudian psychology took sex to be the root of all psychological difficulties and saw the basic sexual problem as repression. It was assumed that loss of desire could only be due to early trauma or to guilt. On an unconscious level, everyone's desire was smoldering; inhibition just kept it out of conscious awareness. This entered pop culture in the sixties, when it was assumed that if you could just let go of your inhibitions, life would be one orgasm after another. Neither Freudian theories, nor their pop version, have much to do with real people's problems. Despite widespread acceptance that sex is a natural and positive part of adult life, many women and men one day find that their desire or their ability to perform has simply vanished. Though guilt or trauma can certainly make sex distasteful, most people with sexual difficulties have neither. For some women I talk to it is almost like a switch has been turned off: They enjoy a satisfying sex life for many years, then one day their sexually feelings simply disappear.

In the past few decades when women's sexual needs have been openly considered, it has emerged that *about a third of women report that their sexuality does not meet their expectations.* While there is no reason to think that low desire is more common, recent cultural changes enable women to feel comfortable in seeking help when sex disappoints. Respectable women are now portrayed openly in the media as wanting and enjoying sex. So complete is this change that women now are more likely to feel ashamed of a low sex drive than a high one.

Female sexual dysfunction (FSD) is not a new problem; what is new is recognition of women's entitlement to their own sexual feelings. With the new openness, many women now look at their sex lives and wonder if they could be better. Studies have shown that most people think that other people are getting more sex than they are. The pervasiveness of sex in the media easily engenders unrealistic expectations, a situation I call MISD—media-induced sexual discouragement. Hormones are essential to sexuality but are not always to blame when the fires subside. Perhaps the most common cause of a lackluster sex life is simply having too many other things to do. I emphasize the role of hormones in low desire because it is now possible to do something about them. But I'll also discuss nonbiochemical factors because there is no point in trying hormonal treatment if the problem lies elsewhere.

Despite more open attitudes, there is still intense social debate about whether low desire in women should be treated medically. Groups that claim to speak for all women imply that a decline of desire is "normal" and should simply be accepted as part of aging. Sadly, this reprises the way doctors often dismiss women's complaints. The implication that women are not entitled to medical help if their sex lives are unsatisfying is in itself discriminatory. No one has argued that Viagra victimizes men—least of all the men who use it.

Another claim on the part of some self-proclaimed "advocacy" groups is that female sexual dysfunction is not a legitimate medical condition but a plot on the part of the pharmaceutical industry to fill their coffers by selling sex-enhancing drugs. Singling out this industry is rather naive. Yes, the pharmaceutical industry may profit from women's sexuality, but so do the lingerie, fashion, cosmetic, and jewelry industries, to say nothing of romantic resorts, psychologists offering therapy for sexual problems, and, yes, publishing too. Augmenting sexuality is not the newest but one of the oldest forms of economic activity. Nor are chemical enhancements a novel idea; love potions are recorded in some of the earliest surviving written records of ancient medicine. In Chinese herbal pharmacies, the largest section is always devoted to sexual tonics—though most are for men. Whatever the risks of hormonally boosting sex drive—and I'll tell you everything that we know about the risks, including ones which have been covered up—they are far less than some of the ancient love potions.

WHAT IS THE RIGHT AMOUNT OF SEX?

Now that women are asking for help, doctors are realizing how poorly their education has prepared them to help patients with libido problems. Perhaps the most basic question is: How much sex is normal? Results vary in different studies, but the overall average for couples seems to be about once a week. For women reporting lack of interest, the average is about half as many sexual episodes—about two per month. Some couples have sex two or more times a week; on the other hand, a surprisingly large number have it only a few times per year. This data does not entitle us to claim any particular frequency of sexual contact is "normal," but is helpful in setting expectations.

Of interest here, couples with children have sex less often. This shows that sexual frequency is determined as much by the difficulty in finding the necessary time and energy as by any other factor. There is, therefore, no "normal range" for sex as there is for body temperature, blood pressure, or lab tests. If sex is often enough to satisfy you and your partner, that frequency is normal. On the other hand, if your level of interest is low and you feel distress over this, then seeking medical help is appropriate.

It seems self-evident that women, like men, are entitled to the sexual expression they want, so long as it is not harmful to themselves or others. It is regrettable that in the twenty-first century, some still question women's rights to sexual satisfaction. Obviously there are ethical issues about sexual behavior, but the propriety of helping a woman who wants to restore her desire is not one of them. How a woman chooses to express her sexuality is really not a medical question. (In saying this, I am assuming that what is done is not harmful to herself or others. Unsafe sex *is* a health problem, just like smoking or driving too fast.)

I hope it will be clear that I don't advocate for any specific sort of sex life. In my endocrinology practice, most of the women I see are serially monogamous, as is true for the American population, generally.

But others have multiple partners, and a few have decided to remain lifelong virgins. The majority are heterosexual, while some are lesbians. The emphasis in much of what follows is on intercourse between men and women for the sole reason that this is the form of sexuality for which women most commonly seek help. Loss of interest in sex by oneself or with a woman partner has the same hormonal basis and can respond to the same treatments.

WHICH HORMONES ARE REALLY SEXY?

For a long time it was assumed that different hormones must stimulate desire in males and females. Though we still do not understand the biological basis of the differences between women's and men's sexualities, it is clear that testosterone can stimulate libido in both sexes. Presumably, the rise of this hormone at puberty is responsible for the turning on of sexual thoughts and feelings in both boys and girls. This does not mean that testosterone works the same way in women as it does in men, nor, obviously, that female sexuality is a mirror image of a man's. One striking difference is that men need much higher levels of testosterone to maintain libido than do women. The average testosterone level for a woman in her thirties or early forties is about 40 ng/dL, while a man of comparable age normally has levels between 400 and 800 ng/dL. Women can be fully sexual at testosterone levels far below those men need. Indeed many women with active sexual interest and response have minimal amounts of testosterone in their blood. With men, on the other hand, when testosterone drops below about 300 ng/dL, lack of libido is common; below 150 ng/dL men stop thinking about sex completely—unbelievable as this may sound—and erections are impossible. So—surprise!—women's desire is biochemically different from that of men.

You may be wondering, if testosterone is important for desire, why do some women feel just as sexual with very low levels. It comes down, once again, to hormonal vulnerability. Some women need more testosterone than others in order to feel sexual interest—they are vulnerable to low testosterone. Other women feel highly sexual with only a drop in their blood.

Women's genital erogenous zones are also less dependent on testosterone than men's. Testosterone does make the vulva and clitoris more sensitive, but for many women, even low levels are adequate. Although clitoral engorgement is comparable to male erection to some degree, since the clitoris does not have to penetrate, it does not matter as much how stiff it gets. Erections and sexual sensation tend to be equated, but are actually separate. Men who are unable to have firm erections may still have sexual sensitivity. Conversely, the harder erections induced by Viagra and other PDE-5 inhibitors do not make the penis more erotically sensitive—which is probably why some men lose interest in Viagra after trying it a few times. If erections are adequate anyway, Viagra does not make sex feel better. One reason that women may need less testosterone than men is the rather obvious difference that women need it only for erotic sensitivity, not for erections.

However, although a few women with elevated testosterone levels due to a hormonal disorder report that their sex drives are higher, the overwhelming majority do not. Increasing the blood concentration beyond normal does not further increase sex drive. Despite some older, rather shoddy research, lesbian and heterosexual women do not differ in their testosterone levels. (Nor, for that matter, do gay and straight men.)

Because the amount of testosterone needed to feel sexy is very individual, testosterone blood levels are of limited value in predicting if a woman will benefit from treatment with this hormone. That said, if you are considering trying testosterone to add zip to your sex life, it is important to do the test. The reason: If you already have high testosterone levels, raising them further by using a testosterone patch or gel may not be a good idea. The test, then, is a safety measure. There is only one way to see if testosterone will restore your sexual feelings: trying it. Before doing so, there is much for you to consider, so I encourage you to read further before making up your mind.

HOW ESTROGEN MAKES SEX POSSIBLE

Testosterone may make a woman interested in sex, but it cannot make her body ready for it; this is the role of estrogen. Everyone is aware of the estrogen-orchestrated changes by which a girl's body becomes a woman's. Just as important are the estrogen effects that no one sees:

lengthening and widening of the vagina, as well as strengthening of the surrounding tissues. Blood vessels expand, so as to permit the increase in blood flow into the vagina and pelvis that is a part of female arousal. Estrogen does not create sexual feelings in a woman's body, but it makes it possible to feel and act upon them.

While the internal changes of puberty are due to estrogen, some of the external ones are mediated by testosterone. Under its influence, the smooth labia majora of a little girl become darker and wrinkled, and the labia minora enlarges. Testosterone also plays a role in making these tissues respond pleasurably to being touched.

PROGESTERONE: THE ANTISEX HORMONE—SOMETIMES

If testosterone is the sex hormone, progesterone is the pregnancy and menstruation hormone. Its sole function is to prepare the lining of the uterus (endometrium) for pregnancy, and if that doesn't occur, for menstruation. Progesterone's main concern is perpetuating the species, although it does other good things, such as protecting the endometrium from cancer. Progesterone levels peak some days after ovulation, when the egg is no longer fertile; intercourse during this late phase of the cycle cannot result in pregnancy. For this reason, it's hardly surprising that progesterone has a slight tendency to diminish desire. For most women, this effect is minimal, but a few may be vulnerable to it, especially if they have other PMS problems. This is not necessarily a direct hormonal effect; if you feel uncomfortable internally, intercourse may not be an appealing prospect. A few women actually feel *more* interest during the post-ovulatory phase of their cycles (weeks three and four), another example of how individual are women's reactions to their own hormones.

PROLACTIN

Just as our bodies have chemical mechanisms for turning us on, they also have ones that turn us off. Serotonin in the brain is one, as we know from the libido-lowering effects of antidepressant medications. The natural antisex factor best studied is the hormone prolactin, which, as its name suggests, promotes lactation. High levels turn off the menstrual cycle and may also put desire on hold. There is a simple biological reason for this: During nursing, it is best for both mother and baby if another pregnancy does not occur too soon. High prolactin is not a common cause of loss of desire but should be checked with a blood test if you are also missing periods—unless the later is clearly due to menopause. If your prolactin is consistently more than about 35 ng/mL, a thorough workup including pituitary MRI is essential to rule out a pituitary tumor as the cause.

SEXUAL PREREQUISITES

Hormones are necessary for a good sex life, but not sufficient. Just so that the other factors, obvious as they are, are not overlooked, I've listed the basic ones in the following sidebar.

WHAT'S NEEDED FOR SEX TO WORK

Hormones doing their thing: enough estrogen, not too much progesterone, and a dollop of testosterone. (Too much progesterone does not occur naturally; it is a result of taking synthetic forms.)

A partner who is affectionate and attractive to you—and also able to do his part by arousing you and having a functional erection himself.

The right things done to arouse you.

Vaginal tissues resilient and able to lubricate.

Comfort during entry and thrusting.

Being able to let go of the day's usual anxieties, from worry about pregnancy to bills.

Security about privacy.

10.

Sex and Women's Lives

Suzanne had actually come to see me not about sex but because at forty-six her periods had become lighter and somewhat erratic. She acknowledged having occasional hot flashes and night sweats, although they were nothing she could not tolerate. She had some vaginal dryness too. As some women do on their first visit to a new doctor, she'd brought a friend along for moral support. After I explained that her symptoms were common ones for women approaching perimenopause (see chapter 24), Suzanne was clearly relieved but then voiced another concern: She felt her sex drive was low and wondered if this might be hormonal. As we talked, I learned that Suzanne and her husband generally had sex about once a week but that she rarely thought about it otherwise. She never initiated sexual activity, although her husband expressed a wish that she would. Once her husband got things started, she became aroused, but it took her a little longer than it used to. Intercourse was pleasurable for her, and she usually had an orgasm. Suzanne talked about her sex life openly but in a rather matter-of-fact way, without the zest that younger women often display.

In fact, Suzanne's sexuality was absolutely normal for a woman her age who has been in a long-term, stable relationship. I told her what most find surprising: that the national average for sexual activity is only once a week. Some couples have more, some much less, but so long as sex is a comfortable and pleasurable aspect of life, there is no reason to force one's sex life to fit some quantitative standard.

Suzanne was concerned that she rarely thought about sex and wondered what that meant about herself and her relationship. I explained that recent research confirms that women can have quite happy sex lives, despite never feeling desire in the sense of thinking to themselves, "Wow, I want it right now!" and dragging their partner to the couch or the bedroom and covering him with passionate kisses. Or even parading in front of him in scanty lingerie. Such things happen in movies or TV but are designed to excite the viewer, not to describe reality. What actually happens behind closed doors is less dramatic, though more satisfying, since it is real rather than fantasy.

What about desire then? Surely it is essential to sex? Of course it is, but for many women it exists as part of their relationship, not something separate from it. If the person one loves makes affectionate gestures, pleasurable emotions arise along with physical events that eventually lead to both emotional and physical readiness for intercourse.

I noticed that all the time I was explaining these things to Suzanne, her friend was nodding—clearly what I was describing applied to her sex life too. Her nod was particularly emphatic when I explained that women can have a good sex life without thinking much about sex except in response to overtures by their partners.

Suzanne had what I have already referred to as MISD—media-induced sexual discouragement. In actuality her sex life was fine. It may have lacked the intensity of a torrid love affair as depicted in a soap, but it was real, a dependable source of pleasure, a way of maintaining closeness with her husband. Common wisdom states that sex loses its excitement after the first years of a relationship. And in a sense it does, but the early excitement is replaced by something better: comfort, ease, tenderness, dependability, security. That is why most opt to stay in long-term relationships and why most married people, again contrary to media depictions, stay faithful to their spouses.

Some women do describe feeling surges of desire that motivate them to go out to find a "hot guy." For many, but not all, this sort of adventure is less tempting as the years go by. This can be viewed as cooling of desire, but just as plausibly can represent the waning of a need for experimentation and a clearer idea of what one really finds satisfying. There are different ways in which women are sexual and different ways the same woman may be sexual at different times of her life. There is no need for any woman to be a critic of her own sexuality based on assumed standards of others.

TAKING THE INITIATIVE

Men tend to think of sex first, then initiate activity; women are more likely to want sex in response to their partner's overtures. This is not true for all women, of course. However, if you don't generally initiate with your partner, don't misinterpret this very usual pattern as a sign that something is lacking.

Many men, it is true, want the woman to sometimes take the initiative. Just as women do, men want to feel desired. If you always leave it to your partner to get things started, it would not be a bad idea to let him know at a comfortable time that you do find him desirable but that you are most comfortable if he begins intimate activity. You can also explain that what most excites you is his expression of desire for you.

As we'll see, many women who use testosterone do feel more frequent desire and are a little more likely to initiate. This is not invariable, and if a woman is satisfied with her sex life, there is no reason to use testosterone or any other treatment just because her partner would prefer it if she made the first move.

Suzanne was much relieved to realize that nothing was lacking from her sexuality. Her friend, who was a nurse, seemed somewhat relieved herself. Media-induced sexual dissatisfaction is epidemic, but easily cured by realistic expectations. This does not, however, mean that you should not pursue help if you are truly disappointed with your sex life. Nonstop ecstasy is an unrealistic expectation; regular, pleasurable sex is not.

Another of my patients, Carolyn, had a story that at first sounded similar to Suzanne's but was actually quite different. She told me that her relationship with her husband was a good one, and I had no reason to disbelieve her. He would have liked to have sex once or twice a week, but even once was too much for Carolyn. Despite her husband's best efforts, nothing happened when he tried to arouse her. Being touched in ways she once found intensely pleasurable, such as clitoral stimulation, was now almost painful. Although Carolyn was still menstruating, she had begun to have a few hot flashes. Never a sound sleeper, she found her insomnia worse than ever. She often awakened worrying about their finances or the children's schoolwork, though they actually had enough money and the children were doing fine. It was Carolyn's suspicion that her fatigued and anxious mental state was related to hormones that led her to consult me. She felt that her life was good, but that she could no longer enjoy it.

Given that she felt anxious much of the time, it would be easy to label Carolyn's problems as psychological. However, there were no specific life events that might account for this. "I've always tended to be somewhat nervous," she told me, "but not like this." Since Carolyn clearly had physical symptoms of perimenopause, it seemed plausible that the recent rise in her anxiety level might have a hormonal basis. Reassured that estrogen posed little risk at her age of forty-six, Carolyn opted to go on hormone therapy (HT). At her return visit two months later, she reported that she was feeling much better. She now felt refreshed after a night's sleep, and her anxiety had subsided to a tolerable level. But she brought up a concern that, now that she felt better, her sexuality had higher priority for her: "You know, my sex drive hasn't come back. Though it was never extremely high, I did enjoy sex when we had it. Now I have no interest at all. I'd just as soon be paying the bills. My husband is great. He's very patient with me, but I know it bothers him. I'm starting to worry about my marriage."

Carolyn's story is like that of many women I see. Her loss of interest had been gradual; she could not date it to any particular moment or event. She had a good, stable marriage and felt close to her husband. As a homemaker with three children in school, she had a lot to do but did not collapse in exhaustion at the end of the day as too many women (and men) do. Her home was big enough that she did not fear that the children would hear when she and her husband made love. In short, there were none of the usual external factors to account for her recent loss of sexual interest. That her anxiety and sleeplessness responded to estrogen was a pretty good indication that these were hormonal rather than psychological issues. However, as is usually the case, estrogen by itself did not restore her sex drive.

Carolyn had a conventional marriage, but loss of sexual interest can occur with alternative lifestyles as well. Women living with men can have the same problem. Single women may not notice loss of libido if they are not dating anyone, but if they are, it can cause worry about keeping their partners' interests. Lesbian women too can find one day that their interest is gone.

Carolyn's story had a happy ending. Treatment with testosterone did restore her sex drive. Before we go on to consider how this new treatment can help, let's look a little more at the issues raised by taking medication to enhance desire.

DO YOU WANT MORE SEX?

First, it needs to be emphasized that low sexual interest is not a disease. Unlike high blood pressure or bad cholesterol, it has no long-term consequences for physical health. If you do not have sexual thoughts and truly do not want them, there is no reason to seek treatment. From a medical or psychological point of view, low interest is not considered a problem, unless it causes distress. The distress may be due to loss of a form of enjoyment, or it may be worry about what will happen to the relationship.

The perfect husband might be willing to forgo sex for the woman he loves, but most husbands are not perfect. Though many will tolerate lack of sex with their wives, few are really happy with this situation. For men, more than for women, sex is necessary to feel an intimate connection with a partner. Women also need physical contact but may be satisfied with more frequent, but less intense forms of contact, such as hugging.

Should a woman have treatment to increase her sexual desire mainly to keep her husband happy? This is a very individual decision, but many women do start treatment from this motive. Some find themselves happier as a result of their restored sexuality, while others are relieved that their partners are more satisfied, even though sex is not particularly important to them otherwise. It may seem unfair that a woman should have to increase her sex drive just for the sake of her partner but, in fact, doing things one may not want for the sake of the other is a daily part of any relationship.

In most of human history, marriage was a basic structural unit of society, a stabilizing factor, a division of labor, a way to ensure children were cared for. While choosing the right partner has always been a concern, it was not assumed, as it is today, that one's primary emotional needs would be met by one's spouse. Nor was it assumed that a man's wife would be his only, or even primary sexual partner. This could reach extremes: In traditional China, men with several wives frequently cheated on all of them at once by going to prostitutes. Women, as now, sometimes sought outside relationships, but at risk of severe consequences.

To expect one's spouse to be congenial company, share domestic tasks, be a good earner, agree about politics and religion, have similar food preferences, like the same movies, and enjoy the same things in sex is expecting a lot. Nonetheless, the institution of modern marriage works surprisingly well, certainly in comparison with the alternative of being alone. True, many couples divorce, but most people remarry or at least want to, so they must still feel it is preferable to being single. Some opt for nonmarital relationships, but issues of partner compatibility still arise. In order to preserve relationships, many compromises, both big and small, must be made. In an important relationship, it can be a reasonable choice to accede to the partner's sexual requests in order to maintain harmony.

Having sex when you don't really want it needs to be thought about carefully, however. Accommodating one's partner does not mean having intercourse despite pain, nor acquiescing to sex if there are serious relationship issues such as infidelity, mistreatment, or substance abuse. Sex is part of a good relationship, not a solution to a bad one. If you have angry feelings toward your partner or other sorts of conflict testosterone is not the answer. Nor is it the answer if the price of enhanced desire is distressing side effects, such as hair loss.

While testosterone may restore sexual interest, it will not change what sort of sexual activity you like. If your partner's tastes incline to the kinky, such as tying you up, spanking you, or wearing your underpants, and these do not appeal to you, testosterone will not change your mind. If you cannot negotiate these things between you, then sex therapy might help, but medication will not.

In my medical practice, I've known couples who did not have sex for years but seemed basically content together. Good sex is a component of many, but by no means all, happy marriages. I've also known cases in which it was the woman who left because her partner's sexual interest was too low. There are many ways to accommodate unmatched desire, but no single way that is right for all couples.

The existence of treatments to enhance sex is empowering to women because it confers choice. It allows a higher level of control over one's sex drive, one of the biological functions that has traditionally been least controllable. Yet it should not be forgotten that using testosterone is a choice. Many women whose sexuality has become dormant will choose it with little hesitation. On the other hand, a few women actually find it a relief to lose their libido because the lack of sexual distraction gives them more time for other activities. To not use medication to increase your libido can also be a valid choice.

SEX, TESTOSTERONE, AND HAPPINESS

We tend to connect sex and happiness. Satisfying sexual activity tends to leave us with a special glow, sometimes apparent to others. Many studies have shown that, in general, those who have regular sexual activity are happier. One study even showed that semen has a mood-elevating effect on women. Clearly, sex is much more than momentary physical pleasure. Although not all need sex to be happy, many do.

Testosterone in itself seems to have a connection with well-being. Men with hypogonadism—the condition in which the testicle is not able to make enough testosterone—show dramatic improvements in mood and generally feel better about life when the missing testosterone is replaced. Women given testosterone in the lower doses appropriate for them also describe enhanced well-being. Both often report an energizing effect when their minds rediscover sex. There is an edgy quality to sexual thoughts, a kind of tension that many feel makes them more productive in other areas of life as well.

It seems then that testosterone, sex, energy, and overall satisfaction with life are somehow interconnected. This is an exciting finding, but it can be taken too far. What worries me is that testosterone will be pushed as a cure-all for women who are tired or unhappy. While I think that the availability of this hormone in a safe form for women is a great advance, I think caution is appropriate; it should not be, as it sometimes is, prescribed as a "tonic" for any woman (or man) who is tired or unhappy.

LEARNING WHAT FEELS GOOD

During puberty, testosterone goes to work to make erogenous zones erogenous. In spite of the differences in the shapes of the relevant body parts, sexual sensitivity in men and women is not totally dissimilar. In both sexes, areas where testosterone induces erotic sensitivity are color-coded—they become darker than nonsexual skin. This is noticeable in the underarms, nipples, vulva, and adjacent areas. (The underarm is perhaps the most underappreciated erogenous zone.) Also in response to testosterone, the labia (lips of the vagina) grow during puberty, giving them a wrinkled appearance. Men's genital skin darkens also.

Men and women can understand each others' pleasure zones better by knowing a little sexual embryology. In the early days in the womb, all fetuses look like girls. Girls obviously keep looking that way. In boys, the scrotum and surrounding skin develops from what would have been the labia majora. These areas on a man are sensitive in the same way as the outer lips on a woman. The skin under the penis, the main location of pleasurable sensations during intercourse, develops from what in a girl would become the labia minora. Mucus membranes are sensitive too: the mouth, labia minora, glans (tip) of the penis, and, for some, the anus.

An old Latin term for the female genitalia is *pudendum,* which means literally, "that of which one ought to be ashamed." Even though recent culture has moved far toward positive acceptance of the body, many women feel some uneasiness about this important area. Some feel it is okay to be touched there by their partners but are reluctant to touch themselves. Others are comfortable touching but not looking. In the early days of the feminist movement, workshops were held for women to look at their own and each others' genitalia with a mirror. The audience reaction to the Broadway hit, *The Vagina*

Monologues, shows that this mysterious place can both embarrass and fascinate. Things are simple for men—the penis is the main area of pleasure, and it is in plain sight. For women, a journey of exploration may be necessary. If you have avoided your private parts and if sex has never felt as good as you had expected, it will help greatly if you can swallow your embarrassment and develop better awareness of what feels good.

Good sex has infinite variety, but a few principles inspire all of it. As just explained, darker skin pigmentation draws attention to places that testosterone has made erotically sensitive. Not all sexual sensations are pleasant, however. Many people have areas where they prefer not to be touched, either because they are too sensitive or because of taboos. Though taboos often become less powerful with more experience, partners need to respect each others' limits.

Sexually sensitive areas have a center and periphery. Just as the nipple is the most sensitive area of the breast, the clitoris is the most sensitive area of the genitalia. This is important because the most responsive areas are also the most delicate. Being touched there may not feel good until you are already aroused. Sex is usually more comfortable if contact starts at the periphery and moves inward. This means touching the outer area of the breast before the nipple. With genital stimulation, caresses can start at the thighs, then the outer lips. Then the inner labia can be touched, first lower down, then gradually moving toward the clitoris. Because these areas are so sensitive, more than very light touch should await the beginning of natural lubrication from the vagina.

I am not suggesting a rigidly invariable sequence; there is plenty of room for creativity. In a sense every sexual encounter is a story and, like a well-crafted story, should gradually work up to a climax. Like fictional narratives, sexual activity sometimes begins in the middle of the action. It can happen that a woman is aroused before being touched—by thoughts and fantasies or even pressure from clothes—and will welcome more intense stimulation at the beginning. Men are supposed to intuit these things but in reality depend to a great degree on hints from you. Sex manuals recommend open discussion—a good suggestion in theory—but it is the nature of sex that talking about it can be more difficult than doing it. Guiding your lover's hand or making your response clear with body language are as good or better than explicit verbal instructions.

When women notice a falloff in sexual interest, genital response is usually lost also. What once felt good, no longer does. Although we separate desire and arousal, they are parts of the same process. When treatment works, it restores both.

11.

Sex Is Much More Than Hormones

This book is about hormones and the problems they cause women. This does not mean that *all* problems, sexual or otherwise, are due to hormones. If sex is losing its thrill, before blaming hormones, you should consider whether other things in your life may be contributing. I've listed some of the more common turnoffs in the next sidebar. None of these necessarily represents anything inherently wrong in a relationship, yet they may dampen one's mood for sex.

MEDICATIONS THAT TAKE AWAY PLEASURE: ANTIDEPRESSANTS, BLOOD PRESSURE PILLS, ALCOHOL, AND OTHERS

If your sex drive has suddenly disappeared, medication is a possible cause. Although the great majority of drugs have no effect whatsoever on sexuality, a few do. The most common culprits are antidepressants, further discussed in chapter 6. One antidepressant, Wellbutrin (bupropion) has the opposite effect: It can help bring back sexual interest. Some blood pressure medications dampen desire, especially the so-called alpha blockers. Newer ones that are more commonly used do not interfere with sex; these include calcium channel blockers, angiotensin

COMMON NONHORMONAL REASONS FOR LOSS OF SEXUAL INTEREST AND PLEASURE

Fatigue

Lack of privacy, such as children, in-laws, or visitors who might hear

Limited relaxed time together

Feeling unattractive, for example, because of weight gain or hair loss

Anxiety or depression

Pain

Conditions such as diabetes that affect nerves and circulation in sexual areas

Debilitating diseases, such as inflammatory bowel disease, heart failure, or chronic lung disease

Medication, especially antidepressants (except Wellbutrin), and some blood pressure medications

converting enzyme (ACE) inhibitors, and angiotensin receptor blockers (ARBs). There are many in each category, and the names are confusing. If you suspect that your blood pressure medication is lowering your libido as well as your pressure, you need to talk to your doctor to find out which category it is in.

Although alcohol is well known for temporarily lowering inhibitions, long-term, heavy use tends to eventually weaken sexual interest and response. Opioids and other strong pain relievers similarly tend to turn off libido. If your libido is low and you are on an opioid or other narcotic pain reliever, it is unlikely that your sexual feelings will return with any treatment unless you can find another way to manage your pain.

A very small minority of women notice slackening of interest with birth control pills; this seems to occur because the pill lowers free testosterone levels. Sometimes a change to a very low-dose pill will help, but more often sex drive comes back only when hormonal contraception is discontinued. For most women, however, OCs have a positive effect on sex because of lessened anxiety about pregnancy.

Medication gets blamed for all kinds of things, not always deservedly. Other than antidepressants, few drugs likely to be taken by women in the hormonal years from ages thirty-five to fifty-five will have any sexual side effects. Antibiotics, allergy or asthma medications, anti-reflux medications, NSAIDs, and most others are sex-neutral. If your desire is not what it once was, checking any medications you are taking to see if they could be part of the problem is an essential first step. Most often, however, the cause will be hormones or the sort of personal factors I cover in this chapter.

COMMON NONHORMONAL TURNOFFS

A wide range of situations can hamper desire, even when hormones are minding their own business. A common one for women is feeling unattractive, often as a result of hormonal vulnerability such as weight gain or hair loss. Some women feel ugly when they have bloating and other effects of PMS and so do not want sexual contact then. Men have difficulty understanding this; they initiate sex because they are aroused and do not find the woman ugly in the least.

What can happen is illustrated by my patient Wendy, who was distraught regarding a weight gain of about twenty pounds, though she was not fat by any means and still had a good shape. Though her boyfriend was still attracted to her, she broke up with him because, as she told me, "Since he still found me attractive even though I've gotten fat, I figured something must be wrong with him." Sadly, Wendy put herself in a lose-lose situation. Perhaps fearful that her boyfriend would reject her, she took action first and ended their relationship, with which she was otherwise happy. My advice here may seem simplistic, but I think it is sound: If your man is attracted to you and wants sex with you, take it at face value and enjoy it. Try not to obsess too much over whatever you think is unattractive about yourself; men are far less critical of women's appearances than women themselves. Having a good time with sex does not require that you be perfect—nor that he is.

ANGER IS NOT SEXY

We tend to think of couple problems as requiring marriage counseling or rather intense psychotherapy. Yet sometimes the cause can be quickly uncovered and harmony restored fairly easily. In my experience, unresolved anger on the woman's part is the most common non-hormonal reason women lose interest. For women, anger tends to block sexual feelings. Men get angry too, but more readily set it aside temporarily rather than miss an opportunity for sex.

Pam was a patient I saw some years ago. She lived in a rural area of upstate New York and had driven several hours to come to see me. Her problem was a complete loss of interest in sex. As she explained, "You have to understand, we live in the country where there's not much to do, so we spend most of Saturday and Sunday in bed. Without sex, our weekends are now a total bore."

When I asked Pam about her relationship, her anger and its cause became clear. Her husband's idea of getting aroused was to sit next to her in bed and watch X-rated videos. Then he would try to make his wife the beneficiary of the ardor elicited by the busty porn actresses.

Not surprisingly, his wife was not pleased to sit quietly beside him as he got turned on by another woman. Pam was tolerant and somewhat enjoyed the X-rated videos but naturally felt jealous. I suggested she make it clear to her husband that she would prefer to be the focus of his attentions. Fortunately, he was quite willing to change, once he understood his wife's feelings, which she had not previously voiced to him. The problem was solved, and their country weekends were no longer boring.

Though not all situations are so easily solved, many are. If you've suddenly lost your interest in sex, it's worth reviewing recent events to see if bottled up anger may be the cause.

DEEPER PROBLEMS

I have emphasized that some sexual problems are simple to counteract the misimpression, foisted by Freudian psychoanalysis, that sexual problems are always deep rooted and require years of expensive therapy to unravel. Unfortunately, however, some really are due to serious conflicts or to deep-seated psychological issues. In such cases, sex may be the least of the problems. Consider Emily's story: She had come for consultation at the urging of her husband who found her hard to get along with and suggested that hormones might be the cause, especially since Emily refused to have sex with him. She seemed somewhat reticent as I asked her about her relationship. Finally, she asked, "Do you want to hear the whole story?" and proceeded to reveal that her husband had recently been released from prison, where he had been sent for drug dealing. Now, Emily was a quite normal-seeming suburban woman; one would never have guessed at this circumstance in her life. Needless to say, her marriage problems had little to do with hormones. Her husband's refusal to see how his drug dealing and consequent imprisonment affected his wife and family was not an encouraging sign for the possibility of restoring their relationship. Sometimes, blaming hormones is a way to avoid other problems. To restate the obvious, if you and your partner are not getting along, it will take more than testosterone to save your relationship.

WHEN TO CONSIDER SEEING A SEX THERAPIST

The term "sex therapist" may conjure up images of sex surrogates and other lurid practices. The reality is different. I've known and worked with many psychologists in this field and have found them as professional as any other specialty in health care. They take sex very seriously and are committed to helping women, men, and couples achieve satisfaction in this area of life. If anything, some take sex *too* seriously. I've sat through many lectures by sex experts who seem to have lost sight of the fact that sex is supposed to be fun. In this light, I do have a few suggestions as to what attitudes to look for in a therapist. First, sex should not be made to seem like a necessary but difficult task, an obligation rather than a pleasure. The best psychotherapists make things seem simpler than you thought, not more complicated. A prominent psychiatrist specializing in sexual difficulties wrote a book called *Sex Is Not Simple*. To my mind, this is the wrong approach. When sex is complicated, therapy should lead to it being straightforward again.

I am not denying the obvious truth that sex is connected to many other areas of life. Sometimes sexual difficulties are so tied in with other life problems that extensive psychotherapy may be the best option. However, most of the women I see in my practice for help with low desire are as normal as any other group. They have problems, as we all do, but not beyond the realm of normal. All in all, I don't find that women whose sexual desire has vanished are different from other women. Nor is it necessarily difficult to find a solution. For this reason, I recommend psychological therapy only when simpler solutions do not apply.

In the following sidebar I list some clues that sexual problems may be better treated with counseling than medication alone.

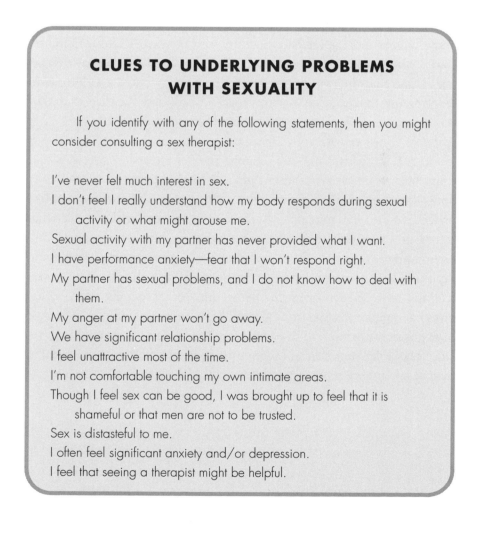

CLUES TO UNDERLYING PROBLEMS WITH SEXUALITY

If you identify with any of the following statements, then you might consider consulting a sex therapist:

I've never felt much interest in sex.
I don't feel I really understand how my body responds during sexual activity or what might arouse me.
Sexual activity with my partner has never provided what I want.
I have performance anxiety—fear that I won't respond right.
My partner has sexual problems, and I do not know how to deal with them.
My anger at my partner won't go away.
We have significant relationship problems.
I feel unattractive most of the time.
I'm not comfortable touching my own intimate areas.
Though I feel sex can be good, I was brought up to feel that it is shameful or that men are not to be trusted.
Sex is distasteful to me.
I often feel significant anxiety and/or depression.
I feel that seeing a therapist might be helpful.

FINDING A REPUTABLE PRACTITIONER

Care should be taken when selecting a therapist to whom you will entrust some of the most intimate aspects of your life. The best way to start is by asking your gynecologist or other physician. Another way is to consult the membership lists of the related professional societies (see the Resources section at the end of the book). While this does not guarantee finding someone who is right for you, it improves the odds. Members are dedicated enough to have joined the society and have met certain minimum educational standards.

WHEN TESTOSTERONE IS UNLIKELY TO HELP DESIRE

Some women have never had much interest in sex. As one told me recently when I asked her about this, "Well, I wanted children . . ." leaving it clear that this was her main motive. Some women go along with sex because that is what is expected and only later realize that they don't enjoy it all that much. If you never had desire—even in your early twenties, when testosterone levels are usually much higher—then it is unlikely that testosterone will change things. Except in special situations, such as a very strict upbringing or past sexual trauma, we really don't know why some women just aren't interested. Some women like provoking men and may dress and act in a very sexy manner, but what they enjoy is not the physical part of the sex but being wanted and having power over men. Men find such women frustrating; needless to say though, they may enjoy showing them off on a date. If your sexual feelings have always been channeled into other outlets than actual physical contact, testosterone probably will not change this. The role of testosterone treatment in our present level of understanding is to restore sexual feelings that have languished; it does not create something that was not there in the first place.

12.

What the New Research Has Discovered About Testosterone and Women's Sexuality

Long a skeptic about the propriety of giving testosterone to women, I have changed my view somewhat, as a result of new research indicating that most women can use this hormone safely, providing the dose is woman-appropriate. While I now believe that testosterone has an important place in the treatment of women's sexual problems, I continue to be troubled by the injudicious way this powerful hormone is often prescribed. The impending availability of forms designed for women should eventually change this, but in the meantime, careless dosing with unsuitable preparations remains prevalent. In this section, I'll explain how you can use testosterone with a reasonable margin of safety, but first I need to provide some background regarding past problems.

THE OLD APPROACHES TO GIVING WOMEN TESTOSTERONE WERE ILL-ADVISED

I feel a strong obligation to disclose the potential adverse effects of testosterone because no other specialist in women's hormones has come forward to do so. For some years I have spoken out in medical conferences and publications against the ways testosterone was being prescribed to women. Often, I was the sole voice pointing out that testosterone has known harmful effects in women and that safety must be proven, not just assumed. My message was not that testosterone should never be used by women but that any such use should be informed by accurate information about possible adverse effects. It seemed to me that this should have been noncontroversial—in all other areas of medicine it is routinely accepted that benefits and risks must be weighed against each other. Yet, my reminders of this elementary principle were not welcomed by the majority of those who appointed themselves as experts in female sexual dysfunction. I became used to being denounced from the floor at the end of my lectures by the uncritical advocates of testosterone. Privately, however, many would approach me during breaks in the program to thank me for being upfront about the safety issues that more vocal colleagues wanted swept under the rug.

Use of testosterone for women got off to a bad start because the first study claiming it could increase sex drive employed doses in the range given to males. Though uncommented upon in the published paper, the blood levels of testosterone produced by this regimen were in the range found in women with severe polycystic ovary syndrome (PCOS) or ovarian or adrenal tumors. As to what adverse effects this misguided treatment caused, there was silence. Few in the female sexual dysfunction field have had training in endocrinology, and so most were not really knowledgeable in evaluating testosterone blood levels, nor in detecting its adverse effects by physical examination. When I challenged the consensus advocating this casual use of testosterone, I was met with antagonism—but not with actual evidence to support safety.

The bad things testosterone can do to women's bodies have been known for more than a century: acne, increased facial and body hair, and scalp hair thinning. I am particularly sensitized to these because I've spent much of my time over the past two decades helping women recover from these destructive effects of their own testosterone. There is nothing esoteric about hirsutism and alopecia being due to testosterone—we all learn pretty early in life that men have less hair on their heads and more on their faces than women. Yet I have seen women who lost hair from taking testosterone, who were told by their doctors that more testosterone would help it grow back. This is inexcusable. No physician should prescribe any medication without being fully aware of all its effects, good and bad. For reasons that still escape me, the monitoring of women on testosterone is often quite lackadaisical.

I felt that research needed to establish three essential points before testosterone could be recommended to women: 1) whether testosterone really does restore sex drive, 2) the frequency and severity of skin and hair effects—and who is likely to be susceptible to them, and 3) whether or not there are adverse effects on metabolism. These three criteria have been largely met by the extensive studies with the testosterone patch. Research does need to continue, especially as regards long-term safety. Though the patch and gel, when used carefully as I describe in the next chapter, can increase libido at a relatively low level of risk, use of other forms cannot be assumed to be safe.

We need better education of practitioners and patients about safe use of testosterone. This section will, I hope, be a useful step in this direction.

CAN TESTOSTERONE HELP YOU FEEL SEXIER? THE EVIDENCE

Until recently, studies purporting to demonstrate that testosterone could boost women's sex drives were scientifically unconvincing. They suggested that it might work but fell far short of proof. Worse, they did not have adequate procedures to detect adverse effects. The situation has changed because we now have some of the results of the large-scale studies carried out by Procter & Gamble to develop their Intrinsa testosterone patch for women. While the FDA is reviewing the product, we can apply the study findings to use current available forms of natural testosterone to get similar results. I emphasize *natural* because several older preparations, which are still commonly prescribed, use synthetically modified forms of testosterone. Most popular are Estratest and Estratest H.S.; both contain a synthetic, methyltestosterone, which is only weakly effective at best. Like all orally absorbed forms of testosterone, it can alter liver function. Older injectable forms are sometimes given to women, but they give uneven blood levels, resulting in excessive levels in the days following each injection.

Compounded preparations are promoted aggressively by some pharmacies; these also tend to produce excessive levels and may vary from batch to batch.

A woman's hormonal constitution is delicately tuned. If testosterone is used, it must be in a way that will not be disruptive. This obvious point has often been overlooked: *To be woman-appropriate, a testosterone preparation must produce blood levels in the normal female range.* The patch was successfully designed to do exactly this. While waiting for the patch, there is another way to get similar blood levels—by using AndroGel, a prescription gel marketed for men that can be adapted for use by women. Although the patch will be much more convenient, the gel can give the same therapeutic result.

I've been involved in some of the early research for the female patch and have scrutinized the available data regarding safety. I base what I say here on data that is now publicly available on the FDA website and in medical journal articles. Anyone interested can consult these sources for herself; I've made every effort to summarize this data in a balanced fashion.

Unlike earlier ways of using testosterone, transdermal application in woman-friendly doses gives blood levels in the normal range for women during their cycling years. Because the Intrinsa patch provides testosterone itself, not a synthetic, the data will apply to any form of natural testosterone that gives similar blood levels. Only with these studies, which included more than 1,000 women in the United States and hundreds more in other countries, do we have adequate data on what happens to women who take testosterone. Let's look in a general way at what this new research tells us about the two key issues: How well does testosterone work, and how safe is it?

HOW MUCH DIFFERENCE DOES TESTOSTERONE MAKE?

As I have emphasized, the average frequency of sexual activity is about once a week. That intercourse happens only once a week hardly means that it is not important to both partners. Women in the patch study had a below average frequency of twice a month. With placebo, this increased to three times a month and with testosterone, to four times a month. Some have questioned whether it's worth taking medication to have sex an extra one or two times a month. However, having sex four times a month meant the women were back to an average level of sexual activity. In any other kind of study, restoring something to normal would be considered a satisfactory result. Most who have expressed doubt that increasing sexual frequency to once a week is enough are men, for whom, notoriously, quantity of sex is more important than quality. The women in the study spoke for themselves; in their responses to standardized questionnaires, they indicated that sex was more pleasurable and satisfying and that they were happier overall. They felt they were sexual beings once again, something very important for self-esteem. The increase in sexual activity to four times a month was the average for the women in the study who received testosterone; some had a bigger increase, and some did not respond at all. As one would expect when hormones are involved, the response was highly individual. What is most significant is not how much more often the treated women had sex, but the strong evidence that it was more satisfying. When the FDA's Advisory Committee met about the patch, a majority agreed that it is effective.

It should be kept in mind that the women in the study signed up because they wanted to improve their sex drives. Presumably sex was important to them, and they missed it. Partner pressure may have played some role as well, of course. Either way, the women still wanted their sex drives intensified. As I already mentioned, no doubt there are women who lose interest in sex, don't miss it, and never ask for treatment.

Is the improvement with testosterone enough? The answer depends on expectations. Most people probably fantasize that their sex lives could be a little better. Testosterone, needless to say, will not make all your fantasies come true. What it can do is restore sex to a normal, satisfying level. If you were not getting what you wanted before your desire waned, testosterone will not change that either. If sex with your partner is not fully satisfying, the answer is to discuss your needs—always hard—or go for counseling. Those who work to help women with low sexual interest all come to feel that what matters to their clients is not how often they do it, but how fulfilling it is. Good sex usually does not mean exotic positions or locales, but emotional and physical intimacy with one's partner.

Not all women in the studies responded to testosterone; their problems were not lack of this hormone but something else. Clearly there are other biochemical factors that regulate desire; unfortunately, we don't know much about them. Though testosterone is not the ultimate treatment for low desire, it is the best one we have now. Research to discover new ones is underway. We may have better ones in a decade, but where sex is concerned, who wants to wait?

Research on use of testosterone for sexual problems has been mostly limited to menopausal women. While it is true that the incidence of low desire starts to rise after the mid-forties, loss of sexual feelings can occur at any time after puberty. Although research has been less extensive, a few studies do suggest that testosterone can restore sex drive in younger women. My clinical experience, and that of other specialists in this area, clearly shows that it does.

HOW SAFE IS TESTOSTERONE FOR WOMEN?

It is clear that when desire takes a holiday, testosterone in female-appropriate doses can bring it back for many, although not all, women. Given this, making a rational decision about whether to use testosterone comes down to safety. Until very recently, hardly any safety data was available. As a result of the patch studies, we now have such data on more than 1,000 women, and it is generally reassuring. Let's look at each of the important safety questions.

First, there is no doubt that testosterone can cause oily skin, acne, increased facial hair, and scalp hair loss in women who are vulnerable to these effects. This is not only theoretical—every day in my practice I see at firsthand the heartbreak these changes bring for women who are vulnerable to their own testosterone. Given that the patch produced free testosterone levels in the normal female range, it would be expected that such effects would be infrequent. The data indeed confirm this hope. At most about 5 percent of subjects reported such changes, which were generally mild when they did occur. I suspect that as women use testosterone longer, a slightly higher proportion will notice such effects.

Skin and hair changes that occur when taking testosterone usually reverse, if it is discontinued promptly. (This is a different situation than when it is your own body's testosterone that is causing the problem.)

So if you do use testosterone, be alert to what is happening to your skin and hair. A slight increase in oiliness or an extra hair to pluck from the chin may be acceptable. But if you start to break out or if you notice dark hairs appearing on your face, you should seriously consider whether or not you want to continue it. Don't let anyone convince you that acne, hirsutism, or alopecia are not due to testosterone or that they will go away by themselves. They are, and they won't.

The most upsetting adverse testosterone effect for women is hair loss. Hair is especially precious to women, and so I suggest being vigilant about yours if you are on testosterone. An increase in hair loss was not described in the studies to date, but I suspect that with longer use, a few women will notice alopecia.

I think the explanation for the low rates of skin and hair changes is that only a subset of women are vulnerable to these effects of testosterone at normal female levels. If you have never had these problems before, this suggests that your skin and hair are probably not very sensitive to testosterone. On the other hand, if you have had acne, hirsutism, or alopecia, there is a definite chance that testosterone will make them worse.

The skin and hair changes produced by testosterone are at least visible; but not all doctors know how to recognize them. What about metabolic side effects that cannot be seen but might affect long-term health? The most common cause of elevated testosterone in women, PCOS, is associated with high insulin levels, increased risk of diabetes, and unfavorable cholesterol levels. This raises concern of whether taking testosterone would give a woman PCOS-like metabolic changes. The studies looked at these possibilities and, fortunately, did not find any grounds for concern. Cholesterol, in both the good (HDL) and bad (LDL) forms, did not change, nor did levels of glucose or insulin. The lack of harmful effects may be due to use of the transdermal route (the patch); it cannot be assumed that oral forms would be as safe.

Breast cancer is, of course, a concern with any sex hormone taken by women. A small number of women in the study did develop it, but review of each case suggests that the cancer was present, but not apparent, before study entry. Some research indicates that women with higher testosterone levels have an increased risk of this form of cancer. Many of these women had PCOS, so the association between breast cancer risk and testosterone may be due to other aspects of PCOS, such as obesity and high insulin levels, rather than the testosterone itself. At this point we have data from two or three years with no increase in breast cancer risk found. Considering that breast cancer is rare in men, although not unknown, testosterone clearly does not cause breast cancer directly. Since the body converts some testosterone to estrogen, some have raised concern that using testosterone might increase breast cancer risk by raising estrogen levels. However, the amount of estrogen produced by woman-appropriate doses of testosterone is minute, a fraction of what a woman's body produces even after menopause. There is no evidence now that testosterone would increase the risk of breast or any other form of cancer in women, but to be absolutely certain will take more years of study on larger numbers of women.

Another concern regarding testosterone use by women is heart disease. Since men become vulnerable to heart attacks about a decade before women do, the possibility must be considered that testosterone might take away this "female advantage." The study did not find any change in risk factors—as already mentioned, carbohydrate metabolism and cholesterol did not change—nor any increase in heart disease in its first two years, but we need to await longer term data. In men with low testosterone levels, replacement of this hormone seems to *lower* heart disease risk, so the male vulnerability to earlier heart disease does not seem to be a direct result of higher testosterone levels. If the difference is caused by hormones, it is more likely due to men's lower estrogen levels. My suggestion is that if you plan to try testosterone, you should do what you should anyway: Have your risk factors, such as cholesterol and blood pressure checked, and get treatment if they are elevated. Nonetheless, at our present level of knowledge, if you are at high risk of heart disease for any reason, I would recommend avoiding testosterone.

Because the encouraging safety data is based on only a year or two of use, any woman using testosterone should stay tuned as more information becomes available. Long-term studies are ongoing. If adverse effects are discovered, we can expect that they will be promptly reported. For this reason, I recommend reassessing treatment at six-month intervals so that your decision will take into account the latest safety information.

THE WRONG WAYS TO USE TESTOSTERONE

I have described the recent research supporting careful use of testosterone by women to improve their sex drives. I want to make it clear, however, that this applies only to preparations of testosterone itself that produce normal free testosterone levels. I've already expressed my concern about the casual prescribing of this hormone. In the context of drug prescribing, I use "casual" to refer to prescribing by doctors who have not fully informed themselves about the relation between testosterone dose and its adverse effects. This nonchalant attitude results in several regrettable practices: doses that are grossly excessive, preparations that are unreliable or unsuited to use by women, or testosterone that was not needed in the first place.

Testosterone is, after all, the male hormone. Even though I have emphasized that it is a normal component of women's hormonal constitution, *testosterone cannot be given to women in the same way it is to men.* I've stressed what should be obvious: Testosterone prescribed for women should produce levels that are normal for a woman. Unfortunately, I have seen many women prescribed testosterone in doses that push their levels way up into the male range. This is completely unnecessary because suitable forms of testosterone for use by women are available now, as I describe in chapter 14.

13.

Testosterone: The Decision

The sidebar on page 199 provides a quick guide to give you some idea of whether testosterone is worth a try. A "yes" answer to all the questions suggests that trying testosterone would be a reasonable choice. On the other hand, a "no" answer to one or more may indicate that there are other issues that may be involved in your loss of sexual interest. The sidebar is intended to give you an idea of whether testosterone might work for you; I'll cover other factors in the decision later in this chapter.

If your answers were all "yes," the next step is to consider how your body is likely to react to this hormone, as covered in the next section.

THE TWO KINDS OF TESTOSTERONE VULNERABILITY

Testosterone may be wonderful or terrible, depending on your body's biochemical individuality. Vulnerability to low normal levels of testosterone can bring about a loss of sex drive; this seems particularly common during the forties and later when levels decline. Vulnerability to high normal levels brings the skin and hair changes already mentioned. What is particularly unfair is that some women have both kinds of testosterone vulnerability. Too little testosterone and sex becomes ho-hum; too much and skin and hair suffer. Fortunately, for most women a dose can be found that livens up sex without dulling complexion or ruining hair. But for a few with very vulnerable skin and hair, the effects of testosterone may not be worth any improvement in sex.

If you don't have oily skin or acne, rarely have to pluck a hair, and your scalp hair is as abundant as it was in your twenties, testosterone is unlikely to cause these problems. However, if you had any of these conditions in the past or have them now, testosterone may make them worse. I do not want to overstate this; if your skin has behaved in recent years, a little bit of skin oiliness or an occasional extra hair on your chin are probably the worst that will happen. They may be a reasonable price to pay for a great sex life. Still, you should keep an eye on your skin—you know it better than anyone else, including your dermatologist—and if it is changing in ways that distress you, you need to reconsider whether you still want testosterone.

If you do develop oily skin and/or unwanted hair on testosterone, they may go away once you stop. If they persist, using spironolactone can speed up your skin's recovery (see chapter 20).

If you have even the slightest degree of hormonal hair loss, as described in chapter 16, my advice is to avoid testosterone. For many women, alopecia is a personal tragedy. No one has ever told me that

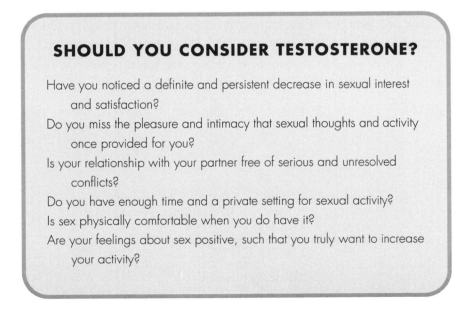

SHOULD YOU CONSIDER TESTOSTERONE?

Have you noticed a definite and persistent decrease in sexual interest and satisfaction?

Do you miss the pleasure and intimacy that sexual thoughts and activity once provided for you?

Is your relationship with your partner free of serious and unresolved conflicts?

Do you have enough time and a private setting for sexual activity?

Is sex physically comfortable when you do have it?

Are your feelings about sex positive, such that you truly want to increase your activity?

getting her sex drive back was worth losing her hair. *If hair loss begins on testosterone, I absolutely do not recommend waiting to see what happens.* A slight increase in shedding that quickly stops within a week or two may be normal. However, if you start to shed more than you ever have before or see less hair when you look in the mirror, then I strongly recommend that you stop it right away. You should also get treatment for the alopecia with a testosterone blocker so as to arrest the hair loss as quickly as possible.

SHOULD YOU USE TESTOSTERONE FOR MOOD OR ENERGY?

There is a current fad perpetrated by a few physicians—who are not trained in endocrinology—of prescribing testosterone and other hormones to anyone who is a little tired or hopes it will give him or her a competitive edge. (The whole idea of "andropause" or male menopause belongs to these suspect practices.) There was even a conference held to define a supposed female "androgen deficiency syndrome." Symptoms in this alleged syndrome included low sex drive, lack of energy, and decreased muscle tone. The problem is that these symptoms are extremely common. Although they often result from hormonal vulnerability, testosterone is by no means the only possible culprit. At this time, the only established reason for taking testosterone is to boost a flagging sex drive. There is no research supporting its use for low energy or depression; almost always these can be helped by more established treatments, as explained in chapter 6. If testosterone has any place at all for depressive symptoms, it is as a last resort.

14.

How to Use Testosterone *Now* to Get the Zest Back in Your Sex Life

When the new testosterone patch, Intrinsa, designed especially for women, is released, it will be the most convenient and precise way for women to use this hormone to rev up their sex drives. The patch is now under review by the FDA. In the meantime, it is possible to get the same benefit and the same safety profile using a gel that is available now by prescription. Use of the gel is a little tricky, so I will explain in clear detail how to do it.

I must emphasize that *transdermal gel is the only way that women can use testosterone that will have the same degree of effectiveness and the same safety profile as the patch*. Only gels approved by the FDA are manufactured with adequate quality-control standards. When used in accord with the instructions that I provide in this chapter, these can give the same blood levels of testosterone as the patch. Oral forms have potential harmful effects on the liver and cholesterol. Injectable forms such as testosterone enanthate (Delatestryl) produce very uneven blood levels. So-called compounded preparations are made up locally by individual pharmacies and are not tested at all before being sold. I have seen many women who developed excessive levels of testosterone from use of compounded preparations of testosterone. Safety of these forms is uncertain, no matter what their promoters may tell you.

I have worked out the method I describe here based on my long experience with the pharmacology of testosterone. Over the past decade, I have carried out research on both gel and patch hormone preparations and have been a consultant on safety issues. This background has enabled me to work out a method that enables women to use a currently available testosterone gel to get normal female levels, similar to those reported for the patch. I have no financial or other interest in the method I describe here; my only concern is that women distressed by loss of libido be able to use testosterone as safely as possible.

The preparation I suggest is testosterone 1 percent gel. Two preparations are now FDA approved: AndroGel and Testim. FDA approval gives assurance that both gels are manufactured in accord with the government's strict requirements. (No quality standards exist for compounded preparations.) Use of gel instead of cream also makes it easier to accurately measure out the small volumes suitable for women.

I am most familiar with AndroGel because several years ago I did research on its use in men, though I have never worked with its current manufacturer. Testim is probably just as good; in fact one study showed it to produce slightly higher blood levels. Other gels are in development, but if you have started on one, I do not recommend switching as absorption may not be the same with a different preparation.

Currently available gels come in three different kinds of packaging, but they are not ideal because they are designed to give the much larger amounts that are suitable for men. However, all can be adapted for use by women using the methods I describe here. AndroGel is available in two forms: premeasured foil packets and a pump dispenser not unlike those used for liquid soap. Testim comes in small squeeze tubes.

Since women's levels are only 5 to 10 percent of men's levels, the amount of gel applied must be only 5 to 10 percent of what a man would use. Here's how to get the woman-appropriate dose.

First, the gel must be measured out carefully using a plastic hypodermic syringe (without the needle). It's important to measure carefully, so you do not get too much or too little. The gel is then applied to the skin of the shoulders, upper arms or lower abdomen. *Like any other hormone cream or gel, testosterone should never be applied on or close to your breasts*. It's sometimes suggested that testosterone gel or cream be applied around the clitoris. I definitely do not recommend this, as accurate dosing is difficult and excessive blood levels can result. In my practice, I've seen several women who consulted me for help with scalp hair loss that occurred because they followed misguided advice to apply testosterone to their genital region. If you apply the gel to your skin as I have just described, it will promptly be absorbed into your bloodstream, through which it will travel almost instantaneously to all places in your body that can benefit from it—genitalia and the brain included. If you want to experiment with enhancing clitoral sensitivity, you can try some of the menthol containing lotions sold in woman-friendly sex shops; these give a tingling sensation some women find stimulating. Sources include Good Vibrations in San Francisco or Eve's Garden in New York (see Resources section). Both also sell their products online.

Gel provides testosterone for only twenty-four hours, so it needs to be applied daily—the patch will be much easier, since it need only be changed twice a week. Some of my patients have found that the gel still keeps their sex drives on alert, even if they apply it only every two or three days. My suggestion is to use it daily for the first two months to get a sense of how well it is working, then, if you want, you can try every other day to see if you maintain the benefit.

When AndroGel is used by men, skin-to-skin contact, or possibly contact with clothes or bed sheets, can result in transfer to the woman; I have seen one patient who got high levels from her husband's use of the gel. Transfer from a woman to a man, however, will not be a problem because his levels will be too high for it to make a difference. However, for the first few hours after application, caution should be employed to avoid skin-to-skin contact with girls or prepubertal boys. There is no need to be paranoid about this—one hug won't transfer enough to affect a child—but repeated contact might.

Though testosterone gel is at this time FDA approved for use in men, women can use it, so long as it is appropriately prescribed by a physician. Because testosterone is technically an anabolic steroid, it is a control drug, meaning its use is more closely regulated than other prescription drugs. For this reason, it should be used only as specifically prescribed for you; it must not be shared with others. While classified as an anabolic, as all forms of testosterone are, the doses recommended here for women will not have the harmful effects that occur in athletes who consume such drugs in mega quantities.

THE SECRET FOR USING TESTOSTERONE GEL: WOMAN-APPROPRIATE DOSING

I've already emphasized that cautious dosing is absolutely critical to avoid possible damage to your skin and hair. There is a tendency with topical medications to just glop them on without thinking much about the exact amount. Don't try this with testosterone—because it is a powerful hormone, this is definitely not a situation of, "If a little is good, more is better."

The secret of accurate dosing is to use a plastic disposable syringe (1 mL)—they are available without a needle—though you'll still need a prescription. For most women, 0.5 mL of gel is the correct dose. Some need a little more, but rarely more than 0.75 mL daily. You should start at the low end—which is just right for most women—and only increase if your blood level has not met its target. After you have been using the gel for about two weeks, have your blood drawn for total and free testosterone. These tests are explained in chapter 19. The blood-draw should be timed so as to be done about two hours after applying the gel. If you are on estrogen in any form, including an oral contraceptive, your total T level will probably be a little above the normal female range because of a high binding protein level. The more important measurement is free T, which is what can actually move out of your blood into your body. Free T should be in the middle to upper half of the normal female range, *but not above it*. This range varies depending on the specific lab, so I cannot give exact numbers here. If your free T is above normal, the dose should be reduced; there is no evidence that a higher level will make you feel sexier, but it definitely increases the chances of oily skin, acne, facial hair, or scalp hair loss.

Sex hormones do not work overnight. It generally takes one to two months for testosterone to make a noticeable difference in sexual feelings. So long as your blood level with the gel or patch is in the target range just described, there is no reason to consider a dose increase until you have been on it for at least six weeks. If you do not notice anything at this point, a slight increase in dose of about 0.1 mL can be considered, for example from 0.5 mL to 0.6 mL. I do not recommend use of testosterone in a dose that produces higher than normal female levels.

If you don't feel comfortable measuring the gel out with a syringe, ask to have a nurse in your doctor's office demonstrate. This method is commonly used to accurately dose for infants and small children; there is nothing unorthodox about it. The best technique is to draw up more than your dose, tap out any large bubbles, and squish out the excess. Be careful to wipe off the tip of the syringe before applying and do not touch any of what is left over. The excess should be disposed of safely so that no one can come into contact with the gel, especially children and pets.

The three different package forms of testosterone gel differ in cost and ease of use. The most important consideration is being able to avoid getting extra gel on your skin. Remember that even a drop of gel contains a lot of testosterone—just a smidgen more than your prescribed dose can lift your blood level above the female range. AndroGel in 2.5 g packets is the easiest to use but most expensive. You simply open the packet and dip the syringe into it, being careful not to squeeze the packet so hard as to get gel on your fingers. Once the packet is opened, you must safely discard the unused amount—you can't use what's left because some ingredients will quickly evaporate. The pump-bottle is more economical because it dispenses only half as much (1.25 g) with each push of the plunger, so the same amount will last you at least twice as long. However you'll need to pump the gel into some sort of container, such as a shot-glass, from which you can draw up what you need. After use, wash the glass very thoroughly without having any skin contact with the leftover gel. Testim in tube form can be used in the same way, with the same cautions. My advice is to start with AndroGel packets. If cost is a problem, you can change to the pump as soon as you've become comfortable in measuring out and applying the gel. If you change to Testim, your testosterone blood levels will need to be rechecked to be sure they have not gone too high.

With all these forms of testosterone gel, you'll be throwing away more than you actually use. For example, with a 2.5 g packet, if your dose is 0.5 g, you'll only use about a fifth of each packet. This is why the patch, once approved, will make testosterone treatment much easier for women. In the meantime, the gel can give the same result, though with less convenience. Even though measuring the gel may sound very complicated, it's quite easy once you've gotten used to it. Doctors, nurses, and pharmacists measure drugs out like this quite frequently; if we can do it, you can too. As I suggested earlier, getting a nurse or doctor to teach you is a good idea if you feel any uncertainty about the procedure.

Testosterone restores sexual pleasure for many women, but not for all. If you have tried it for three months, checked your blood level at least twice, and found it in the target range, but nothing has happened, there is no reason to continue. Other possible treatments are discussed later in this chapter.

WHY TRANSDERMAL IS THE ONLY WAY WOMEN SHOULD USE TESTOSTERONE

As we grow up, we become used to applying creams for skin problems, but to some people, the idea of applying medicine to the skin to affect internal function still seems a little strange. Yet, for many medications, the transdermal route, in which the active ingredient travels from a patch or gel through the skin and into the blood, is ideal. Transdermal administration has at least two advantages: First, it permits steady blood levels rather than the peaks and valleys that usually occur with oral administration. Second, since the hormone or drug does not pass through the liver all at once, there is less potential for harmful effects on this vital organ. Although patches and gels look pretty ordinary, they depend on surprisingly complex technology. For this reason, good preparations of medicines for transdermal use have only been available for the last ten to fifteen years.

Testosterone itself has very little activity if it is taken orally. For women, the oral and injectable forms are obsolete. Despite this, one oral form is still commonly used, methyltestosterone, which comes combined with estrogen in a preparation called Estratest. Although this is the only form of testosterone for women that is FDA approved, it is far from ideal. In fact, it makes my list of the worst hormone replacement preparations. (See the appendix to chapter 26.) Not only are there side effect issues, it does not work very well.

Now that we have gel, with the easy-to-use patch on the way, there is no place, in my view, for women using oral or injectable versions. The patch will be the best way, since getting the correct dose takes no more effort than removing the backing and pressing it on the skin. The gel, if used carefully as I have detailed, will give the same blood level as the patch and, therefore, affect the body in the same way. As I have stressed, those from compounded pharmacies are not reliable—I've seen them produce blood levels that are ten times higher than they should be for a woman. Even after release of the patch, gels will be a good option for those few women who get skin irritation from patches.

A testosterone vaginal ring is also under development. This works on the same principle as the contraceptive ring—the hormones are readily absorbed through the vaginal mucosa, and, as with application to the skin, the liver is bypassed. The important questions are how closely the testosterone blood levels will mimic normal female ones and how steady they will be. Though the ring is promising, we need to await more details.

TESTOSTERONE, MENOPAUSE, AND ESTROGEN THERAPY

Most of the testosterone studies reported to date have used this hormone in combination with estrogen. This raises a question: Can testosterone be used by itself? The answer is an individual one and depends on whether the vagina is moist and resilient enough for comfortable intercourse. If your periods are normal and you have no symptoms of estrogen deficiency, such as hot flashes and vaginal dryness, then you will not need estrogen in addition to testosterone. On the other hand, if what used to feel good now just makes you sore, there may be reason to consider adding estrogen together with testosterone to maintain the vagina and surrounding tissues in a youthful state. (The many issues regarding estrogen therapy are covered in detail in Part VI.) Low estrogen is far from the only reason for pain during sex, so don't ignore your body's signals—if sex is starting to hurt, a check by your gynecologist is in order. This is particularly true if you experience bleeding after sex. In fact, you should have had a recent gynecologist check before starting on testosterone. If it was prescribed by your gynecologist, presumably he or she will note the conditions of your pelvic tissues during your exam. Just the same, it is a good idea to ask if your vaginal tissues look sufficiently estrogenized for increased sexual activity to be comfortable.

If you are on birth control pills, they will provide enough estrogen for sexual comfort. Even on the pill, if your ovaries are slowing down, you may feel dry during the fourth week of inactive pills. If lubricant doesn't restore comfort, then an estrogen supplement such as a 0.1 mg Climara patch usually will.

Another factor is your partner. If he starts using Viagra, Levitra, or Cialis, or you have a new partner whose erections are firmer, you may experience discomfort. Some women notice pain with some partners but not others. This is probably a result of how well a particular man's penis fits your internal anatomy, something no one has yet found a way to measure—though MRI scans are now being used to study how the penis moves within the vagina.

KEEPING SEX COMFORTABLE

In the previous section, I mentioned that estrogen is needed to keep vaginal tissues resilient. Dryness occurs with lowering estrogen levels, but some women with adequate estrogen levels notice dryness even when fully aroused. In this case, lubricants can usually help. There are basically two sorts: jellies such as K-Y and liquids such as Astroglide. Both forms are available in cheaper generic versions. The liquids are less gooey but more likely to run down onto the bed. It is just a matter of trying the different types until you find what is most suitable. Special lubricants, including ones which supposedly taste good, are sold at sex shops, such as Eve's Garden and Good Vibrations.

Condoms increase the possibility of irritation, since the vaginal walls were not designed to be rubbed by latex. Only lubricated condoms should be used, but some women need extra lubricant in addition. Vaseline and similar oily or greasy lubricants should be avoided; they prevent your tissues from breathing and may damage condoms. Lubricants make things slipperier but do nothing to build up the vaginal tissues. If sex is uncomfortable, despite use of a lubricant, then dryness is not the entire problem. Either the vagina is irritated, for example from infection, or falling estrogen levels have made it less resilient. To tell the difference you need to have an exam.

WILL TESTOSTERONE MAKE A WOMAN A SEX FIEND?

Sexual desire and its fulfillment are among the greatest satisfactions of human life. Yet if desire is too strong, it can be disruptive. There is no need to worry that testosterone will make your sex drive too strong— I have never heard of it making a woman into a nymphomaniac or otherwise out of control. Such is the stuff of fiction.

A widespread misconception about testosterone is that it increases aggressiveness. While it is likely that testosterone exposure in early life has something to do with programming males to be more aggressive, there is no evidence that later exposure to higher levels affects behavior. "Steroid madness" due to taking anabolics is a myth. Rather, those who take " 'roids" to improve their athletic performance are likely to be aggressive anyway. Who has ever heard of a pacifist football lineman? In my practice, I see many women with elevated testosterone due to adrenal or ovarian conditions. I have not noticed any particular personality differences between these women and those with normal or low levels. So no one need worry that using testosterone will alter her personality.

We don't know whether testosterone will slightly boost desire, that is normal to begin with, because research has been done only with women who have sought help for waning desire. This is partly because of politics. Pharmaceutical companies are nervous about a backlash if they market a drug to make normal sex better. I don't see any reason to use testosterone if your sex life is working well, but some women probably will try it anyway. My guess is that some will notice a slight enhancement; however, it's hard to be sure this is not a placebo effect. We do know something about the effects of very high testosterone levels from women whose bodies make greatly excessive amounts. Most often there is no significant effect on sexuality. Those few whose sexual feelings are stirred up often find it uncomfortably distracting. Pleasurable as sex is, it cannot occupy all of life. Few truly want to spend most of their time having sex. (Romantic getaways or honeymoons may be exceptions, but they do not last forever.) The value of testosterone is to give sex its rightful place, not to make it take over one's life.

CONSIDER POSTPONING TESTOSTERONE IF:

Your partner has erectile dysfunction or another condition that makes him unable to have intercourse. In this situation, both of you will need treatment, though it need not be from the same doctor. Nonpenetrative sex is a reasonable alternative, of course.*

You have more than mild or occasional pain during intercourse. This needs to be evaluated and treated before you do anything to increase the frequency of intercourse.

Your skin and hair are vulnerable to testosterone. Most women can take the modest amount of testosterone contained in the patch without developing acne, unwanted hair, or scalp hair loss. But if you have these problems already, testosterone will likely make them worse.

You have significant relationship problems. Taking testosterone will not solve these.

You are pregnant or trying to be. The small amount of testosterone in the patch is probably safe for the fetus, but it is best not to take any chances when the health of a future child is involved.

---

*Taking testosterone is perfectly reasonable if you simply want to restore the ability to masturbate. I emphasize sex with a partner simply because this is usually a concern of the women who consult a physician about low sexual interest.

If you feel sexual yearnings and enjoy it when the opportunity arises, there's no point in trying testosterone. But if the thought of sex is no more exciting than doing household chores, trying it is a reasonable option, even if you are not approaching menopause.

SOME REASONS NOT TO TRY TESTOSTERONE RIGHT AWAY

If you have read this far, you may be very eager to start testosterone to spice up your sex life. I don't want to put a damper on anyone's ardor, but I do need to offer a reminder that with testosterone, as with everything else in life, timing is critical. The sidebar on page 210 lists situations that you might want resolved before you try it.

OTHER TREATMENTS FOR SEXUAL DYSFUNCTION

Viagra (sildenafil) is perhaps the world's best known pharmaceutical, which testifies to the interest sexual enhancement holds. Some women have complained that with the great research effort devoted to male sexuality, they were left out. This was certainly not intentional. Viagra has been studied in women and the research expenditures for developing woman-suitable testosterone have been enormous.

Viagra was discovered entirely by accident. It works by vasodilatation—opening up blood vessels so that more blood flows through them. Originally, it was tried for treatment of angina, a common heart condition in which coronary artery blood flow is inadequate. Men who used it in the studies discovered that their erections improved, and so it ended up being developed as an erection drug. (Viagra inhibits an enzyme, phosphodiesterase type 5, which breaks down nitric oxide [NO], a potent vasodilator produced in tissues. With Viagra, NO accumulates and improves penile blood flow. Drugs like Viagra are referred to collectively as PDE-5 inhibitors.)

Not long after it was released, Viagra was tried in women. This may seem odd until one remembers that female arousal also depends on increased blood flow to the genital area. Large-scale studies did not find an overall benefit, but Viagra does seem to help some women. To understand who might benefit, it is necessary to consider the difference in how testosterone and Viagra work.

In men there is a clear difference between desire and performance. Men with erectile dysfunction (ED) feel desire, but their equipment does not do what is necessary—they want to have sex, but cannot. Viagra makes erections firmer so that men with ED can act on their desire. For women, the most common sexual problem is lack of desire, and Viagra does not help this. There are a few women who still feel desire but find that not much happens when their partner tries to stimulate them or they try to masturbate. If you feel like sex but being touched no longer evokes a pleasurable response, then Viagra or a related medication might help.

Two new PDE-5 inhibitors have been approved for men, although women can use them if prescribed: Levitra (vardenafil) and Cialis (tadalafil). Levitra is rumored to be slightly stronger, but the difference is small. Cialis is different in that it lasts for about thirty-six hours compared with about six for Viagra and Levitra. Dubbed "le weekend pill," it has been touted as more woman-friendly because it need not be timed so closely to intercourse. Since men more frequently initiate, timing Viagra may be awkward for women.

Women complain about PDE-5 inhibitor side effects more often than men do. I suspect that men are so happy to be able to have erections once again that they keep their mouths shut about any problems for fear that their doctors will want them to discontinue the medication. The most common side effect is headache—not surprising when one recalls that migraine is related to dilatation of blood vessels in the head. With Viagra at least, a few notice a sort of bluish discoloration of their vision. These side effects wear off as the effect of the medication does. Though there have been reports of PDE-5 inhibitors causing blindness, no cause-and-effect relationship has been proven. Such events are exceedingly rare.

If you feel desire but don't respond to stimulation as you once did, Viagra is worth a try. If it works but does not last long enough, you might want to switch to Cialis. The Viagra dose is 50 or 100 mg. You can try 50 first and then increase to 100 only if 50 does not work and does not cause side effects. Unlike testosterone, which has a gradual onset over about a month, Viagra either works within an hour or two, or it does not work at all. It does not affect sexual thoughts, only genital sensation. If you do not notice any effect with Viagra after several tries, it probably will not work, nor will Levitra or Cialis.

The antidepressant Wellbutrin (bupropion) helps restore sexual thoughts and desire in women taking SSRIs or who have lost sexual interest without any clear cause. It does not work for everyone, and a few do not like how they feel on it. Nonetheless it is the best alternative to testosterone for low desire. The effect of bupropion on sexuality seems to be unrelated to its antidepressant effect, so you don't have to be depressed for it to help you feel sexier.

Herbs are promoted for enhancement of sexual desire, though their marketing has been mainly toward men. I have not seen evidence that any are effective. Traditional Chinese medicine offers an abundance of sexual tonics for men. I once saw one in a Chinese pharmacy whose label read "Golden Gun Pills" in English, then in Chinese, "May your Golden Gun never droop." Such offerings are quaint, but given the high incidence of toxic heavy metals in Chinese patent medicine, I do not advise trying them. One widely used by Chinese women to "supplement yin" is called White Phoenix Pills. I do not recommend this either and for the same reason. China has an immense herbal pharmacopoeia that I believe will one day have much to offer. Unfortunately, purity needs to be assured before it will be safe to try them.

15.

Getting the Most from Your New Sexuality

This book is not a sex manual; it does not discuss exotic positions or other ways to spice up your sex life. This sort of information is available in many other books but is not of much use unless you feel desire in the first place. The role of medicine is to keep the biochemical and physical prerequisites of sex in working order. Although hormones may be less exciting to read about than sexual techniques, they make excitement possible.

The previous chapters have described virtually everything that is now known about the treatment of low desire. To experience the reawakening of sexuality is a wonderful thing but can bring new questions in its wake. This chapter offers advice about some of the concerns that can arise as your sex life revives.

TELLING YOUR PARTNER ABOUT TESTOSTERONE

Men who use Viagra often keep mum about it with their partners, unless they are in a long-term relationship. In some cultures, using male sex-enhancers is a macho thing, and men will boast about it. For a woman, the issues are more delicate because some still feel a little awkward admitting that they are deliberately augmenting their sexy feelings.

Sex is supposed to happen of its own accord, not as a result of technology. In case you feel reticent about discussing your use of testosterone with your partner, I'll make some suggestions for handling the issue, based on how men are likely to feel about it. The matter is actually pretty simple. None of my patients on testosterone have reported any negative reactions from partners. A husband will welcome its use if he understands that you have started it because you want to be more sexual with him. Like initiating sex, it shows you are attracted to him. If anything, the problem is that starting testosterone may engender unrealistic expectations on the man's part. As I have emphasized, it restores sex drive to a normal level, not insatiability. Nonetheless, men are generally happy for any improvement in their partner's sexual availability.

If you are dating, things are a little more tricky. Many women do not like to be so open about the details of their sexuality until they have been with a man long enough to feel some degree of trust and comfort. My personal view is that in a dating situation, privacy is still each partner's right, unless the matter affects the other directly, for example, infection with an STD. Testosterone gel is invisible soon after application and transfer to an adult male will not be harmful. (However, it might be to a man being treated for prostate cancer. This special situation often brings sexual problems of its own. If your partner has this form of cancer, both of you will need specific medical advice regarding sexuality.) So if you are dating, there is no reason to tell, unless you want to. If you are living with someone, it is of course much harder to keep use of the gel a secret—especially if you are discovered measuring it out with a syringe. Most likely he'll be aware that your interest in sex has waned, and things will be more comfortable if you explain that you are using testosterone.

I doubt most men will care much one way or the other about your use of testosterone. If he senses that you are attracted to him and are sexually responsive, he is unlikely to analyze matters further. When testosterone is started in a long-standing relationship, he may be apprehensive that you will become sexually more demanding. For most men, even though they know better, being asked for sex more often than they are able to perform seems to challenge their masculinity.

Providing general reassurance that testosterone may restore your sexual feelings to the way they were before, but will not change them otherwise, should be sufficient.

Since testosterone typically takes about a month to start working, if your husband will be away for a week or two, or even a little longer, it does not make sense to stop during that short time. If testosterone has reactivated your sexual appetite, it is best to stay with it, rather than let your libido wind down and then have to reactivate it. If you need to explain to him why you are continuing to use the testosterone, you can point out that where hormones are concerned it is best to not change them around too often. You can add that it will keep thoughts of sex with him on your mind and make you especially eager for his return.

While testosterone gel disappears a few minutes after application, a patch will be visible when you are undressed. (Though the patch is not available at this time, once it is released, many women will prefer it over the gel because of its convenience.) In an established relationship, this presents no problems—I have never heard a woman using estrogen patches report that it bothered her husband or boyfriend. If you are dating and you prefer not to explain the patch to a new lover, you can simply say it is a hormone patch. Few men will be able to tell an estrogen patch from one with testosterone. Indeed, many men find the subject of women's hormones somewhat intimidating and will be happy to avoid the subject. It may be that with media coverage of the patch, some men will suspect an estrogen patch of being testosterone. Here the easiest course may be to say that your doctor told you that you were deficient in estrogen and should use the patch for replacement. But I make these suggestions only if you feel shy about explaining it. In most cases it is not a problem.

If you are using the patch and want to avoid the issue altogether with a new partner, there is a simple solution. Take it off just before you'll be undressed with him and put a new one on once you are by yourself again. (You'll probably need a new one, as patches tend to shrivel up when removed.) Just as the effect of testosterone comes on gradually, it wears off slowly as well. Even if the patch is off for a few hours, it will still be doing what you want it to do. If the patch leaves a dark ring, you may want to use an alcohol swab to remove that, but once he gets to the point of seeing all of you, the meaning of a smudge on your skin will be the last thing on his mind.

In case your partner wants to know more about how testosterone may affect you, I've provided a sidebar itemizing the essential information. You can use this as a basis for your explanation to him, or you can simply show it to him. For that matter, if he wants to know more, he can read this entire section. Some men will want to understand why you are ready for more sex; most will simply want the sex.

WHY A WOMAN TAKES TESTOSTERONE

About a third of perfectly normal women experience a loss of sex drive.

The cause of decreased sexual interest in women is not fully understood, but hormones clearly play a role.

When a woman loses interest in sex, it need not mean that she finds her partner less attractive or that she feels less affectionate toward him.

For many women, sex drive returns with use of testosterone.

Testosterone works gradually; it can take from one to three months for sexual interest to come back. If there has not been much sex for a long time, it may take awhile for it to become relaxed again.

Testosterone does not change the nature or direction of a woman's sexual interest, nor will it make her more aggressive.

SEXUAL CHANGE IN LONG-STANDING RELATIONSHIPS

When testosterone is started, expectations may be high on both sides. Both may feel some anxiety as to what the other will expect or whether testosterone will alter sexual tastes. This is true even between partners who have been together for many years and know each other very well. Sexual activities tend to fall into a pattern that becomes comfortable for both. When this changes, both partners may feel awkward because how they have sex needs to be renegotiated. Especially if you have covertly set up your routine to make it easier to avoid sex, you'll have to change this. If sex has been infrequent in your relationship for a long time—by infrequent, I mean only a few times a year—then doing it more often will require many subtle changes in routine. Testosterone will not make up for fatigue, proximity of children, different work schedules, frequent travel, or other modern hindrances to sexual bliss. Eventually comfort will be reestablished, but the transition may have awkward moments. Open discussion is always recommended, but some couples find this difficult to achieve—after all, sex is very much a matter of nonverbal messages. The most important thing is to keep trying. Testosterone does greatly improve sex for many women and their partners, but the changes will not occur overnight.

WHAT TO DO ABOUT TESTOSTERONE IF YOU ARE BETWEEN RELATIONSHIPS

To be eligible for the patch studies, women had to be in a relationship with a partner for at least several months. As it turned out, the average length of the relationships of the women in the study was nearly twenty years. However, you don't have to be in a relationship for any particular length of time to use testosterone. Some women who are dating find lack of interest in sex particularly worrisome because they fear, not unreasonably, that the man will not stay interested very long if physical intimacy does not develop fairly quickly. Testosterone is also suitable for a woman in this situation.

Many questions arise that the testosterone patch research was not designed to answer, such as what to do if you suddenly find yourself without a sexual partner. Several things are at stake in this situation. First, since testosterone takes a while to start working, if you discontinue it and later find yourself in another relationship, there may be a lag before it starts to work again. Perhaps even more important, it's probably not a good thing to have sexuality turned on and off repeatedly. So unless you are having side effects, it's generally better to stay on the gel or patch. After all, sex is not just what you do with a partner.

Many value sexual thoughts and feelings for their own sakes, even at those times when they cannot be fulfilled in physical activity with or without a partner. As one patient of mine, a very hard-working executive, expressed her dismay at loss of libido, "Sexual thoughts energize me, even at work when I cannot act on them. Without them I feel something is missing from my life." Western culture is highly goal-oriented, and so sexual desire tends to be thought of as what leads to intercourse and then to the intense pleasure and release of orgasm. This ignores the obvious fact that sexual feelings are pleasurable in themselves even when there is no prospect of any actual contact. Many women, after all, despite being happily married and without any interest in extracurricular sex, still love to flirt. Men notoriously get pleasure from looking at women, even though most are unattainable. These purely mental forms of sex are so common that they are hardly thought much—until they are gone, when they are missed. If the patch simply makes you feel more energetic and alive, these are reasons to consider continuing it, even when you are without a partner. Another question is the role of masturbation in your life. Some women virtually never masturbate, while others do so frequently. If this has been a source of sexual pleasure for you, and testosterone has enhanced it, this is another reason to continue to use it.

If your sexual feelings mainly occur in response to intimacy with your partner and they are otherwise not important in your life, then there is no definite reason to continue testosterone if a relationship has ended and you are not seeking a new one. I'd make one exception; however, it may sound strange at first. If your relationship has ended because of the death of your partner, it might seem disloyal to him if you continue the patch even though you have no thought of starting a new relationship. However, testosterone does have an antidepressant effect, and so it is possible that it might help you keep going during this very difficult time. There is certainly no research about testosterone and bereavement, but it seems to me prudent not to do anything that might make coping harder. This can also apply to any traumatic breakup that leaves you depressed.

A final point needs emphasis: Testosterone does not restore libido in all women. If you have not noticed any difference in how you feel on the patch—after a fair trial of two to three months—and if your blood level is in the target range, then there is no reason to continue it, whatever your relationship situation.

WHAT MEN WANT—AND DON'T WANT— IN AND OUT OF BED

Neither women nor men automatically know what the other wants sexually. Sex education has narrowed the gap, but not completely. My view is that what men want is actually closer to what women want than women usually realize. Affection is equally important to both, but there are differences in what counts as affection for men and women. While it is true that men can enjoy sex without any real caring, at least in the short term, the converse is not true—by which I mean that affection for men must usually include sex. Many women, on the other hand, particularly in a long-standing relationship, can be satisfied by physical contact that does not lead to intercourse.

Ultimately most men sooner or later come to find sex without love unsatisfying, which is why they eventually seek stable relationships. Variety is sacrificed for things of greater value: affection, comfort, dependability, and knowing a fellow human on a deep level. Women often assume that men want sex for physical pleasure and fail to realize that for men sex is also a primary way of experiencing love. Most men want sex to be with the woman they love. If they simply sought the physical sensations of intercourse, it would be easy enough to find them elsewhere. Some men do wander, of course, but most do not: They want physical intimacy from their wives or long-term partners. This usually means intercourse but can mean oral sex or other means of release. Women, on the other hand, tend to see sex as added onto the relationship but not absolutely essential to it. Much tension can be avoided by appreciating that for men, sex means far more than physical pleasure.

Having said this, not all men need regular sexual intimacy. There are happy marriages in which sex is infrequent or never happens. If both partners are satisfied without sexual contact, there is nothing wrong with this. Sex is one element of marital satisfaction, but far from the only one.

WHEN YOUR PARTNER NEEDS HELP: THE WOMAN'S QUICK GUIDE TO COMMON MALE DIFFICULTIES

When the woman's interest in sex increases, any problems her partner has may come to the fore. If you are considering treatment for low desire, but your partner has erectile dysfunction, he may need treatment as well. There is not much point in stirring your own desires if your partner cannot respond. It is sensible for him to try Viagra or another PDE-5 inhibitor—such as Levitra or Cialis—to be sure it will work for him before you start testosterone. If he still cannot have functional erections, there's little reason for you to try to increase your own sex drive, unless you have another outlet than penetrative intercourse.

Premature ejaculation is more often a problem for men in their twenties, although it can happen to older men. A common side effect of SSRI antidepressants such as Prozac, Zoloft, Paxil, and others is to slow arousal; for this reason they often help premature ejaculation.

WHAT IF HE'S THE ONE WHO DOES NOT WANT SEX?

Women partners of men uninterested in sex usually find the situation distressing, even if they do not miss the sex in itself. They feel that something is missing. As one patient whose husband never touches her put it, "He's affectionate toward me, but it is like the affection you have for a child or a pet dog." What she missed was the intensity of male interest she had experienced in earlier relationships.

Lack of desire is far less common in men and harder to treat. Low testosterone is one cause, but the majority of affected men have normal levels. A simple blood test will quickly tell if the problem is hormonal. If not, adding more testosterone does not help. Counseling is the appropriate step to deal with the resulting marital issues but does not usually change the man's sexual interest.

TESTOSTERONE AND SEX FOR LESBIAN WOMEN

Like heterosexual women, lesbian women are diverse in their sexual attitudes and preferences. Having said this, I have not found any fundamental difference in sexual interest problems between my lesbian patients and those who are heterosexual. Loss of desire is common and can be distressing for both groups of women. Imbalance in sex drive between partners can still create tension. When this happens, testosterone is a reasonable option and can work, just as it does for heterosexual couples. Testosterone is like the volume control on a stereo; it changes the intensity but not the composition. The large studies of the patch included lesbian women, but no separate results have been published at this point.

Low desire seems to be at least as frequent in lesbian as in straight women. What is more common is for *both* partners to find their desires waning. Since low sexual interest is more common in women, it is more likely in a lesbian relationship that both will be affected. Reactions to this so-called "bed death" vary. Some, but by no means all, lesbian couples are content with little sexual contact leading to orgasm. In this situation, there is no need for both to use testosterone, unless both miss the intensity of sexual encounters. But if both want more sensuality, testosterone can help lesbian couples just as it does heterosexual ones.

There does not seem to be any basic difference in how hormones affect sexuality in straight and lesbian women. Most of what I have written in this chapter applies just as well to the concerns of lesbian women. I have generally, it is true, referred to male-female interactions, but this is simply because it is the most common pattern.

IS MEDICATION FOR LOW DESIRE A QUICK FIX?

It's no secret that Americans are busier than ever. A standard criticism of almost any medical advance that simplifies treatment is that it is a "quick fix," particularly if the condition is one involving the mind as well as the body. Thus antidepressants are a quick fix, or Viagra. Even Lipitor has been branded a quick fix for cholesterol. A group calling itself FSD-Alert has aggressively pushed the claim that using testosterone is objectionable because it ignores the complexities of human sexuality. Maybe, but psychology can create complexities where there were none to begin with. There is an odd sort of puritanism here that implies that there is something wrong with curing a condition directly with medication instead of months or years of psychotherapy. My own view is that the best treatment for any condition *is* the easiest one, so long as it works and is safe. Before Viagra and now testosterone for women, there were no treatments for sexual problems other than counseling, a time-consuming and expensive undertaking that was ineffective much of the time. The assumption that all sexual problems are psychological is clearly refuted by the success of Viagra in men and testosterone in women. Of course, the effectiveness of these treatments does not imply that sexual problems are never psychological. Some are, and need to be treated accordingly.

Psychological treatment is not inherently better than medication. Nor is it without potential adverse effects. An incompetent therapist can create confusion that makes problems worse, at least until a better therapist is found. For many, psychological approaches feel invasive, since the process requires revealing all sorts of intimate matters. Some prefer to keep these private; others welcome the chance to discuss the ups and downs of their sex lives in a safe setting. It is really for you to decide what form of treatment to pursue.

All parties to the debate have economic self-interest at stake. Physicians and pharmaceutical companies make their money by providing medication as some psychologists are quick to draw attention to. On the other hand, effective medical treatments draw clients away from psychotherapists. Competition between treatments has the same benefits as competition in other contexts: It stimulates development of better methods. However, for the consumer, the contending voices may create confusion. The only answer is to look into both modes of treatment and choose what is most comfortable for you. If what you choose first does not give the hoped-for result, there is no reason not to try another.

Earlier in this chapter I listed some factors that would make seeing a psychologist or psychiatrist sensible as the first step. If none of these applies to you and you do not feel that your problem is psychological, my suggestion is that you try medication first—unless of course you have a contraindication. If it solves your problem, you've had a quick solution and can go back to enjoying sex. If it doesn't, then the next step is to consider counseling.

CONCLUSION: SCIENCE IS MAKING SEX BETTER

The generations now in their forties or beyond have assumed that sexual pleasure should continue throughout life. Given this expectation, it can be a shock if, one day, sex stops working. Once thought to be entirely psychological, it is clear that many sexual difficulties are organic. We are now on the threshold of a new era in which it is possible to keep on having great sex for many more years. Thanks to both cultural change and scientific advance, sexual pleasure does not have to stop in the prime of life.

PART V

The Most Visible Part of Your Body May Be the Most Vulnerable: What Hormones Can Do to Skin, Hair, Weight, and Metabolism

A NOTE ABOUT TESTOSTERONE
AND ITS PLACE IN YOUR LIFE

When they are working right, hormones give a fresh, feminine glow to the complexion. When they are being contrary, they can undo your best efforts at skin care and makeup. Most of the common complexion and hair problems are due to the ill effects of hormones or, more specifically, to skin's vulnerability to them. The culprit for most of these problems is testosterone. The general term for medical conditions caused by testosterone and related hormones is *androgenic disorders.*

In this part, you'll find chapters explaining hormonal hair loss, increased hair growth, and acne. Then I provide separate chapters describing the necessary lab tests and the details about effective hormonal treatment. By putting workup and treatment together, I avoid repeating similar information for each condition so I can use the space to tell you how you can have clear, smooth skin and a full head of hair.

Like estrogen and progesterone, testosterone is decidedly a mixed blessing. Women—and men—need all three of these hormones, yet all can be troublemakers. Some of the trouble caused by testosterone is welcome: the pleasant agitation of sexual desire. Testosterone can be a near-miracle for women who want to recover the zest for sex that has mysteriously vanished. Yet testosterone has other effects that can be heartbreaking for women afflicted with them. That testosterone can help sexual pleasure must not blind us to its shadow side: the damaging effects it can have on appearance. The function of hormones is to carry messages, but the messages borne by testosterone are decidedly mixed.

If you have a testosterone problem, proper treatment can be life-changing. The paradox is that some women's lives are transformed by taking testosterone to raise their levels, while others are transformed by having their testosterone lowered or blocked. By now, you'll have figured out why: It depends on individual hormonal vulnerability.

Testosterone has a dysfunctional relationship with many women's bodies, and like other dysfunctional relationships, this one can be confusing. As with difficult family members, many women's feelings toward their own testosterone are both love and hate. If you don't let yourself become discouraged, it really is possible to come to terms with your testosterone. What's needed is frank talk about this exasperating hormone so you can make sense of what it is doing to you and find effective treatment. I've summed up the good and bad news about testosterone in the sidebar on page 229. (If I talked about hormone effects as "good or bad" in a scientific meeting, I'd be laughed out of the room. Scientists are supposed to use neutral, objective language. Yet the effects of hormones are far from neutral. Sometimes, seemingly unscientific language is the most accurate way to talk about them.)

HOW THIS PART IS ARRANGED

Although hair loss, facial and body hair, and acne look quite different, their underlying cause is similar: excess effect of testosterone, due to high levels or to hormonal vulnerability—or both. Because the causes of these conditions are similar, the workup and treatment are too. Each does have specific, usually nonhormonal, treatments that are fully explained in the separate chapters on each condition.

My suggestion is that you first read the chapter on those skin and hair problems you have, then the chapters on testing and treatment. You may want to go back to earlier chapters to help you make decisions about what treatment is best for you, especially regarding choosing between hormonal and nonhormonal approaches—or combining them. Although this does involve some going back and forth, I promise your effort will be rewarded with clearer, smoother skin and more abundant hair.

TESTOSTERONE AND WOMEN

Good Things:

Sexy thoughts and sensations

Strong bones

Muscle power

Vitality: good mood and ample energy

Many women have all of these despite relatively low levels of testosterone.

Bad Things:

Oily skin

Dull, sallow complexion

Skin aging

Acne

Rosacea

Facial and body hair

Thinning of scalp hair (alopecia)

16.

The Most Heartbreaking Hormone Problem: If You're Starting to Lose Your Hair

Roxanne had come all the way from Texas to New York City to see me and had asked to have an appointment as soon as possible, not even wanting to wait a week or two to get a cheaper airfare. Roxanne was suffering from alopecia—hair loss. Men's hair always thins; though none of us likes it, most of us just accept it. For women, thinning hair is not an anticipated life event, and even the most self-possessed woman can lose her nerve when her scalp starts to show. Oddly, considering the distress it causes, not only medicine but also the women's media have virtually ignored female hair loss. (One of my patients suggested this may be because the women who write about health and beauty find the idea too disturbing to even think about.) Alopecia is quite common—about 20 percent of women are affected by age forty; the percent keeps going up after that. Physically hair is useless; emotionally, it is essential. A full head of hair symbolizes youth, vitality, attractiveness, and femininity; a woman with alopecia may feel that she is losing all of these along with her hair. Because women with alopecia can become deeply depressed, it is, in my opinion, an urgent medical problem.

Roxanne had been to several doctors locally. Two did not see that losing hair was a problem at all. One even said, "I've got patients who have cancer; why are you worrying about your hair?" Although Roxanne was grateful that she did not have cancer, this did not make her feel any better about losing her hair. Another doctor, a dermatologist, conceded that her hair was thinning but remarked, "You're healthy; don't worry about it. Anyway, there's nothing that can be done; you'll just have to learn to live with it."

I wish I could say that the response Roxanne got from the doctors she consulted is atypical. Unfortunately, it is not. Most of the women I see in consultation for alopecia have been subjected to similar patronizing attitudes. For Roxanne, not only were the dismissals hurtful, but also the advice she received along with them was wrong. Female hair loss is definitely treatable. Although there are a variety of causes of hair loss, by far the most common is hormones. Follicles overly sensitive to testosterone can shed their hairs when exposed to even a whiff of this hormone. A dip in estrogen can have the same effect. Roxanne was thirty-six, an age at which most women's ovaries make plenty of estrogen. In her case, the problem was testosterone. Though her levels were actually normal, her hair follicles couldn't handle even tiny amounts; they were hormonally vulnerable.

WOMEN AND HAIR LOSS

Alopecia is simply the medical term for hair loss; calling hair loss alopecia says nothing about the cause. Women seeking help for this condition are often frustrated that no one believes them. Friends may not notice or out of politeness pretend that they can't see any change. Few doctors are trained to properly examine the hair and scalp, and so most cannot recognize the early stages of hormonal hair loss. If you are wondering whether you are starting to lose hair, check out the next sidebar.

THE WARNING SIGNS OF HORMONAL HAIR LOSS

Losing more than 100 hairs a day

Thinning at the temples, crown, and vertex. (The vertex is the pointy part at the back of the head.)

Widening of your part or thinning of your ponytail

Scalp becoming visible on top

Your hairdresser no longer thins your hair when you have it cut

Itchiness, burning, or sores on your scalp

Presence of other hormonal skin changes: persistent acne, increased facial and body hair

Irregular periods

Difficulty controlling weight

WHAT DOES IT FEEL LIKE TO HAVE ALOPECIA?

A renowned but unsympathetic dermatologist once said to me, chuckling, "We know hair is totally unnecessary." Some just cannot understand why hair matters to women. It's true that hair is not necessary for survival in the way the heart or kidney is, but human life is more than survival. I've already said something about the symbolic meanings of hair. To these I'd add youthfulness, not meaning any particular age but a sense of freshness and enthusiasm for life. This has no age limit—my patients in their sixties value their hair quite as much as do twenty-five-year-olds.

Hair is the only part of the body that can be frequently and painlessly altered and shaped. Styling and coloring hair are forms of self-expression. Even the choice to do nothing with one's hair but wash and comb it or to shave it off completely is still a way of showing one's individuality.

Most women take their hair for granted and have no particular reason to reflect on what it means to them. When it starts to fall out, however, everything changes. Women with alopecia tell me that they are embarrassed and humiliated that their hair is thin. There is no reason for shame—alopecia is not anyone's fault—yet such feelings are nearly universal when hair starts to thin.

Nor have I found any notable cultural differences in how women react to losing hair. My patients with alopecia are as diverse a group as can be imagined. In age they range from teens to sixties and older. Some have advanced academic degrees; others left school to go to work early. They come from all over the United States and many foreign countries. Some have careers; others are homemakers. One affected a punk look and shaved her head, yet she was embarrassed that the stubble was less dense on top than on the sides. Even though she chose to shave off her hair, she wanted it to be there.

I see some Muslim women who always cover their heads with scarves, yet still feel self-conscious that their hair is thin. The same is true for Orthodox Jewish married women whose own hair is concealed by wigs. I emphasize these diverse cultural practices to demonstrate that distress over alopecia is not specifically American, not neurosis, not vanity; it is simply the way women react when faced with the loss of a part of their bodies.

Married women are as bothered by alopecia as those who are single. It is perhaps harder on single women because they worry it will make them unacceptable to men. Dating is hard enough without this additional source of insecurity. Yet most men seem not to notice when their wives or girlfriends have thinning hair and are not much bothered by it if they do notice. Women with alopecia find this hard to believe, but I base it on hearing the stories of several thousand women with this condition. Men's concern is usually about the distress it causes to their partner. Sometimes, it is the patient's partner who has heard of me and comes along for the first visit. This is never because the boyfriend or husband minds the alopecia; always it is that they want her to find a way to get her hair back so that she'll be happy again.

Alopecia occurs in all ethnic groups. Asian women are commonly affected, and Chinese herbal pharmacies do a brisk business in hair loss remedies. Black women may be particularly vulnerable because their hair is naturally more fragile. Perhaps this is a factor in styles like cornrows that add hair. However, these styling methods can be hard on the hair follicles, creating a dilemma. I have not found any relationship between skin and hair color and risk of alopecia. However, it may be more visible if someone has dark hair and light skin.

Men's reaction to their own hair loss is more varied than that of women. I will not say much about it because this book is not about men's problems. Though some men are only moderately embarrassed by hair loss, others are just as anguished as women. I do treat some men for hair loss, though only when the standard measures dermatologist prescribe have not worked. Therapy for men is more problematic; here women have the advantage because more treatments are suitable for their hormonal makeup.

For women with androgenic alopecia, the fear that others will notice becomes a near-constant presence in their lives. Some come to avoid social occasions and settle into a life of going to work and staying home the rest of the time. This seems like an overreaction, but it is a common one. Psychologists sometimes misattribute this social anxiety to neurosis, but this is incorrect. One of my first alopecia patients told me she would never go to the theater because she feared everyone would stare at the back of her head. I must admit that at the time I thought this behavior was neurotic. Yet once her hair got better, she started going out, got married, had children, and now is quite content with her life. She was right all along; her only problem was her hair. Psychotherapy is not the answer to distress over hair loss. Several patients have said to me: "My other doctor said I should go to a psychiatrist, but I don't see the point. Talking to someone won't give me my hair back and that's what I want." I cannot argue with this. Regrowth of hair as a result of psychotherapy has never been reported. (Counseling won't make anyone not care about her hair, but sometimes it can help a woman cope while she waits for treatment to work.)

Yet despite all these fears, most of the time no one else notices. This is not always reassuring to women with alopecia because they worry that someone *might* notice. And if your hair is thinner, *you* notice, just as *you* notice the extra hair in the drain. Appearance is not just for others; pleasing oneself comes first.

Lesbian women seem to feel the same way as heterosexual women about alopecia. I once treated both partners of a lesbian couple. They had not lost their attraction to each other; each wanted her hair back for herself.

HOW I CAME TO TREAT FEMALE HAIR LOSS

Over the past two decades, I have seen more than 5,000 women with alopecia, probably the largest number of any endocrinologist in the world. I must admit, however, that in the early days of my medical education, when I dreamed of being a doctor making rounds in my white coat, I never envisioned concerning myself with hair problems. And in my earlier years, I spent much of my time caring for children with growth disorders, brain tumors, and other "serious" problems. However, I'd always had a particular interest in puberty because it was so often the start of body issues that could last a lifetime. A detailed understanding of the endocrinology of puberty, I soon recognized, can give essential insights into how hormones and the body's response to them evolve throughout adulthood. As I started to care for more and more adults, I realized that the developmental changes these hormones produce do not end with the onset of menses, nor with being old enough to vote, nor with pregnancies, nor even with menopause but continue in subtle ways throughout life. Adolescence is a very dynamic time hormonally, but so are the decades that follow it.

For coming to understand female alopecia, I am greatly indebted to Wilma Bergfeld, M.D., a dermatologist with whom I collaborated throughout the 1980s while I was at the Cleveland Clinic. Dr. Bergfeld has had a distinguished career, being world-renowned and the first woman to be president of the American Academy of Dermatology. During the many years she had strived to help women with alopecia, Dr. Bergfeld had never found anyone else who was willing to take female hair loss as seriously as she did. Indeed, the attitude of many of her colleagues toward her interest in this condition was patronizing.

I still recall our first meeting in the doctor's cafeteria. I'd recently heard Dr. Bergfield lecture on androgenic alopecia and so joined her at lunch to discuss it further. At first, I have to admit, I was skeptical that hormones had anything to do with hair loss, despite my long-standing interest in testosterone problems in women. At that point, my knowledge of what testosterone could do to women's scalp hair was minimal—

endocrinology training programs barely mention it. (This has changed somewhat since then because I do teach doctors-in-training about alopecia.)

Alopecia caught my interest immediately because it is a problem of body image, and mind-body relationships had always seemed among the most intriguing areas of medicine to me. I was fascinated as I listened to Dr. Bergfield explain this condition and was honored to accept her invitation to work with her in trying to help women who were losing their hair. The first patients I saw with this condition surprised me in two ways. First, although their hair appeared normal to me at first glance, I paid attention to their descriptions of how it had changed. Also I knew that Dr. Bergfeld had examined them and determined that they did indeed have hair loss. Involuntarily, I started to look at the heads of women when I was out in public, which raised my consciousness about how common alopecia is in women.

Medical training tends to emphasize severe and life-threatening conditions. Obviously doctors need to know about these, but we also need to know about problems that, though they never kill anyone, destroy their quality of life. In endocrinology training, we are taught that very high testosterone levels can induce male pattern baldness in women, but the far more common and much milder forms that result from hormonal vulnerability are never mentioned; indeed, most endocrinologists don't know about them. Textbooks sometimes show dramatic—and tragic—pictures of women with only a thin band of hair around the edge of the scalp, like a bald man's. This sort of very severe hair loss in women is, fortunately, extremely rare; I've only seen it a few times. The problem is that these pictures condition the mental image doctors have of what hormonal hair loss looks like. Being schooled only about the extreme forms, it's no wonder they fail to recognize alopecia in its milder, but far more common, forms.

Dr. Bergfeld's patients were far from being bald. Yet, as I listened to these women's stories, I came to realize that their hair thinning, although subtle, was both very real and very distressing. Many women cried when telling me about how their hair had changed. When they repeated the insensitive remarks they'd endured from other doctors, I was shocked and embarrassed for my profession. I rapidly came to disagree with the mainstream of the medical establishment, which regards alopecia as unworthy of attention. It seems obvious to me that any bodily change that causes so much unhappiness must be taken seriously.

STARTING TO TREAT ALOPECIA

When I began to treat women to help them get their hair back, there was almost no precedent. Dr. Bergfeld had begun prescribing spironolactone, still a mainstay of treatment, but felt that it would be best to do a hormonal workup first—which is where she invited my collaboration. It was logical to use spiro, a drug I knew firsthand to be safe because I'd been prescribing it for increased facial and body hair. And so I began prescribing it for women with alopecia, carefully explaining to my first patients that there was a good scientific basis for expecting it to work, but that only time would tell if it really did.

I must say I was happily surprised some months later when my early patients came back for follow-up visits and reported that they were starting to see some improvement. Now, twenty years later, I am still happy to hear that treatment has worked, but I am no longer surprised—though patients often are. Since I first found that spiro, a testosterone blocker, can help alopecia, I have discovered additional treatments, including other ways of protecting hair from testosterone and the importance of estrogen for hair health. As a result, I am able to help a much higher proportion of women with alopecia than I was twenty years ago.

In a way I could never have anticipated while a medical student, I find this very satisfying. I am not saving anyone's life—yet in a way, I am. No woman dies from alopecia, but for many, losing hair takes the joy out of life, leaving them with a sense of just going through the motions. I've already mentioned the sad fact that some women with alopecia retreat from life. They stop dating, stop going out to restaurants or theaters, and put plans to further their education or careers on indefinite hold. Put in medical terms, alopecia causes serious disability. For this reason, treating alopecia is as important as treating any other incapacitating condition.

ALOPECIA AND THE MEDICAL ESTABLISHMENT

Alopecia falls in between medical specialties. Because hair is part of the skin, it is included in dermatology. Yet the cause of the most common form is hormones, which are the focus of a different specialty—endocrinology. Dermatologists can recognize it but lack a background in the internal hormonal causes. Endocrinologists understand hormones, but most have not been trained to recognize and treat their effects on skin and hair. Most often the connection between hormones and hair loss is not made, leaving women with alopecia without help.

My point is not to reproach dermatologists or endocrinologists. Most are conscientious and give great help to patients with conditions in their areas of expertise. This is scant comfort, however, for women with alopecia who are frustrated in their efforts to keep their hair. There are still very few physicians who treat alopecia. Unless you can consult one of them, you'll need to study up on it yourself and come to your doctor with suggestions for workup and treatment. Some doctors are annoyed by such assertiveness, but many appreciate that patients want, and are entitled to, an active role in their own care. This and following chapters will prepare you to work with your doctor to get alopecia under control.

DIAGNOSING HAIR LOSS

Obviously, to treat a condition, you have to find out what is causing it. Since few physicians, even dermatologists, are really expert at diagnosing hair loss, it's a good idea to have some notion of possible causes before you see your doctor.

Dermatology textbooks distinguish between scarring and nonscarring alopecia. They tend to go into more detail about the scarring forms, but these rather rare forms are easily recognized and diagnosed by scalp biopsy. Unfortunately, standard texts give little practical guidance about the nonscarring forms, which account for all but a few cases of women's hair loss.

The incidence of hair thinning in women has not carefully been studied. A reasonable estimate is that about 20 percent of women in their thirties and at least 40 percent in their fifties experience hair thinning.

WHY DERMATOLOGISTS— AND MOST ENDOCRINOLOGISTS— CAN'T TREAT ALOPECIA

- Alopecia is a skin condition, but its causes are internal.

- Dermatologists are not taught about hormonal factors affecting hair growth.

- Endocrinologists know about hormones but not hair.

- Dermatologists are taught that nothing can be done for alopecia, and this fallacy becomes self-perpetuating because they don't even try.

- Most doctors misinterpret normal tests because they do not know about hormonal vulnerability.

- Many doctors are uncomfortable with alopecia patients because they do not understand why hair loss is so upsetting to women.

By the time they are seventy, almost all women have lost some of their hair. Invariably, this is the end result of a process that started decades earlier. I've heard thirty-five-year-olds tell me that they won't care how they look when they are seventy, but I've never heard a seventy-year-old say this. The message is stark: Hair loss tends to progress over time, so it is best to seek treatment as soon as you notice it.

How do you tell if you are starting to lose your hair? My answer may sound simplistic: If you think your hair is thinning, it probably is. You know your body better than anyone else and so you are best at recognizing any change. Not all shedding presages alopecia. It's normal to have intervals of slightly increased shedding during which you may notice more hair on your clothes or in the shower drain. However, if this continues for more than a week or so, and especially if you have less hair when you look in the mirror, something is definitely happening. More specifics are given in the sidebar, "The Warning Signs of Hormonal Hair Loss," provided on page 232.

If you have concluded that you are experiencing hair thinning, the next step is to convince your doctor. A common frustration for alopecia patients is having no one believe them. I've had women cry with relief when I tell them I can see that their hair really is thinning because no one else would even admit they could see the change. Friends or doctors may think they are being kind by denying that the hair loss shows, but the result is to make the person feel isolated and hopeless: How can you find treatment if no one admits you have a problem?

Recognizing that hair loss is real is the first step; next is to determine what kind of alopecia it is. There are three important terms that apply to common forms of female hair loss: *androgenic alopecia* (AGA, also referred to as *androgenetic alopecia; telogen effluvium* (TE); and *alopecia areata*. I'll explain areata first because it is quite different from the other forms and not really due to hormones.

ALOPECIA AREATA

Alopecia areata occurs when the immune system turns against the hair follicles and rejects them as if they were a foreign tissue. This form of alopecia has a very distinctive appearance that is quite different from hormonal hair loss. With areata, as the name implies, some areas have no hair at all. There are shiny, bald patches, while the surrounding hair is entirely normal. Although areata can be diffuse, this is unusual. In diffuse forms, the thinning is usually most pronounced around the edges; hormonal hair loss has the opposite distribution, as I'll discuss shortly.

The course of alopecia areata is unpredictable. Usually, the hair grows back over the next few months. Occasionally, however, the affected area enlarges sometimes to the point where all hair is lost from the scalp, in which case the condition is termed *alopecia totalis*. The most extreme form is *alopecia universalis* in which all body hair is completely lost, including eyebrows and lashes, legs, and even pubic and underarm hair. Fortunately, these more extreme forms of alopecia areata are uncommon. Most areata involves only small areas and goes away by itself.

Treatment of alopecia areata is less than satisfactory. When small areas are affected, injections of a cortisone-like medication, usually triamcinolone, into the scalp sometimes help. When the entire scalp is affected, injections are impractical, as well as painful. Oral steroids such as prednisone may restore hair, but the side effects are even worse than the alopecia: weight gain, severe stretch marks, and loss of calcium from bones. When the steroid is stopped, hair loss resumes. Because of these side effects, *oral steroids should never be used to treat any form of alopecia areata.*

ALOPECIA AND THE THYROID

Areata is sometimes associated with a common thyroid condition known as Hashimoto's thyroiditis. This is also autoimmune—white blood cells migrate into the thyroid and gradually damage it, eventually causing it to become underactive. There is usually mild swelling, which can be detected on physical exam by a physician experienced with thyroid conditions. If you have alopecia areata, you should definitely have blood tests to see if you have Hashimoto's and whether your thyroid is slowing down. (The tests are TSH, the most sensitive test for an underactive thyroid, and antithyroid antibodies, which test for immunity against your thyroid.) An underactive thyroid can affect your energy and also pregnancy outcome, so checking your TSH periodically is essential if you have ever had areata.

When areata and hypothyroidism occur together, treating the thyroid aspect does not help the hair, unfortunately. There is little point in taking thyroid medication for hair loss unless your tests show a definite abnormality. Except for the noncausal association with Hashimoto's, areata is not related to hormones. However, hormonal hair loss is so common that some women have both alopecia areata *and* hormonal hair loss. When this occurs, it is best to get both forms addressed, the areata with scalp injections and the AGA with treatment directed at the underlying hormonal cause.

Many articles and texts list thyroid disorders as causes of hair loss. This is misleading. Though areata can be accompanied by an underactive thyroid, thyroid medication does not in itself help the hair loss. Severe over- and underactivity of the thyroid can affect hair, but these are rarely seen nowadays because much improved diagnostic tests permit very early diagnosis. Still, it is prudent to have a thyroid check if you have alopecia of any kind just to be sure it is not a contributing factor.

If you are taking thyroid medication such as Synthroid, Levoxyl, Unithroid, generic levothyroxine, Cytomel, or one of the pig-source forms, such as Armour thyroid, it's important to be sure your dose is not excessive. Your TSH should not be below 0.5 mU/mL (or the lower limit for the lab you used) because an excessive dose may make alopecia worse—and adversely affect the heart and bones as well. I have seen some women who were treated with excessive doses in the mistaken hope that it would help their hair, so be careful to avoid this. (The TSH result can be confusing because it moves in the opposite direction as the activity of the thyroid. A high level means an underactive thyroid and a low one means overactivity or an excessive dose.)

HORMONAL HAIR LOSS

Hormonal hair loss is usually called androgenic alopecia (AGA). (Androgens are the family of hormones that includes testosterone.) The name implies that testosterone is *always* the hormonal factor causing AGA, but my experience has taught me that estrogen is a critical factor as well. For this reason, I now prefer the term *hormonal alopecia* (HA). Dermatologists usually do not refer to hair loss as hormonal, but as AGA or TE (see below). Dermatologists tend to downplay the role of hormones in regulating hair growth, another reason that the dermatology establishment has not been of much help to women with alopecia. I'll return to this matter later.

Hormones cause hair to be lost in a characteristic pattern, one that is quite different from alopecia areata. With HA, hair thinning is greatest on the temples, top, and vertex. The sides may thin also, but less than the crown. Hair may become very thin, but in contrast to what can occur with areata, hair is never completely lost.

Testosterone affects women's hair less severely than it affects men's, probably because of the protective effect of estrogen. While men's hairlines nearly always recede noticeably, women's rarely change more than very slightly. More common is to have the hairline stay in its proper place but to have slight thinning just behind it. The temple is another common area affected by HA—many women have some mild thinning here, typically in a triangle-shaped area with the point facing backward. This slight change can occur in women who have no alopecia elsewhere. Some worry that the loss at the temples will extend backward to involve most otheir scalp; fortunately, this never happens.

Everyone's hair is thinnest at the vertex—the "pointy" end of the head—and this area also tends to be most affected in HA. Women can usually style their hair to conceal this, though it is, of course, better to get your hair back. All in all, female AGA tends to be much milder than male hair loss, although this is not much consolation for the women who experience it. Women believe, not unreasonably, that they have a right to fuller hair than men have.

HAIR AND HORMONES

Two of the hormones you've been hearing about throughout this book are the main players in the drama of hair: estrogen and testosterone. Regarding hair, it's clear who is the hero and who the villain: Estrogen is good for hair, while testosterone is bad. Estrogen nurtures hair just as it nurtures breasts, uterus, blood vessels, and many other tissues in a woman's body. Under its influence hair grows faster and stays on the head longer—producing a more luxuriant head of hair. The hair-friendly action of estrogen is why so many women notice that their hair becomes fuller during the second half of pregnancy—estrogen levels go through the roof. Unfortunately, this effect of pregnancy is temporary. As soon as the baby is born, estrogen plummets; a few weeks later the extra hair bestowed by estrogen starts to fall out.

Testosterone sends hair follicles into a slump—their metabolism slows down, and hairs get smaller and smaller until they virtually disappear. The visible result: less hair. Within the hair follicles, testosterone is converted to a more active from called DHT (dihydrotestosterone). While it is commonly believed that it is DHT, not testosterone itself, that inactivates the follicle, based on my experience treating women with hormonal hair loss, I think both DHT and testosterone itself are involved. An implication of this, which I'll discuss in more detail later, is that medications designed for men that block formation of DHT do not work very well as sole treatment for women.

ESTROGEN NURTURES HAIR

The importance of estrogen in female alopecia is really my discovery, one that has enabled me to help many more women get their hair back. Because hair gets fuller during pregnancy, when estrogen levels are high, and sheds afterward, when levels drop, it's been known for a long time that estrogen improves hair growth. The shed that occurs some weeks after delivery makes it pretty obvious that drops in estrogen are not good for hair. Perhaps because of the general indifference of medicine regarding alopecia, no one had connected the dots to recognize that when estrogen falls at other times, it can also trigger hair loss. Events in a woman's life when her estrogen levels fall include not only giving birth but also stopping birth control pills, rapid weight loss, and perimenopause/menopause. Sometimes women have a decrease in estrogen for no reason that we can discover. Remember that each month estrogen is made by a new ovarian follicle, and for this reason, each cycle is not quite the same as any other. We do not entirely understand the reasons for these subtle hormonal variations, but fortunately we can do something about them.

When I first began to treat women for hair loss, I assumed that testosterone was always the culprit. However, this did not explain why some women whose hair had always been healthy suddenly began to lose it in their forties when testosterone levels are actually lower. This led me to recognize that the cause was not testosterone but falling levels of estrogen. More specifically it is having hair follicles that are vulnerable to lower estrogen levels. Some women need more estrogen than others to maintain abundant hair.

Even before any definite signs of perimenopause, some women have subtle symptoms that suggest estrogen levels are on their way down. The lab is of limited help here because levels of estradiol, the main estrogen, fluctuate widely during each cycle. Also, different parts of your body need different amounts of estrogen. If you are having normal periods, this means your ovaries are making enough estrogen to stimulate your uterus and, if you lubricate adequately, enough for comfortable sex. Your bones are almost certainly getting enough because they seem to need relatively little to stay strong. (Normal estrogen is not a guarantee against osteoporosis; bone health is discussed in chapter 27.) Hair seems to need more estrogen than these other organs, at least for women who are hormonally vulnerable. Clues that low estrogen may be a factor in your hair loss are listed in the following sidebar.

I've stressed the importance of estrogen for hair health because it has been ignored in the past. Identifying low estrogen as a factor in alopecia is a great step forward because many more women can now be successfully treated.

CLUES TO HORMONAL CAUSES OF ALOPECIA

Signs of Low Estrogen

Onset in late thirties or after

Perimenopausal symptoms, even quite mild ones, such as hot flashes or vaginal dryness

Being very slender

High level of aerobic exercise

Light periods (if not on birth control pills)

Dry or delicate skin

Fine, dry hair

Signs of Testosterone Problems

Onset between teens and mid-thirties

Oily scalp, hair, and/or skin

Itchy scalp

Acne

Increased facial and/or body hair

Being overweight

Periods that are irregular but often heavy

TESTOSTERONE'S VENDETTA AGAINST HAIR

The effect of testosterone on hair is pretty obvious to anyone who compares men's and women's heads. That men have less hair because of higher testosterone has been known for ages. Although normal women's levels of this hormone are less a tenth of men's, even this minute amount can turn off follicles, if they are vulnerable enough.

With testosterone, as with estrogen, the lab only tells part of the story. Most women with androgenic alopecia have normal levels; the problem, as you have probably figured out for yourself by now, is hormonal vulnerability. This vulnerability is genetic, and both men and women are affected. Bald men do not have higher testosterone levels than those who keep their hair; rather, they inherited vulnerable follicles. The same genes in women also predispose to alopecia, although to the milder female form.

Though it's usually normal, testosterone can be elevated with androgenic alopecia, especially those with PCOS. For this reason, your level of both total and free testosterone need to be checked because elevated levels need to be brought down. Even with a normal level, lowering testosterone helps protect vulnerable follicles. Determining whether testosterone is the culprit with alopecia depends in part on guilt by association. If you have other skin and hair problems that are caused by testosterone, your hair loss probably is too. Less commonly, both testosterone action and diminishing estrogen contribute to alopecia; in such cases, both aspects need to be addressed in treatment.

There is no real doubt about the roles of estrogen and testosterone in female alopecia. Nonetheless, a few dermatologists still deny that hormones have anything to do with hair loss. Ignoring what we know about the cause of alopecia means refusing to treat it. If you encounter this form of hormonal pessimism, all I can suggest is that you seek a more enlightened physician to help you.

THE NATURAL HISTORY OF HORMONAL HAIR LOSS

If you've noticed that your hair has started to shed more than usual or that there is less of it when you look in the mirror, you will naturally be apprehensive as to what the future holds for your hair. The news here is mixed. Without treatment, HA is likely to increase over time. On the other hand, it never progresses to complete baldness the way men's hair does. The rate of thinning is hard to predict, except that brisk shedding suggests that progression will be more rapid. Slower shedding is not reason to be complacent, however, because it can still result in hair getting progressively sparser. Nonetheless, there is a limit to how quickly hair is lost. Some women with HA wake up at night with scalp discomfort and fear that all their hair will be gone when they look in the mirror in the morning. Fortunately, this never happens.

Although I prefer to look at the positive side of things, I cannot be completely reassuring about HA because, if untreated, it usually gets worse over time. Waiting to see if it gets better by itself is usually not a good idea. If you do have alopecia, I encourage you to read this chapter and then seek out a physician willing to treat you.

THE TELOGEN EFFLUVIUM FALLACY

Many women I see who actually have hormonal hair loss have been told that they have something called telogen effluvium (TE). This term sounds impressive and implies a profound diagnosis. In fact, as I shall explain, it is almost meaningless. Let's look at the derivation of the term. The hair cycle has three phases: First is anagen, the time of active growth; next is catagen, during which the follicle shrivels up and becomes inactive. During the final phase, telogen, the hairs linger on for awhile but cannot grow anymore. Telogen hairs always fall out, generally after two to four months, but sometimes sooner. This lag between the follicle becoming inactive, and the hair's actually falling out makes it harder to determine the cause of a particular episode of shedding. When a hair falls out, whatever triggered it may have faded from memory—unless it was something dramatic such as childbirth or major surgery. Another effect is to cause a delay in the initial response to treatment; those hairs already in the telogen stage have to fall out before any improvement can become apparent.

Effluvium means an outflow. So "telogen effluvium" is simply a fancy way of saying someone's hair is falling out. To announce to a patient that she is having TE is no more than telling her that she is losing hair, which she knew already. There is a so-called hair pull test for TE in which the dermatologist tugs at your hair to see how many come out. However, if you are having increased shedding, the pull test will be positive, no matter what the cause. Most of us had enough hair pulling when we were in grade school, I see no reason to go to a dermatologist to have it done.

I once heard a learned dermatologist claim that the pattern of hair loss can distinguish between AGA and TE. As I recall, AGA affected mainly the top—which is true—and TE also involved the top but affected the sides more. I know from my experience treating thousands of women for alopecia—on virtually all of whom I obtained hormone levels to that such subtle differences in the pattern of hair thinning cannot distinguish hormonal hair loss from so-called TE. In fact, this is a classic distinction without a difference. Nearly all female alopecia, other than areata or scarring forms, is hormonal. I have no doubt that there are other factors regulating hair growth that have not yet been identified, so it is likely that estrogen and testosterone are only part of the story. Unfortunately, we cannot treat what we don't know and so must focus on the hormones whose role in alopecia is fully confirmed.

The implication of labeling increased hair shedding as telogen effluvium is that it will be temporary and that the hair will grow back. The dogma about TE is that hairs fall out because they are being pushed out by new ones. If true, this would be reassuring because new hairs should appear. Unfortunately, I see many women who were told they had TE and so waited months for new hair that never appeared, only to lose more in the interim. Some hair loss really may be temporary, for example, that following childbirth or major surgery. Far more often, though, once hair starts to thin, it just keeps on getting thinner because the cause is hormonal. The progression may be gradual or rapid, but the longer before treatment is started, the thinner the hair becomes. If you're having progressive hair loss, don't let yourself be put off by the TE ruse.

WEIRD SCALP SENSATIONS

Many of the women I see for alopecia are also troubled by scalp discomfort. Because they fear it will sound crazy, some women are reluctant to mention this symptom. Indeed abnormal scalp sensations—

dysesthesia—are sometimes wrongly attributed to psychological factors, but they too often accompanies alopecia to be imaginary. Some women worry that the sensation is due to hair falling out; this anxiety is understandable but unnecessary, since scalp discomfort is not a sign that alopecia is getting worse.

Scalp itching often occurs with AGA, which is hormonal hair loss due to testosterone. With this form of alopecia, the scalp discomfort is due to excessive stimulation of the oil glands by testosterone, a condition termed seborrhea or seborrheic dermatitis. Facial oiliness and acne are often present as well. When seborrhea occurs on the scalp, there may be crusting, especially around the ears and the back hair line, though sometimes elsewhere. Pimple-like lesions may appear. Though dermatologists sometimes deny the hormonal basis of seborrhea, there is no question that testosterone is the inciting factor.

Scalp seborrhea improves dramatically when testosterone is lowered or blocked. When AGA is treated with a testosterone blocker, the oiliness and the itchy discomfort usually resolve within weeks. If the seborrhea is very bothersome, a topical steroid lotion applied to the irritated area will clear the scalp within a few days. Once the testosterone blocking treatment begins to work, the steroid lotion should be discontinued; prolonged use for many weeks or months can cause thinning of the skin.

HA due to low estrogen can also be associated with scalp discomfort, but this feels somewhat different from the intense itching of testosterone-induced seborrhea. More common with falling estrogen levels is a burning sensation; touching the hair or scalp may be surprisingly uncomfortable. This sensitivity seems to be related to the general sensory changes that occur with estrogen deficiency and can happen to women in menopause, even without any hair loss. (This sort of sensory change as an effect of estrogen deficiency is discussed in chapter 23.) Treatment with estrogen nearly always helps this form of scalp discomfort, though it may take several months to resolve completely.

SCALP BIOPSY

Biopsy is very valuable for many conditions in which the microscopic appearance of the tissue can give exact diagnostic information. It is essential for tumors, but has other applications. Unfortunately, when done for alopecia—unless there is scarring, which is rare—biopsy gives no information on the key question: Is the hair loss due to vulnerability to testosterone, to estrogen, or to both hormones? I've reviewed hundreds of biopsy reports on women with alopecia and am hard put to think of any case in which this test has helped anyone get her hair back. Scalp biopsy is safe and harmless, just not very informative.

LAB TESTS FOR ALOPECIA

Measurement of total and free testosterone is essential in the workup of alopecia. DHEA-S should usually be measured as well. These tests are discussed in detail in chapter 19. Excessive levels indicate that the problem is due to androgens, but *women whose follicles are vulnerable to testosterone may have alopecia with entirely normal levels of testosterone and DHEA-S.* In fact, this is the most common situation. It's essential to have your testosterone measured if you are having alopecia, but don't despair if it is normal. *AGA is treatable whether or not your testosterone is elevated.* Don't let anyone try to persuade you otherwise; too many women lose their chances of recovering their hair because they think normal blood tests mean nothing can be done.

Measurement of estradiol is useful in some situations, but because this hormone fluctuates widely during a normal cycle or during perimenopause, a single level may not be representative. Another pitfall is that levels are normally low in women on the pill, not because estrogen is deficient, but because the estrogen from the pill does not show up on the test. Because of these and other possible sources of confusion, estradiol levels need to be interpreted by an expert.

HORMONAL HAIR LOSS CAN BE TREATED

The first question many women ask me is whether alopecia is treatable at all. Given how easy it is to become demoralized if you have alopecia, it is regrettable that so many women encounter negativity everywhere they turn for help. Doctors either are unfamiliar with it or declare it untreatable. The Internet contributes, too. Although chat rooms at their best are sources of support, some women become embittered at not finding help and post negative messages about every possible treatment, even those they have not tried. If you surf the net about hair, remember that those who find successful treatment usually find other ways to spend their time and so stop posting, leaving the disgruntled few to fill up cyberspace.

TREATMENTS FOR HORMONAL HAIR LOSS

We've seen that her inherited response to two hormones, testosterone and estrogen, decide for a woman how full her hair will be. Treatment derives quite logically from knowledge of the effects of these two hormones. Basically, it involves thwarting the injurious action of testosterone and enhancing the nurturing properties of estrogen. The relative importance of each depends on the extent to which each hormone is contributing to the hair problem. (The sidebar on page 245 summarizes the clues that point to testosterone or to estrogen.)

PROTECTING YOUR HAIR FROM TESTOSTERONE

It's time to return to the story of Roxanne, one of my alopecia patients who'd traveled a long way to get help. Fortunately, she responded well to the first treatment we'd tried: a hair-friendly birth control pill and a medication to protect her follicles from testosterone. After four months she noticed definite slowing of shedding, and, after a year on treatment, there was some filling in on her crown and temples. She no longer woke up at night with the desperate apprehension that when she looked in the mirror in the morning, she'd find that all her hair would be gone. While her hair was still not as full as it had been five years earlier, Roxanne now felt comfortable with her appearance, and no longer was apprehensive whenever she was in public.

Not everyone responds to the same medication. Spironolactone is usually the simplest and safest. However, if it does not work after several months, assuming that the dose is sufficient, another testosterone blocker can be tried or a 5-alpha-reductase inhibitor can be added.

Use of medication to combat testosterone is discussed in more detail in the next chapter, so I suggest that you refer to that. Here I need to emphasize the caution that treatment must be individualized for you. I've given guidelines for deciding treatment, but I cannot cover all the factors, so guidance from a knowledgeable physician is essential.

ENHANCING THE HAIR-NURTURING EFFECTS OF ESTROGEN

Estrogen has become a scare word due to the extensive publicity surrounding the WHI study, which supposedly showed that estrogen increases risk for breast cancer and heart attack. In fact, it has been widely misinterpreted, as covered in chapter 22.

Prior to menopause, oral contraceptives are the easiest way to safely raise your estrogen. Issues concerning OCs and hair are covered in the next section. If you are in perimenopause, the pill may still be the most convenient way to go. For women definitely in menopause, patches are usually the best form of estrogen. These are described, together will a full discussion of safety issues, in Part VI.

THE PILL AND HAIR

For most women in their thirties through menopause, the best way to enhance estrogen is by using birth control pills. Now I know that some of you reading this want to tell me that birth control pills *caused* their hair loss. This question of OCs and hair is a vitally important one, so I'll do my best to clarify it. First, it matters greatly what OC you take. In chapter 4, I discuss differences between pills and the fact that some contain a progestin, levonorgestrel, which has considerable testosterone-like activity. While experts debate whether this is enough to cause adverse effects, it seems to me common sense to avoid pills with this ingredient, if you are having problems related to testosterone. The critical variable here, as with so many other women's conditions, is hormonal vulnerability. Many women take OCs with levonorgestrel and have no problems at all with their skin. However, if you have hormonal alopecia, you are definitely vulnerable to testosterone, and the last thing you need is more of it. So if you think that OC use set off your alopecia, one possible reason is that you were on a pill that had some testosterone-like activity. Fortunately, these are prescribed less and less these days.

Some women notice hair loss beginning a few weeks or months after the pill was stopped. When this happens, it seems as if the pill caused the hair loss, but it was actually *stopping* the pill that did it. Hormonally, going off an OC is a little like giving birth because estrogen levels suddenly plummet. Since estrogen is good for hair it follows that falling levels are bad. Of course all women who use the pill stop it sooner or later, and most of the time, their hair is fine. Those women who experience this post-pill alopecia have follicles that are more dependent on estrogen than average.

If you are on the pill now, you may be thinking, "What happens when I decide to stop so I can become pregnant?" The good news here is that pregnancy is one of the best things for hair. Of course, I certainly do not suggest having a baby simply to treat alopecia. My point is that there's no need to worry about going off the pill to have a pregnancy. It's a good idea, however, not to go off the pill too soon. Waiting one to two cycles before trying to conceive is optimal. There are other variables, however, so such decisions should be discussed in advance with your OB.

Many women with alopecia feel that the pill has not helped. Indeed, the alopecia may begin while someone is on an OC. There are two reasons that the pill by itself may not be adequate to treat or prevent alopecia. First, although the pill lowers free testosterone, to fully protect hair, a testosterone blocker is usually needed also. The second reason brings us to the special way the pill should be taken, if you have alopecia. Most OCs are set up in twenty-eight-day cycles in which the first twenty-one days have pills with estrogen and progesterone in them, but the last seven are completely inactive. The drop after day twenty-one is good for triggering a period but not so good for keeping your hair on your head. (Women not on the pill may also have a sharp drop as menstruation begins, especially if they are in perimenopause.)

There is a simple way to avoid these monthly estrogen crashes: Use the pill on a schedule that avoids the seven days of inactive pills. Two OCs available now are set up for this. With Seasonale, the seven days off hormones come every three months, instead of every month; periods occur four times a year. Seasonale is conveniently set up for this but, unfortunately, it contains levonorgestrel, the progestin I've already fingered for its testosterone-like activity. For these reasons, I do not recommend this for women with alopecia, unwanted hair, or acne. A better option is Mircette (generic: Kariva), which has no testosterone-like effect and has only two days without estrogen each cycle, instead of seven. Periods occur every four weeks. As discussed in chapters 5 and 8, it is also good choice for women who suffer from migraine. The disadvantage for treatment of alopecia is that the estrogen dose is low— 20 micrograms of ethinyl estradiol. OCs with 30 or 35 micrograms are just as safe and may be better for alopecia. Mircette can work, though, so it is still a reasonable choice, especially if you feel nauseous or have sore breasts on OCs with 30 or 35 micrograms of estrogen. (OC selection is detailed in chapter 4.)

The best way to use the pill for alopecia is a customized regimen that I devised. Using Yasmin or another nonandrogenic OC, one takes active pills continuously for twelve weeks, then takes four days off. Usually the four pill-free days allows an adequate period. I've been recommending this approach for the past two years, and it clearly is more likely to work for alopecia than the standard schedule. The only adverse effect is a higher chance of spotting. It will not affect your ability to become pregnant, nor will it affect your cycle once you come off. More details on use of OCs on an extended schedule is given in chapter 4.

If the twelve by four regimen does not work, a remaining possibility is to use higher-dose pills that contain 50 micrograms of estrogen. These are still available but are rarely prescribed because they have a slightly higher risk of causing potentially serious blood clot problems. They are only to be considered if nothing else works and hair loss is completely devastating.

WHAT ABOUT MINOXIDIL?

If you've been to a dermatologist, odds are that you were advised to use minoxidil (Rogaine), and by now you must have noticed that I have not mentioned it. Minoxidil was developed as a blood pressure medication, but patients complained because it caused hair to appear all over their bodies. This accidental discovery led to its being developed as a topical for thinning scalp hair. Minoxidil does have a place in treatment of female hair loss, but it is a very limited one. It is certainly not the first choice because of three significant problems: applying it twice a day is inconvenient, scalp irritation is usual, and, last but not least, it usually doesn't work. Let's consider each of the drawbacks in turn.

Most women are in a rush to get to work in the morning or to get their families ready for the day, or both; to have to also apply a liquid through one's hair onto the entire scalp is difficult. The treatment was originally designed for men, whose hair is almost always thinner and shorter than women's—even women with alopecia. Most women who try minoxidil find getting it onto their scalp difficult. Some also find that minoxidil makes their hair look gummy or that it leaves dandruff-like flakes.

The women's minoxidil that is marketed for women is 2 percent, while that intended for men comes in both 2 percent and 5 percent formulations. The 5 percent is far more likely to be effective; unfortunately it is also more irritating to the scalp, sometimes intolerably so. A useful compromise is to use 2 percent in the morning and 5 percent at night. The reason there is no 5 percent preparation packaged for women is that it will stimulate facial hair growth. This definitely can happen, especially on the forehead but sometimes on cheeks as well. Remember, though, that the same vulnerability to testosterone that causes AGA can also result in increased facial hair. Sometimes the minoxidil is blamed for hair that is really due to hormones. When applying minoxidil, the best way to minimize spread onto the face is to apply it an hour or two before bed, so it will be absorbed before your head moves around on the pillow during sleep.

Minoxidil produces satisfactory hair improvement only about 10 percent of the time. The major drawback of starting minoxidil early is that if your hair improves while on minoxidil in combination with other medications, there is no means to tell how much it contributed. This means, as a practical matter, that you'll be stuck with the scalp irritation and inconvenience for years to come. This is why I consider it only the last resort, to be tried only if nothing else has worked.

WHAT CAN YOU EXPECT FROM ALOPECIA TREATMENT

Here's the all-important question: Does treatment really work? We have no formal clinical trials of treatment for alopecia, except for minoxidil, for the simple reason that no granting agency will fund research on hair loss. However my own experience—extending more than twenty years with more than 5,000 women whom I have treated using the methods I describe in this chapter—indicates that about 80 percent of women with HA get stabilization, by which I mean their hair stops getting progressively thinner. No medical treatment works equally well for everyone. For a few women with alopecia, treatment seems to slow progression but does not arrest it completely.

It is very important to realize that even if you are destined to get a great result, your shedding will not slow overnight. This lag in response is not due to limitations of the medications but to the biology of hair growth. Remember that before falling out, hairs enter an inactive phase called telogen, which typically lasts two to four months. Telogen is irreversible; these hairs will fall out no matter what. At any moment in time all of us have hairs that will shed over the next few weeks. This has to run its course—the same two to four months—before any benefit from treatment can be noticed.

Treatment also helps the body and texture of the hair; in fact, this is often the first improvement noted. Even before shedding has slowed, the hair usually starts to look fuller, feel stronger, and even becomes easier to style. The next event is stabilization, when hair loss slows down so that it is balanced by appearance of new hairs. Most women with alopecia get stabilization after the first few months on treatment. Many, but not all, eventually have some regrowth, but this can take a year or longer to become apparent. Although hair is unlikely to go back to the fullest it ever was, many women have enough improvement that they are once again happy with their hair. They stop obsessing over it and can devote their energy to other matters in their lives. This is not to say that hair anxiety goes away completely; there may be a lingering fear that alopecia will come back. Still, this is far better than watching your hair get thinner before your eyes.

HOW LONG IS TREATMENT NEEDED?

I generally encourage women to continue alopecia treatment until they are happy with their hair for at least one or two years. After that, if hair is back to normal, it is reasonable to try gradually tapering testosterone-blocking medication. Some women can maintain the benefit off medication, but not all. When hair gets thin as part of perimenopause or menopause, realistically, if estrogen is stopped hair loss will probably resume. A decision has to be made as to whether to stay on estrogen or not. Most women opt to stay with treatment, but not all. Given present uncertainties regarding hormone therapy for menopause, there is no one answer for all women regarding how long to take estrogen—or even whether to use it at all. In chapter 24, I give some guidelines for making a decision you will be comfortable with.

ALOPECIA TREATMENTS THAT DON'T WORK

In doing research for my earlier book *The Good News About Women's Hormones*, I came across thousand-year-old hair loss treatments from ancient India, proving that hair loss is not new and women in ancient times were no happier about it than modern women. Nor is hope of finding a remedy specific to a particular culture. My wife often shows me ads for hair loss treatments from her Hong Kong newspaper, and sometimes there are stories of women who have been ripped off for thousands of dollars for hair loss treatments that don't work.

So far as I can tell, no over-the-counter topical products or vitamins work for hair loss. Only a limited number of ingredients are used in such products, and none of them helps hair. Sometimes a hair treatment will be offered on the Internet with a guarantee. The guarantee is often a scam—by the time users realize that it has not worked, the seller is long gone.

A Chinese herb, shou wu (literally, head black), is supposed to keep hair youthful, but I have never met anyone who said it had helped her. Again, because many Chinese herbs are adulterated with hazardous chemicals, I do not recommend them at this time.

Many health food stores sell supplements for hair. Generally, these are merely expensive ways to get the same vitamins that are already in your standard multi. Some believe biotin is helpful, and it is reasonable to try, but it does not substitute for the treatments I cover in this chapter.

One possible exception is saw palmetto, an herb that inhibits 5-alpha-reductase, the enzyme which activates testosterone to DHT. This might, in theory, help alopecia due to testosterone vulnerability but, as with other herbs, potency of specific preparations is indeterminate. If blocking 5-alpha-reductase is indicated, I suggest using the more consistent and potent prescription forms. These can be used by women—see chapter 20—but work best in combination with other medications. I suggest saw palmetto only if you cannot find a doctor who will prescribe more effective medications. The possible risk of saw palmetto, as well as prescription 5-alpha-reductase inhibitors, to interfere with the genital development of an unborn male child needs to be stressed. They absolutely must not be taken if there is any chance you will become pregnant on them.

Revivogen is a nonprescription product that may have some benefit, based on some isolated reports by people who have tried it, but it's hard to be sure about it. The problem in using unresearched remedies is that, given the lag before you can tell if they are helping, much time can be wasted. The approaches I have explained in this chapter, which are based on the underlying hormonal cause, are still the best bet.

Some of my patients have been sold topical concoctions by dermatologists. A popular one is minoxidil combined with tretinoin (the active ingredient in Retin-A and several others). This can be even more irritating that minoxidil alone, and I am not impressed that it works any better, but there is at least a rationale for its use. The same cannot be said regarding other potions that some of my patients show me. A popular ingredient of late has been metformin. This medication in oral form is valuable for PCOS (see chapter 21) but will do nothing for hair loss not associated with this condition. Even with PCOS, applying Metformin to the scalp is pointless because its site of action is the liver. Except for Minoxidil, no topical has been proven to be effective for hair loss.

A popular line of products for thinning hair is Nioxin. Although the shampoo is excellent, this and the other products are quite expensive. They contain many vitamins and supplements but in minute amounts. There is no evidence that Nioxin will stop alopecia.

The laser comb was introduced recently with considerable publicity. Solid information on this has been hard to come by; but so far as I have been able to find out, any positive effect of the laser comb is temporary. It is quite expensive and, given its uncertain effectiveness, I do not recommend it at this time.

Women often wonder if their hair loss is related to their nutrition. While very rapid weight loss of more than thirty pounds over a few months or malnutrition, as occurs with anorexia nervosa, can result in shedding, inadequate diet is generally not a factor in alopecia in the developed world. Many worry that their protein intake is inadequate, but anyone who eats dairy, fish, or meat will get more than enough protein for their body's needs. Some of my patients have been told that eating red meat will be good for their hair. This is highly inappropriate because there is no evidence at all for a benefit to hair and much evidence for deleterious effects on cardiovascular health. I am perhaps biased because I am vegetarian, but you can be reassured that if you have cut down on your meat intake for health or ethical reasons, your hair will not suffer.

Another inappropriate dietary recommendation for alopecia is restriction of carbohydrate. This is based on a fallacious rationale similar to that for metformin. PCOS benefits from low carb intake and is a cause of alopecia. For women who do not have PCOS—and the majority with alopecia do not—lowering carb will not benefit their hair. There are advantages to low carb diets for women who are overweight, but it is far from clear that nonobese women will get any benefit. There may be health benefits from low carb for some women, but better hair isn't one of them.

HAIR TRANSPLANTS

Spencer Kobren, a consumer advocate for people with hair loss, founder and president of the American Hair Loss Association, and a good personal friend, runs a radio show, *The Bald Truth,* about alopecia. Because he hears from thousands of people who call in to discuss the results of treatments they have tried, Spencer is one of the world's most knowledgeable people about hair loss. Here is what he has to say about hair transplants for women.

> Contrary to the marketing efforts of many in the hair loss industry, hair transplantation is rarely of any benefit to women suffering from androgenetic alopecia. In fact, the trauma from the procedure itself can cause the native hair surrounding the grafts to shed, leaving the woman in an even worse position than before.

Spencer goes on to explain that for transplant to work, the hair taken from the sides and back must be resistant to the damaging effect of testosterone. In women with alopecia, hair from this area is usually sensitive to testosterone. In other words, in women with alopecia, all the follicles are hormonally vulnerable. Transplant is said to work for a few women—although, I must state that I have never seen a good result. You need to exercise caution with hair transplant because the procedure is a big moneymaker for some plastic surgeons and dermatologists. Many are conservative in recommending surgery, but not all.

HAIR EXTENSIONS, ADDITIONS, AND WIGS

I never suggest wigs, additions, or other artificial forms of hair because women with alopecia want their own hair back. The big problem with these contraptions is that all of them pull on your hair and increase breakage. This means that if you use any of them, you'll end up with even less of your own hair. Once you begin, you more or less have to continue to use it or your hair will look even thinner. Maintenance can be very expensive, often more than the upfront cost.

An addition in which a partial wig is fitted into your own hair gives the most natural look. These are a reasonable option, but only if all efforts to grow back your own hair have failed.

HAIR CARE

Especially if your hair is hormonally vulnerable, proper care is essential to preserve youthful abundance and brightness. Most advice available on hair care comes from cosmetologists or companies that want you to buy their products. Some of this advice is sound, but much is not. I will conclude with some medically based guidelines for hair health. Since some women inadvertently do things that are bad for their hair, I've listed some harmful hair care myths in the sidebar on page 262.

If your style requires pulling your hair back, as with a ponytail, braids, or corn rows, any tugging should be as gentle as possible. Hair is delicate and when handled comes out more easily than you might think.

If you're like many women with alopecia, you dread washing your hair because it's depressing to see how much comes out. Actually, though washing makes you more aware of shedding, it does not cause it. To keep your hair in good shape, you should wash it every day, or at least every other day. Unwashed hair accumulates oil and grime that can irritate your scalp and possibly damage the hair you do have. Avoiding washing just makes matters worse.

If your scalp is oily or irritated, an antiseborrhea shampoo can help. One that works well, even for delicate hair, is Neutrogena T-Gel (regular strength). The smell of this shampoos is rather medicinal, but it dissipates almost immediately. For best results, wet your hair, rub the T-Gel in gently, leave it in for five minutes, then rinse out and repeat—you don't need to wait five minutes with the second shampoo application. If your hair is not oily or your scalp itchy, then you can choose whatever shampoo leaves your hair looking good. Conditioner is okay to use with alopecia and can improve your hair's body.

HAIR CARE MYTHS

Myth: Brushing 100 strokes every day keeps hair healthy.
Truth: Brushes pull out hair. Throw away your brush and use only a loose comb. Never tug at tangles: Separate them gently with your fingers.

Myth: Using high heat from the blow dryer is a good way to save time.
Fact: Hair is more fragile when hot. Either turn the heat off or handle your hair with extreme care when drying it. As for irons, they are for clothes, not hair.

Myth: Stale beer or raw eggs are good for your hair.
Fact: Stale beer will make you smell as if you were at a fraternity party. As for eggs, your hair doesn't need the cholesterol anymore than you do.

Myth: It's bad to wash your hair too often.
Fact: Washing every day, or at least every other day, is best. Washing gets rid of the oil and the chemical pollutants your hair picks up during the day. Modern shampoos will not harm your hair. If you see more hair in the shower drain, it is not caused by washing; the hair would have fallen out anyway.

Myth: Having your hair cut makes it grow faster.
Fact: Your hair grows at its own rate. Cutting does not make any difference.

Myth: It's bad to go outdoors with wet hair.
Fact: You may not like the look of wet hair, but it will not harm your health. Colds are caused by exposure to viruses, not wet hair.

Myth: Coloring hair will damage it.
Fact: Dyeing your hair to make it darker is safe. Bleaching, however, can weaken already vulnerable hair. Light highlighting is okay.

Myth: Thinning hair is caused by stress.
Fact: There is absolutely no scientific evidence for this old cliché. The culprit is hormones or, less often, the immune system.

CONCEALING ALOPECIA

Because all women with thinning hair do their best to hide their condition, some who are affected imagine that they are alone in their misfortune. It is also a reason why pharmaceutical company executives, most of whom still are men, take no interest in developing medications for alopecia—they never notice it in the women around them. Ironically, while women with alopecia fear others will notice, they generally succeed so well in hiding it that there is little awareness among health care professionals.

Hiding one's scalp is not a substitute for getting your hair back but can reduce self-consciousness while you wait for treatment to work. Since thinning is greatest on the top of the head, styles which bring hair back over their crown are usually effective in preventing scalp from showing. Mousse and other hair products that add body can give hair a fuller appearance—which is why they sell. One product that is effective in making scalp invisible through hair is Toppik, which consists of flakes of fibrous material which you sprinkle on. It really does conceal alopecia very effectively.

There are other products in the Toppik line such as hair spray. Although they are good products, I am not convinced that they are any better than standard brands available in retail stores. Toppik is easily ordered online. (See Resources Section.)

THERE *IS* HOPE FOR ALOPECIA

If you have androgenic alopecia and were told that it is untreatable, don't believe it. Finding a doctor who is knowledgeable about alopecia and willing to help can be difficult, unfortunately. Astonishingly, only a few physicians in the United States specialize in this condition even though more than twenty million American women suffer from it. Some doctors simply dismiss hair loss as insignificant—as if you don't have a right to be distressed by a change in your own body. Others are more open-minded. Here you need to be your own advocate. If you find a doctor who is understanding and you tactfully educate him or her, he or she may be willing to prescribe the effective treatments I describe in this book.

17.

Peach Fuzz and Worse:
Hormones and Facial Hair

If you are one of the millions who have to remove unwanted hair, you probably feel demoralized when you look at the countless photos in women's—or men's—magazines showing ladies with absolutely smooth, hairless skin. You may think you are the only woman who grows hair on her face, chest, or abdomen. Be reassured; you aren't. Many of these seemingly perfect women, like you, remove or conceal unwanted hair, but you can be sure they don't own up to this when interviewed. Some celebrities are comfortable talking about their breast implants or face lifts; virtually none will admit to extra hair.

Our cultural trichophobia is historically novel. In ancient Indian love poetry, a line of hair down the lower chest, called the *romaraji*, was considered a mark of great beauty. No more; contemporary fashion allows women less and less hair. Now not only leg and underarm hair but also pubic hair fall victim to wax or the razor. Real women's skin does not usually accord with the vogue for hairlessness—fully half of all American women remove facial hair on occasion, and 10 percent do so at least twice a week (this does not include eyebrow plucking).

Many ways have been devised to remove unwanted hair, ranging from primitive—tweezers—to high tech—lasers. All these methods have serious drawbacks. Tweezers and lasers can permanently injure skin. With high-tech removal methods, cost can quickly mount up because hormones can stimulate unwanted hair to grow back too fast for removal to keep up. Used right, such methods can be a godsend—I'll cover them in more detail later in this chapter.

A few unlucky women have so much facial hair that they have no choice but to resort to using a razor each morning. Even so, many fear that toward the end of the day they'll have a visible five-o'clock shadow. I've even been told by some women that they keep their problem secret from their husbands. Each morning they get up first, tiptoe to the bathroom, and secretly shave.

No woman should have to live with the embarrassment of visible facial hair, and no woman has to because there are effective treatments. In fact, there are too many; given the proliferation of hair removal methods, women need a guide to help them choose what will be most effective, safest, as well as affordable for them. One or a few hairs on the corner of the upper lip or the chin can be handled easily with local removal. But when simple measures do not give effective concealment, medical treatment can make a great difference. Extra hair on a woman's body—*hirsutism* in medical jargon—is, like acne, the result of testosterone acting on hormonally vulnerable skin. It can be dramatically reduced by medications that protect a woman's skin from testosterone, as discussed later in this chapter.

WHY DO SOME WOMAN HAVE FACIAL AND BODY HAIR?

Actually, we might ask the opposite question: Why don't women have as much hair as men? The answer, obviously, is that women have much less testosterone. A typical adult woman in her mid-thirties will have a testosterone level around 35 to 40 ng/dL. A man the same age will have a level of 400 to 800 ng/dL, sometimes even higher. Women's levels are therefore only 5 to 10 percent of men's. This is a huge difference and is part of the reason men and women look so different. Yet men's and women's bodies have the same hormones, just different amounts, and so the genders overlap somewhat in physical traits. Thus women usually have some facial or body hair, just a lot less than men. Most have leg hair, removal of which is routine. Pubic and underarm hair are, of course, normal for women; they appear at puberty because testosterone rises in girls as well as boys at this phase of life. Also common is a row or two of long dark hairs around the areola (the edge of the nipple). These periareolar hairs are part of normal development; like pubic and underarm hair, they mark a sexually sensitive area. Women understandably dislike having hair in this location because breasts are feminine, and chest hair is masculine—or so our culture decrees. Actually many men have a small nubbin of breast tissue under their nipple and even more have a mammary fat pad. This is rarely seen because men willing to bare their chests are usually those who are muscular with little fat on their upper chest. Lest we imagine that some swelling on the upper chest on a man is inherently unattractive, next time you are in an art museum, take a look at ancient Indian sculpture; you'll see breast-like protuberances on nearly all the male figures. In a different place and time, this was considered attractive and not at all unmanly.

Now I am certainly *not* trying to convince you that women should be happy to have body hair or men to have breasts. Rather my point is that our assumptions about how our bodies should look are as much cultural as biological. There is nothing biologically unfeminine about some facial and body hair, nor unmasculine about some extra fat in the mammary region. Since we live as much by culture as by biology, we tend to be uncomfortable with aspects of our bodies that do not conform to cultural norms for our gender. Though androgyny is fine in theory, all but a tiny, though visible, minority want to look entirely female or male. If something about oneself seems gender discordant, it is natural to want to correct it. This does not simply involve acceptability to the opposite sex—we want our bodies to match our sense of our own identities.

Dislike of body hair has gone beyond being solely a gender issue in our culture. Hair is now considered unattractive, though it is obviously biologically quite normal. I have no explanation as to why hair now disturbs us. A heavy five o'clock shadow is considered vulgar, even though it has nothing to do with a man's hygiene level. Many of the clients of electrologists and laser specialists are men who are uncomfortable with their body hair. The Mexican artist Frida Kahlo made use of the disturbing aspect of hair in her expressionist paintings, which brilliantly represent the physicality of her injured body in disquieting ways.

Whether hair is normal for a woman or not, it is not accepted by our culture, and so it is quite reasonable to get rid of it. Fortunately, medicine and technology have given us good ways to do this.

HOW TESTOSTERONE AFFECTS HAIR

The cause of increased facial and body hair is always testosterone. Or almost always; certain drugs can do it, although none is likely to be taken by basically healthy young women. They include cyclosporine, used to suppress the immune system; dilantin (phenytoin), an anticonvulsant; diazoxide, used for low blood sugar; and minoxidil, rarely employed in oral form because it causes hair to spread everywhere. Medications commonly used by women in the hormonal years, such as antibiotics, allergy medications, birth control pills, stomach soothers, cholesterol-lowering drugs, and antidepressants will not affect hair growth. For practical purposes, then, increased hair is always due to the effect of testosterone. The main exceptions are eyebrows and lashes whose growth is not affected by hormones.

Supposedly, testosterone does not increase the number of hairs; rather it stimulates the nearly invisible vellus hairs to turn into terminal hairs—the kind of dark, thick, stiff ones that no woman wants on her face. There is also a transitional state in which hairs are just barely visible. Generally referred to as "peach fuzz," these hairs are soft, thin, and translucent, invisible except under special lighting conditions. Many women have some peach fuzz on their face and do not find it too bothersome. If peach fuzz is stable, it need not raise concern. However an increase or darkening may be the first sign that actual hirsutism is developing.

How much an individual's hair follicles respond to testosterone is genetic. East Asians, both male and female, have less visible hair than Caucasians. Blacks are intermediate but can have visible hirsutism. Within the white population, those of Mediterranean origin—Italian, Spanish, Greek, Middle Eastern—have more conspicuous hair growth. Yet under the influence of testosterone, even those with light skin and fair hair can have noticeable hirsutism.

Ethnicity should not be a reason to be denied workup or treatment. I've had more than one woman tell me that when she expressed concern about unwanted hair, the reply was, "You're Italian (or Greek, etc.), what do you expect?" Since ideas about how women should look are now international, being Mediterranean does not necessarily make hirsutism less bothersome, especially if you live in the United States. In the past leg and body hair seem to have been more acceptable in Europe than North America, but this seems to be changing. The increasing worldwide trichophobia is unfortunate for women since most have at least some facial and body hair. It's easy for me to criticize the increasing intolerance for normal amounts of hair, but this will not change society. Given the importance of a positive body image, medical treatment is a reasonable way to reduce hair to a comfortable level.

DOES MY UNWANTED HAIR MEAN I HAVE A HORMONE PROBLEM?

This is an important question, of course. Is the extra hair something normal, though embarrassing, or does it represent a medical problem? To help you with this, I've provided a sidebar that lists the usual places on a woman's body where testosterone can induce extra hair growth. Hair in these places may be unwelcome but is not of itself abnormal, unless it is extensive. The second sidebar gives some guidelines for when medical evaluation is indicated. Some of the signs listed, such as irregular periods and difficulty with weight suggest the possibility of polycystic ovary syndrome (PCOS) covered in detail in chapter 21.

I want to stress very clearly that *while PCOS is a common cause of hirsutism, most women with unwanted hair do not have PCOS.* They may have a slight increase in testosterone, but normal ovaries; or they may simply have hair follicles that are vulnerable to testosterone.

Most women with unwanted hair have normal lab tests. As a result, many are brushed off with comments like, "Everything's normal; there is nothing wrong with you." The pithy comment of one patient sums up why this is fallacious: "I was told nothing's wrong. But I have to shave twice a day. No one can tell me that is normal for a woman."

She was right, of course. Lab tests for testosterone problems are covered in detail in chapter 19, including the paradox of normal tests with increased hair.

COMMON PLACES FOR UNWANTED HAIR

Upper lip, especially the outer corners
Chin
Sideburn area
Around the nipples
Midline of chest and abdomen
Extension of pubic hair: sideways, upward toward the navel, and down
    over the upper thighs
Lower back above the buttocks and sometimes the buttocks themselves

WHEN UNWANTED HAIR NEEDS MEDICAL EVALUATION

Large areas covered, especially if the hair growth extends toward the
    sides of the body
Recent or rapid increase
Need for daily removal of facial hair of more than a few hairs
Presence of other androgenic changes: acne and/or alopecia
Irregular periods
Weight gain
Voice change
If you have more facial or body hair than you are comfortable with

TREATMENT FOR UNWANTED HAIR

There are basically two ways in which hirsutism can be treated. The most obvious is to physically remove the hair. This includes home methods such as plucking, waxing, and shaving as well as technological ones such as electrolysis and laser. The second approach is to use medication to lower or block the testosterone that has sent the hair follicles into overdrive. I'll cover both approaches: removal in this chapter and counteracting testosterone in chapter 20.

LOCAL REMOVAL (DEPILATION)

Half of American women remove hair at least occasionally. The most commonly used, plucking, is also the worst. I've been admonished by aestheticians to refer to this miniaturized violence as tweezing, but I choose to call it plucking to emphasize the aggressive nature of this form of depilation. Each pluck tears a hair out by its root, producing a tiny trauma to the skin. If plucking is infrequent, the skin recovers without visible ill effects. Done on a regular basis, however, plucking results in a lumpy, irregular appearance to the skin accentuated by little patches of redness. If you only need to pluck a few hairs from your chin once every few weeks, use of tweezers won't harm your skin. But if it has become a daily event in your life, I recommend you find a more skin-friendly method.

Waxing is a sort of super-all-at-once plucking. It does give a wonderfully smooth feel to the skin because not even tiny hairs are left behind. If you do it once a year on legs or bikini area to get ready for the beach, waxing won't harm you—though it does hurt. Done frequently waxing has the same injurious effects as plucking.

Depilatories are creams applied to the skin to dissolve the hair. They work well and do not damage the underlying skin—provided that you follow the instructions meticulously, and *do not leave them on too long.* If your skin is irritated after depilatory use, a single application of hydrocortisone cream 2.5 percent right after washing off the depilatory will minimize subsequent inflammation.

Which brings us to the device specifically designed to remove hair—the razor. Women are comfortable enough shaving their legs but naturally find using the same method on their face unsettling because shaving is, in our culture, a symbol of masculinity. However in other cultures—Japan and the Middle East are examples—removing facial hair is a normal part of women's grooming. I'm not suggesting that razors will take on a feminine image any time soon. What I do suggest, modestly, is that use of a razor may be a reasonable stopgap until medication or high-tech methods get the problem under control.

Women who do shave understandably try to get the process over with as quickly as possible, but it is better for your skin to do it carefully. First acquire a high-tech razor such as the Gillette Venus, next wet you hair for three minutes to soften it, then apply a shaving gel. Don't shave against the grain—while this leaves the skin smoother, it makes ingrown hair (pseudofolliculitis barbae, or PFB) more likely. Also, don't use a blade on your face that you used on your legs—it will be too dull.

PSEUDOFOLLICULITIS BARBAE (PFB)

This is the medical term for ingrown hairs. Sometimes as hairs grow back in, they get stuck under the skin, where they produce irritation and foster bacterial growth. The result is a breakout that looks much like acne. As with acne, scarring and darkening can occur as PFB heals. African Americans are particularly vulnerable because curly hairs more easily become trapped under the skin.

Although PFB looks like acne, its cause is different and so antiacne measures will not work for it. One OTC product, Tend Skin, which is applied after hair removal, definitely helps some women with a tendency to PFB. Other than this, the best way to minimize PFB is to not pull hairs out by the root or use a razor against the grain. Though this means more frequent removal, and for some, greater insecurity that it will show, it will reduce breakouts after removal.

VANIQA (EFLORNITHINE)

This cream directly inhibits hair growth within the follicle. I was involved in its development and believe it is an excellent, but underused, product. To get the benefit from Vaniqa, it's important to understand what it does and what it doesn't do. Vaniqa simply slows the growth of the hair shaft. It does not lighten or soften hair, nor does it make it fall out. For this reason it supplements, but does not replace, local hair removal. If you do remove, you can do so less often if you use Vaniqa; even more important, you can have greater confidence that the hair will not grow back so quickly as to be detectable late in the day. The cream is applied to the entire area of concern twice a day. Vaniqa is intended to be used only on the face, not on the body. It takes about two months to begin to see a noticeable result.

ELECTROLYSIS AND LASER

Laser depilation has been around for little more than a decade but is already the most widely used method. A variety of laser devices are available, and the technology is advancing quickly, so there may be new ones by the time you read this. Several treatments are needed at about two-month intervals because new follicles become active over time. From my viewpoint, laser hair removal is a mixed blessing. It does remove hair quickly and effectively, but doing so may lead women to defer medical evaluation for the underlying hormone problem.

The laser energy is absorbed by the pigment in the hair. This means that optimal results occur with dark hair and light skin. When skin is dark, it absorbs more of the energy, causing pain, and, sometimes, pigmentary changes that can be permanent. Dark-skinned individuals therefore need lower settings on the laser, which means treatment is slower and less effective. White or very pale hairs will not be removed by laser. Electrolysis is a much better option for these nonpigmented hairs. Setting the intensity of the laser is an art: too low and more treatments are needed, too high and pain and skin injury may occur. The moral of this is that it is important to choose a laser specialist who is really expert in the technique—usually a dermatologist or plastic surgeon.

Unfortunately, laser has been a moneymaking gimmick for doctors and others who have no real interest or expertise. If you are considering laser hair removal, be sure to pick a doctor who is really committed to the procedure. In New York City there are ads on the subway for laser hair removal; this is not a good way to pick the person to whom you'll be entrusting the most visible part of your body. Also be sure you've been told what the real cost is likely to be. The initial course is typically four treatments, but if you have a significant hair problem, you will almost certainly need touch-ups at least twice a year. Pricing of electrolysis is more straightforward, based on the time spent by the electrologist.

Electrolysis is more than one hundred years old, though it has advanced greatly over its primitive beginnings. It is slower than laser, but most electrologists usually have a real commitment to helping women— and some men—troubled by increased hair. Laser removes hair from an entire area at once, while electrolysis goes hair by hair. A single electrolysis treatment is usually much cheaper than a single lasering, but more are needed. Be sure to pick someone who is a member of the International Guild of Hair Removal Specialists, many of whom offer both laser and electrolysis, or the American Electrology Association, whose members do electrolysis only.

GETTING RID OF UNWANTED HAIR:
THE PLACE OF MEDICATION

You may be wondering, if there are so many ways to remove hair, why would anyone consider using medication for this purpose? The reason is that direct removal by itself does not always produce a complete result. If you have only an occasional unwanted hair, then any of the several local methods will be all you need. But for more troublesome unwanted hair, there is no single method that gives perfect results for everyone. I've listed the main reasons for using medication in the sidebar on page 275.

Although electrolysis is billed as "permanent" and laser as "permanent hair reduction," many women notice that the problem recurs or that prolonged treatment is necessary to keep it under control. This is not really a fault with the procedures, rather if there is an underlying hormone problem, such as high testosterone; as in PCOS, or vulnerability of the follicles to testosterone, new hairs soon take the place of the previous ones. When there is continued hormonal drive to hair formation, what often gives the best result is to combine laser and/or electrolysis with treatment directed at the hormonal cause. The medical part greatly reduces hair but does not necessarily eliminate it. Combining medication with hair removal often gives the best result.

WHEN TO CONSIDER MEDICATION FOR UNWANTED HAIR

You want to deal with the underlying hormonal cause.

You have other androgen-related problems, such as acne or alopecia and want help with these also. Medication will also help skin and scalp hair; electrolysis or laser only affect unwanted hair.

Local removal, such as plucking or razor takes significant time from your day and does not leave you confident that your secret is safe.

Local removal causes breakout (PFB) or is otherwise hard on your skin.

Despite high-tech methods (electrolysis and laser), the hair just keeps coming back.

Cost: Medication is usually covered by insurance but electrolysis and laser are not.

A LAST WORD

If you have never had hair removal treatment, I recommend beginning medical treatment first, then starting laser or electrolysis six to twelve months later. Once the obstreperous hormones have been tamed, less extensive laser or electrolysis will be needed.

I have tried to give you the facts you need to make informed choices among the many methods for controlling hirsutism. Because there are so many options, you can find one or a combination that will solve your problem. Medical treatments to counteract the adverse effects of testosterone are covered in chapter 20.

18.

Acne: Not Just for Teenagers

Peggy had a problem that seems trivial to people who do not have it: adult acne. Because her husband was a politician, she had to accompany him at social events nearly every night. Peggy felt quite awkward about her blemishes during these functions and even felt guilty—she believed that her appearance was important for her husband's career and feared that she was letting him down by having imperfect skin.

All the times I saw Peggy, she was carefully and neatly dressed. Her skill with makeup enabled her to hide her acne while still looking natural. For Peggy to reveal her acne, even to a doctor, was extremely embarrassing. She said, "You know, maybe if I'd had acne at the normal age, I'd have gotten used to it. But in high school when the other girls were having a bad time with their skin, mine was perfect. I don't think I ever had more than two or three pimples in all of high school."

But then at forty-three, Peggy noticed that her skin had become much more oily, and she began breaking out with large red blemishes. She'd tried many things: giving up chocolate, which she'd never eaten much anyway, washing with special cleansers, applying creams, and, finally, oral antibiotics. A topical retinoid gel prescribed by a dermatologist she'd consulted helped her skin at first, but then made it red and sore.

Peggy's skin was now hormonally vulnerable. Adult acne like Peggy's is all too common. Teenagers with acne are routinely told that they'll grow out of it; problem is, many don't. Although acne eventually goes away, it may be decades before it does.

At her first visit I measured Peggy's levels of androgens, the family of hormones that trigger acne. Her testosterone was on the high side of normal, enough to trigger her oversensitive oil glands. The answer for Peggy was spironolactone, a medication that blocks the effect of testosterone on the skin. Over the next few weeks her acne cleared, and her complexion brightened. Her uncharacteristic social unease vanished. Treatment such as this, which is directed at the hormonal cause of acne, is far more effective than the commonly prescribed creams and antibiotics. It is explained in this chapter with further details in chapter 20.

Women know that acne is related to hormones because it fluctuates with their cycles. Unfortunately many dermatologists ignore this obvious hormonal link. This is lamentable because the key to clearing acne is combating its hormonal cause: testosterone. The standard dermatological treatments—that immense repertoire of creams, gels, and cleansers, as well as oral antibiotics—may reduce the number of blemishes, but they rarely get rid of them completely.

Don't let anyone convince you that you can't have completely clear skin. You can, and this chapter will tell you how. Unfortunately many doctors do not really exert themselves with acne. Because it is not life-threatening, the medical establishment tends to dismiss breaking out as a "vanity" disorder. Some reasons many women do not get effective treatment from dermatologists are listed in the sidebar on the next page.

HOW HORMONES TRIGGER BREAKOUTS

You probably remember the perfect skin of your childhood. Then, in your teens, just as you were becoming more self-conscious about your appearance, you may have been one of the unlucky ones whose hormones took over and messed up your skin. For most, acne is only a mild embarrassment, but for girls whose skin is vulnerable to testosterone, the teens can be a time of heartbreak. Too often, when acne is supposed to go away, it doesn't. Or perhaps your skin made it through your teens unscathed, only to erupt later. I often see women like Peggy whose acne first appears in their thirties or forties. Some have it even after menopause.

WHY DERMATOLOGISTS CAN'T TREAT ACNE

- Dermatologists are experts in treating the skin. Though acne shows itself on the surface, its root cause is internal: hormones carried in the blood. Testosterone travels from deep within the body to the skin, where it stimulates oil production. This oil gets trapped in the pores, where bacteria flourish, making the redness even worse.

- Medications applied to the skin don't even start to work until after blemishes have gotten started. Oral antibiotics work even later.

- Acne is best stopped *before it starts* by decreasing or blocking testosterone. Even when dermatologists' treatments have failed, hormonal treatments almost always clear the skin.

- More and more dermatologists are pushing expensive procedures such as chemical peels and injection of lesions. These usually need to be done over and over because they do not counteract the underlying cause.

Acne may be a disease of youth, but it doesn't make one feel youthful to have it. Worse, it is a persistent case of blame-the-victim. Many assume that acne sufferers do not eat right or have poor hygiene. Research has effectively refuted this: Diet plays no role in causing acne. Burgers and greasy french fries may not be good for your heart, but they don't do anything to your skin. Nor does chocolate cause acne. The oiliness that goes with acne is not due to uncleanliness, but to sebaceous glands that are in overdrive. Washing does remove the oil, only for it to reappear shortly afterward. Regular use of a facial cleanser, such as Purpose, helps, but by itself cannot restrain overenthusiastic oil glands.

The perpetrator of acne is testosterone, which activates the oil glands. The last week of the cycle is blemish week for many women because at ovulation, there is an upward blip in testosterone that soon shows up as oil and zits. Making matters worse, pores plug up, trapping the excess oil within the skin. Bacteria grow happily in this oil, resulting in inflammation and exudation—the redness and pus-like yellow liquid that make acne so ugly. If things get really out of hand, the pimples enlarge and become hard due to inflammation—nodules—or fill with fluid—cysts. These are not only embarrassing; they can be quite painful as well and may take weeks or months to heal—or not heal at all.

Which brings us to the next stage of acne: wound healing. Acne represents an injury to the skin, and nature has provided us with mechanisms for healing this. The immune system eventually gets rid of the aggravating bacteria, although at the price of redness and swelling. As the infection subsides, the area heals—but also at a price. As happens with other kinds of skin injury, the healing of acne can leave scars. Pitting occurs when the damaged area does not completely fill in. The increased blood flow that helped cure the infection may persist in the form of reddened areas. To add insult to injury, as the skin heals, pigmentation increases. For someone with very fair skin, the difference may not be noticeable; but for anyone who is dark complexioned, the blotches need to be covered up with makeup.

It's been hard for me to convince gynecologists and my fellow endocrinologists to take acne seriously. Acne is not trivial; several studies show that it can cause significant depression—which will hardly come as a surprise if you have acne. It is one of the oddities of many in health care that they don't believe something if a patient tells them directly, but do believe it if they read it in the pages of a prestigious medical journal. Perhaps the most important study on the social effects of acne is one showing that unemployment rates are about 50 percent higher in both women and men with acne. On reflection, this is not much of a surprise since acne is disturbing to look at. Many feel uncomfortable being around people with physical problems, and so try to avoid them. Acne in a sense is a handicap, and it brings discrimination with it. Fortunately for those burdened with acne, it can be reversed.

DON'T BE DISCOURAGED!

So far I have said many negative things about acne, not to discourage you but to get out into the open what acne sufferers go through. When I lecture doctors about acne, I show a series of pictures illustrating what acne can do to skin if left uncontrolled. Then I conclude by saying that I regard acne as a sort of emergency in that it may cause irreversible scarring if not cleared up ASAP. My point is that acne should be treated without waiting to see if it goes away by itself.

Acne can almost always be cleared. You may find this hard to believe if, like most of the women I treat for acne, you've been to dermatologist after dermatologist, only to have your oral antibiotics and topical creams or gels shuffled around without noticeable benefit. Or you may have taken Accutane, most likely reluctantly, and discovered, contrary to what you were promised, that the acne came back.

I assure you that your acne can be cleared. The secret is to direct treatment at the underlying internal hormonal cause.

THE SECRET OF CLEAR SKIN REVEALED

The key to clear skin is applying the brakes to testosterone. Because this hormone initiates the chain of events leading to acne, countering it stops acne before it begins. The principles of lowering and blocking testosterone that work for alopecia and hirsutism work as well or better for acne. Nonandrogenic birth control pills contribute by cutting free testosterone levels by about half. Some women come to believe that the pill does not work for acne. I think this is because it reduces acne but does not eliminate it. For this reason, results are dramatically better when the pill is combined with a testosterone blocker, usually spironolactone. This drug can be truly miraculous for skin, not only clearing acne but also conferring a youthful feminine glow. An alternative if spiro does not work out is Androcur (CPA or cyproterone acetate), available in Canada and almost every other country in the world except the United States.

It takes some time for any acne treatment to start to show results. This is because existing lesions need to heal, a process that can take several weeks and even longer if you have hard nodules or large cysts. With antitestosterone treatment, such as an OC and spiro, improvement is usually apparent at two months and skin nearly clear by four months. With extensive inflammation, improvement may be more gradual.

Lowering and blocking testosterone takes away the biochemical stimulus that keeps the sebaceous (oil) glands in overdrive. In about a month, skin stops being oily. As the old blemishes disappear, fewer and fewer new ones appear to take their place. Although an occasional zit may still appear, especially before your period, this treatment usually produces a lovely clear complexion.

Full details on antitestosterone treatment are provided in chapter 20.

Many women I see in my practice have come because they were told they need isotretinoin (Accutane), an extremely potent drug that can cause birth defects if taken during pregnancy. Antitestosterone treatment is gentler than Accutane and makes the skin look better overall. For those few who really do need Accutane, it can be made safer and more comfortable, as described later in this chapter.

THE PILL AND ACNE

Something needs to be said about birth control pills and acne. Since I was the lead investigator for the original OrthoTri-Cyclen acne study, this is a subject close to my heart. The pill really does help a lot, but on average it gets rid of only about half the blemishes. For some women with mild acne, this may be enough. But if half as many zits are still way too many, its time to add a testosterone blocker to get rid of the rest.

The best OCs for acne are those with no testosterone-like activity. Picking the best pill for your skin and body is fully explained in chapter 4. Here I'll simply list the best ones for acne, which are Yasmin, Ortho-Cyclen, Ortho Tri-Cyclen, Desogen, and the Ortho Evra patch. If you are on a different OC, but your skin is clear, there is no reason to change. If your pill isn't helping your skin, changing to one of these may be a step in the right direction. Adding a testosterone blocker, however, is what makes the greatest difference.

CONVENTIONAL ACNE TREATMENT:
TOPICALS AND ANTIBIOTICS

The women I see in my practice for acne have become disillusioned with the standard dermatologic repertoire of topicals and oral antibiotics. They report going from dermatologist to dermatologist and being switched from one cream or antibiotic to another without seeing any change for the better. Such experiences give a bad name, not entirely undeserved, to conventional acne treatments. Topicals and antibiotics work best as adjuncts to antitestosterone treatment. By themselves they are sufficient only for very mild cases.

If you have only the odd pimple before your period, then it is reasonable to start out with one of these standard acne therapies. However if topicals and/or antibiotics have not worked for you, then rather than wasting time switching around yet one more time, the best thing is to address the underlying hormonal cause.

Since conventional acne treatment can still play a role, I'll give some inside information on some of the better preparations.

Topicals These fall into three groups: antibiotics, benzoyl peroxide, and retinoids. Benzoyl peroxide (BP) is available over-the-counter in 5 and 10 percent strengths. It is mainly antibacterial and can definitely help mild acne. A currently popular form is Proactiv, which some of my patients have liked. Topical antibiotics probably work better than BP, but require a prescription. Both erythromycin and clindamycin are used; I think the former may be slightly safer. Topical antibiotics will not work as well as oral ones (see below) and so are mainly for very mild acne.

Retinoids are related to Accutane, but without the serious side effects since they are not taken internally. They work by reducing the plugging of pores, which is the second step in acne formation. Retinoids are particularly good for getting rid of comedones (whiteheads and blackheads). Their main limitation is their tendency to make skin red and sore after a few weeks of use. For some, this is as bothersome as the original acne. Fortunately, there is a very simple way to prevent this. Instead of leaving it on overnight, wash off the cream or gel about thirty minutes after you apply it. The results will be as good, and irritation is usually minimal.

To work, acne topicals must be applied faithfully every day. They are preventive treatment and don't work nearly as well if you wait until you are broken out to use them. Good products include Differin, Retin A Micro, and Tazorac. Differin comes in cream, gel, and lotion forms and is the least irritating. Gels are generally slightly more drying and irritating, so creams are better if the hormonal treatment of your acne has gotten rid of the excess oiliness. Tazorac is both more effective and more irritating than the others, so it is the one to try if the milder ones have not done the job.

Oral antibiotics These block growth of bacteria in acne lesions. They do not stop pimples from appearing, but limit swelling and speed healing. Several antibiotics are used for acne. All need to be taken daily; once you've broken out they speed healing only slightly. The one most commonly prescribed by dermatologists is minocycline (Minocin), a member of the tetracycline family. It may be slightly more effective than others, but has two potential problems: photosensitivity and a tendency to cause yeast infections. Many women take it without any problem, but if you're out in the sun a lot or tend to get yeast infections, it's not the best option for you.

Erythromycin is less likely to cause side effects than minocycline. Although high doses can cause stomach ache, lower doses of 250 or 333 mg twice a day rarely do this and are quite adequate for acne. Erythromycin does have some interactions with other drugs, so if you are taking others, check with your doctor to be sure they are compatible.

Trimethoprim-sulfa (Bactrim, Septra, and others) is an additional alternative, but allergies to sulfa are common and sometimes serious, so I'd rate this a rather distant third choice.

SKIN CARE FOR ACNE

I have not emphasized skin care because most women with acne become pretty conscientious about it without having to be told by a doctor. Special cleansers such as Purpose are better than soap, but the difference is not great. Regular washing is the important thing.

If you have acne, cosmetics are unavoidable. So long as you choose noncomedogenic ones such as Clinique or Prescriptives, they will not make your acne worse. Anything oily should be avoided. Some cosmetic products sold for acne actually are not good for your skin. Astringent lotions do temporarily reduce the grease, but they also remove the natural moisturizers your skin needs. Even worse are grit-containing cleansers—they don't rub off the pimples, but they do irritate the skin and can cause rashes.

Good skin care is simple: Wash your face regularly and avoid products that may irritate it. While it helps maintain skin health, washing will not by itself cure acne.

THERE IS STILL A PLACE, THOUGH A LIMITED ONE, FOR ACCUTANE

Accutane, once touted as the ultimate acne cure, has a fearsome reputation but is neither quite as effective nor quite as dangerous as its reputation suggests. This drug is a potent derivative of vitamin A that acts by completely drying out oil glands. As would be expected, generalized dryness of skin, lips, and eyes, is a usual side effect and may be uncomfortable with higher doses.

Accutane (isotretinoin) is now available in several generic forms: Amnesteem, Claravis, and Sotret, which are cheaper and just as effective. I will continue to refer to Accutane since that name is most familiar, but I don't endorse any one brand.

The great danger of Accutane is the high probability of severe birth defects if an unborn child is exposed to it. *For this reason, either abstinence or absolutely reliable contraception must be practiced while taking Accutane or its generic equivalents. If there is any chance you might get pregnant while on Accutane, you should not take it.* At the time Accutane is prescribed, you should receive detailed information about pregnancy risks and contraception. Pregnancy tests are required before starting. The safest course is to use double contraception—OC or patch, plus condom. If you have any doubts about contraception, it's best to visit your gynecologist first so that you can be sure your method is completely reliable. Once you have completed the course and allowed time for the drug to get out of your body, it will not affect the health of future pregnancies. I recommend waiting two months after stopping Accutane before attempting to get pregnant.

Much has been made in the press of a supposed suicide risk with Accutane. In my practice, I have not found it to cause or aggravate depression. Nonetheless, any degree of depression should be under some form of treatment before beginning Accutane. My suspicion is that the suicides reported of people taking Accutane were either unrelated or due not to the drug but to the psychological effects of living with terrible acne.

Liver problems can also occur while taking Accutane, so simple blood tests for the liver should be done before you start and at intervals after that. There are many other side effects and contraindications, so if you opt for Accutane, you should be under the care of a physician who is experienced with this powerful medication.

You may be wondering now: Why would anyone ever take Accutane? The reason is that occasionally it is the only thing that will work. Also, despite the scary sounding side effects, most have a pretty easy time while taking it. Nearly everyone experiences some dryness, usually mild, of the lips and, less commonly, the eyes. Moisturizer generally takes care of any skin or lip dryness.

For many women starting Accutane, the biggest worry is the supposed risk of temporary exacerbation—in other words, your skin getting worse before it gets better. If acne is out of control to begin with, the prospect of it becoming even more unsightly is indeed daunting. I've seen this early exacerbation only once among the hundreds of women I've treated with this medication. This is because starting antitestosterone treatment before Accutane almost always prevents this getting-worse-before-you-get-better syndrome. If testosterone has been blocked, the early worsening of acne does not occur. For this reason, I rarely recommend Accutane by itself—but only in the infrequent cases in which blocking testosterone is not sufficient.

ACCUTANE VERSUS HORMONAL TREATMENT OF ACNE

If conventional treatment with topicals and antibiotics does not clear your skin, the next step, in my view, is not Accutane but hormonal treatment. I've seen hundreds of cases of all degrees of acne clear virtually completely when skin is protected from testosterone. Often this will be a birth control pill plus spironolactone, but sometimes other combinations are preferable. Not only is this safer and more comfortable than Accutane, but also puts a healthy-looking glow to the skin, something Accutane does not. In my experience, this approach achieves excellent results more than 90 percent of the time. Accutane need only be considered if you are one of the few who have a suboptimal response.

MAKING ACCUTANE EASIER: LOW-DOSE THERAPY

Although higher doses of Accutane are supposed to produce a permanent cure, in actuality, benefits are often temporary. Skin may stay clear for a few months or even for a few years, but then the acne comes back. Fortunately, when Accutane is combined with a testosterone blocker, small doses are usually sufficient. Side effects are milder, so if necessary, low doses in the range of 10 mg once or twice a day, or sometimes only three times a week, can be taken for an extended period. The pregnancy caution still applies, of course.

HIDRADENITIS SUPPORATIVA (HS)

This distressing condition has some similarities to acne, but is actually a different process, one involving sweat glands. I cover it here in the acne section because many with HS at first think it is a bad form of acne. In HS, abscesses (boils) form in the intertriginous areas, which are those places where skin rests against skin. Most often it is the underarms and groin that are affected, although I have seen it occur under the breasts. These boils are painful and usually drain pus-like material, which can have a noticeable odor. Needless to say, having pus around intimate areas is extremely disturbing as well as inhibiting to sexual activity. Many HS sufferers never even tell their doctors because they find the condition too embarrassing. As a result, many doctors have never heard of HS, nor seen a case.

Research on HS is sadly lacking, and so I can only go by my own experience evaluating and treating women with the condition. It does seem to me that testosterone plays a role in HS, although there must be other, unknown factors. It is clearly associated with PCOS, though only a minority of women with PCOS also have HS. Since HS occurs mainly in testosterone-sensitive skin and begins after puberty, it would seem to be a form of vulnerability to testosterone. Testosterone levels are not necessarily elevated, however.

HS is treatable by the same principles that work for other testosterone-dependent skin problems, but treatment needs to be more intensive than is usually required for acne. Androgen blockade makes the most difference and should be maximal. This is discussed in chapter 20. Unless contraindicated, an oral contraceptive to help lower testosterone should be part of the regimen. Although not all agree, I think long-term antibiotic use can help. I recommend erythromycin 333 mg twice a day or minocycline 100 mg twice a day. Realistically these measures are not likely to completely eliminate HS, but they may reduce the number and size of boils and the amount of drainage. It is definitely worth getting treatment rather than suffering in silence.

Accutane might seem useful because it dries out the skin. Yet because it increases the number of sweat glands, it should not be used for HS.

Most sources discourage surgery for HS. Some get a seemingly good result, only to have more boils form later. It's important that the surgery not remove so much skin that motion of the arms and legs is restricted. I see surgery only as an absolute last resort, if at all.

YOU CAN HAVE CLEAR SKIN!

It makes me sad when I see women on the street or other public places with acne too conspicuous to hide because this is entirely unnecessary. Treatment of the hormonal cause of acne nearly always clears it. The problem is finding a physician familiar with this form of treatment. There are some out there, though it takes some effort to track one down. As with alopecia, if you find an open-minded physician, you may be able to convince her or him to treat you in accord with the principles in this chapter. It's important to spread the word so that the day will come when all women enjoy clear complexions.

19.

Making Sense of Your Testosterone Results

Modern medicine would be unimaginable without the help of the laboratory. At the same time, with so many tests available, many of which require considerable background for correct interpretation, lab results can confuse as well as clarify. Many of the women I see in my practice have had pages and pages of lab work that was never integrated into a coherent explanation of what was wrong. Most often, what is needed is not more tests but astute interpretation of standard ones. For this reason, this chapter focuses on the few essential tests for testosterone problems rather than presenting a lengthy catalog of exotic ones that are helpful only with rare conditions. I have never forgotten the advice of one of my teachers in medical school that most difficult diagnoses are not rare diseases but unusual presentations of common ones. This is definitely true with women's testosterone problems.

USING THE LAB TO CLARIFY WHY YOU HAVE ACNE, HIRSUTISM, OR ALOPECIA

The sidebar on page 289 lists the tests that are essential for the basic workup of acne, hirsutism, and alopecia. The remainder of this chapter explains what these tests measure and how they can help get to the root of your problem. Equally important, I will point out some of the common pitfalls in laboratory diagnosis. Many of the women I see in my practice have not received the best treatment because the meaning of their lab results was not properly understood. Correct interpretation is just as important as having the right tests ordered. This is particularly so if you are hormonally vulnerable, in which case *it is essential that tests be interpreted in the context of what is happening in your own body.*

I cannot cover all tests that may be useful in every circumstance because there are just too many possibilities. Nor is this list intended as a substitute for medical consultation, but rather to give you the background to get more from discussion of your results with a knowledgeable physician.

THE BASIC TESTS FOR ALOPECIA, HIRSUTISM, AND ACNE

Total and free testosterone—the following are the most important:

DHEA-S—Elevated levels may add to your body's testosterone.
FSH and prolactin—needed only if your periods are irregular or you may be approaching perimenopause/menopause.
Estradiol—the main estrogen. Helpful in some situations to assess estrogen status. Generally not necessary nor helpful if you are under forty-five and have regular cycles, are taking an OC, or are clearly postmenopausal.
TSH—the most sensitive test for thyroid function and usually the only one necessary.
Blood count (CBC) and chemistry profile—part of any health evaluation.
Iron—deficiency may contribute to alopecia.

If you want to refresh your memory on what hormones do, you can refer back to chapter 2, which explains these matters.

TESTOSTERONE TESTS AND THEIR LIMITATIONS

Testosterone can be measured in several ways; unfortunately no single one tells the whole story.

Total and free testosterone Testosterone is the sole trigger of hirsutism and acne and the main cause of alopecia when it begins before age forty. (Low estrogen can also contribute to alopecia as explained in chapter 16.) Testosterone levels are so commonly misconstrued that I suggest never accepting a blanket statement that this test is normal. To understand how testosterone levels are properly interpreted, you need to know some things about this hormone that most doctors do not know, although there is nothing truly arcane about them.

Testosterone (T) is measured in three different forms. The total T sounds as if it would be the most important one, but actually is least useful because most of what it measures is inactive. Most T in the blood, about 98 percent, circulates attached to a protein called SHBG (sex hormone-binding globulin), which also carries estrogen. When hormones are bound to SHBG, they are out of the action because this protein keeps them safely trapped in the bloodstream, rather than letting them escape into tissues. Only about 2 percent of testosterone is not attached to SHBG and therefore free to diffuse into tissues, including oil glands and hair follicles. This is referred to as free testosterone (FT) and is what actually affects your body. Labs offer assays for FT, but unfortunately many are inaccurate, so the result gives only a very general idea of the actual level. SHBG can be measured, but this information is less useful. Another test, bioavailable testosterone, gives about the same information as FT.

SHBG is made in the liver and is itself controlled by the two sex hormones that attach to it. Estrogen signals the liver to make more SHBG, which results in less testosterone being in the free form. This is the main way that estrogen counters testosterone—it keeps it in the bloodstream, out of harm's way. Testosterone lowers SHBG so that more T is able to escape into the tissues. Testosterone thus exerts a double whammy effect on women—as levels go up, more and more is free to slip out of the blood into the tissues, where it wreaks its havoc.

Who decides what's normal? The next problem in making sense of testosterone levels is that different labs give different normal or "reference" ranges. Since they never tell us how they decide on these ranges, we cannot be sure they are really correct. In different laboratories, the upper normal for total T ranges from 55 to 120 ng/dL. This would suggest that a level of 100 ng/dL, which would be very high in one lab, might be normal in another. My experience—and this is based on seeing testosterone results in nearly 10,000 women over twenty years—is that when the level approaches or exceeds 50 ng/dL, unwanted effects such as acne, hirsutism, and androgenic alopecia are common. The unmeasured variable is, of course, individual vulnerability. The more sensitive your oil glands and follicles are to testosterone, the lower the level at which it can adversely affect your skin and hair.

Like everything else hormonal, testosterone fluctuates Release of testosterone, like that of other hormones, is far from steady; blood levels sway up and down, depending on whether a secretory episode has just occurred or not. Because there is no means for predicting the timing of these peaks and troughs, they create much uncertainty when test results are interpreted. If blood happens to be drawn during a low point, the result will be normal for a woman who might have high levels at other times. Testosterone levels tend to be highest in the morning, so the best time to have the test is between 8:00 and 10:00 A.M. Even levels obtained later in the day can be helpful, however.

What's really normal? Before accepting a result as normal, we must ask, "Normal for what?" This is a particular point of confusion with respect to hormone tests. A testosterone level within the normal range means that the ovaries and adrenals are not overproducing this hormone. When the level is definitely elevated it is essential to find out the source and cause of the overproduction and to correct the condition. Possible causes of a significantly elevated testosterone include PCOS, late-onset adrenal hyperplasia, thecal cell hyperplasia, and tumors, which fortunately are extremely rare. PCOS and its variants are explained in chapter 21.

When testosterone is not elevated, this is good news because we can be reassured that the function of ovaries and adrenals is relatively normal. (There can be exceptions with PCOS.) The most important things to bear in mind—and unfortunately this is not widely known— is that *for women who are hormonally vulnerable, "normal" levels of testosterone can still damage skin and hair.* This is because the test only tells us what ovaries and adrenals are doing; it says nothing about how the body responds. For some women even a borderline-high TT level of 50 ng/dL will not cause noticeable effects. For others who have the bad luck to be ultrasensitive to testosterone, even a much lower level will leave its mark on skin and hair.

How testosterone changes over time In women (and men, but that's another story) both TT and FT levels peak in the late teens and early twenties, then gradually decline. Despite this, lab-reference ranges rarely include a breakdown by age. This further obscures the meaning of the test because you need to know what the level means for a woman your age. If you are forty, you want a normal level for a forty-year-old, not a twenty- or sixty-year-old.

The length of exposure to high levels of testosterone is another critical variable. The more years your T is near the top of the range, the worse for your hair. A total T level of, say, 50 ng/dL that lasts for a year is far less damaging than a level of 45 ng/dL that persists for a decade. Of course there is no way to measure past levels, but an experienced physician can often infer them based on your present level, menstrual history, and careful physical examination of skin and hair. That is why I emphasize that tests tell part of your hormonal story, but not all of it.

Is it worth measuring testosterone at all? At this point you may be worrying that testosterone is too complicated to be tested for. Fortunately not; the tests give very useful information about where you stand with this hormone. The most important thing to bear in mind is that a "normal" testosterone level does not mean that this hormone is not the cause of acne, hirsutism, or alopecia. Sometimes women are disappointed when their result is normal because they think that it means the cause cannot be found. Actually, a normal result is always a good thing. *With testosterone-induced skin and hair conditions, a normal testosterone level tells you that your problem is hormonal vulnerability.*

This sidebar gives a quick guide to pitfalls in testosterone interpretation.

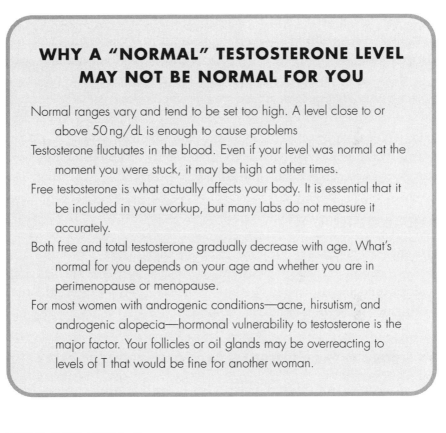

WHY A "NORMAL" TESTOSTERONE LEVEL MAY NOT BE NORMAL FOR YOU

Normal ranges vary and tend to be set too high. A level close to or above 50 ng/dL is enough to cause problems

Testosterone fluctuates in the blood. Even if your level was normal at the moment you were stuck, it may be high at other times.

Free testosterone is what actually affects your body. It is essential that it be included in your workup, but many labs do not measure it accurately.

Both free and total testosterone gradually decrease with age. What's normal for you depends on your age and whether you are in perimenopause or menopause.

For most women with androgenic conditions—acne, hirsutism, and androgenic alopecia—hormonal vulnerability to testosterone is the major factor. Your follicles or oil glands may be overreacting to levels of T that would be fine for another woman.

DHEA AND DHEA-S

These hormones are invariably referred to by their abbreviations, DHEA and DHEA-S, because of their tongue twister full names, dehydroepiandrosterone and dehydroepiandrosterone sulfate. The two forms are nearly identical; the -S, or sulfate, version is the better one to measure because its levels in blood are more stable. The two can be considered together. DHEA seems to be inactive in humans but can be converted to testosterone—high levels therefore suggest the possibility of increased testosterone production. Sometimes both testosterone and DHEA are elevated. In this case the increased testosterone may be coming from the adrenal, but this is not always the case.

Even more than testosterone, DHEA-S levels are age-related. Although some lab-reference ranges give the upper as 300 µg/dL, levels up to 400 are common for women in their twenties, and some women have levels in this range into their mid-thirties. There is no reason to be concerned if your DHEA-S level is a little above average for your age. DHEA-S should be measured as part of the workup for any androgen problem; if it is very high, further testing is indicated.

DHEA supplements have been heavily promoted in the past as a youth-preserving treatment and to enhance sexual desire. Because DHEA is converted into testosterone, it is the last thing you want to take if you have androgenic skin and hair changes. Nor is it a good way to raise your testosterone to enhance sex. The only reasonably safe way to do this is detailed in chapter 14.

ANDROSTENEDIONE

Another tongue twister hormone, it can be called delta-4, or more simply and intuitively, andro or A. Andro is a main precursor for both testosterone and estrogen. This test is needed only in unusual situations, such as hereditary adrenal disorders.

17 HYDROXYPROGESTERONE AND OTHER EXOTIC TESTS

A shorter name for this is 17 OHP. It is a marker for late-onset (also called acquired) adrenal hyperplasia. As the name suggests, this is a form of overactivity of the adrenals. The wrong balance of enzymes in the adrenals causes them to make excessive amounts of testosterone. In the much more severe congenital form, both boys and girls can have testosterone levels above those of normal adult men. The late-onset form is much milder—and much less well understood—but it is one of the causes of high testosterone levels in women. For rarer forms of adrenal enzyme blocks, a variety of other steroid metabolites can be measured, but these conditions are so rare that the tests are mainly useful for children suspected of having a congenital form of one of these conditions. Workup of any form of adrenal hyperplasia needs to be done by an endocrinologist with special expertise in androgenic conditions.

THE DEXAMETHASONE SUPPRESSION TEST

If your testosterone is more than mildly elevated, this test can determine if it is coming mainly from the ovaries or adrenals. Dexamethasone (dex), a form of cortisone, is taken for six to eight days. Testosterone is measured before and after. If the T is coming from the adrenal the level drops sharply, while that which is made in the ovary is unaffected. Interpretation is usually straightforward. Suppose you have a testosterone level of 60 ng/dL that drops to 20 after taking dex. This means that two-thirds of your T is from the adrenals and one-third from the ovary. When T does not drop much at all, the ovary is the main source of T, usually indicating a diagnosis of PCOS. Rarely, it can mean that it is coming from an adrenal tumor—especially if the T level is very high—so the dex test should be interpreted in the context of your other results by a physician experienced in androgen excess conditions.

There is another kind of dex test in which cortisol is measured rather than testosterone. This is often used by psychiatrists since depression can cause levels of cortisol to be high. For this test, dex is given as a single dose in the evening, and a single blood sample is taken the next morning. My view of this test is that it is of academic interest only. If someone is depressed, they are depressed, whatever an esoteric blood test shows. This one-day dex test is useless for testosterone problems.

The dex test is needed only when T is clearly high. Similar information can be obtained if you will be starting on an OC by measuring your testosterone again during the middle of the third pill cycle. If the level goes down to normal, the ovary is the source of the extra testosterone, and the pill is adequately suppressing it. If testosterone remains high, further workup is necessary.

SALIVA AND OTHER UNORTHODOX LAB TESTS

To be useful, a medical test has to be validated, a process that involves trying it out on several hundred people, both normal and those with particular diseases. Without such studies, a test is uninterpretable. Getting a number is not enough; there needs to be hard data to demonstrate that it is reliable and specific. In recent years, a variety of alternative labs have sprung up offering tests that are neither FDA approved nor validated. Saliva tests have been especially popular. This is an unfortunate trend because such tests rarely do anything but confuse. Measuring a hormone in saliva has no advantages over determining it in blood and, as usually performed, is far less accurate.

Hormonally vulnerable women are often victims of those who proffer such dubious tests, which can be tempting if your problem has been brushed-off with: "All your tests are normal; there's nothing wrong with you." If this has happened to you, the answer is likely to be found by seeking more sophisticated interpretation of the tests you have had, rather than by having additional tests whose meanings have never been established.

20.

Effective Treatments for Hormonal Skin and Hair Problems

We have seen how testosterone, while it is good for bones and for sex, is not so good for skin and hair. Testosterone tends to extremes; there seems to be either too much or too little of it. In this way, testosterone functions quite differently in women from men. Men's levels are so high that a small change up or down makes no noticeable difference. Not so for women, whose levels are close to critical thresholds and whose normal range is much narrower than men's. When testosterone is behaving and the body responding as it should, there is just enough for sexual interest but not enough to harm skin and hair. A relatively small drop may make sex blah, while an upward blip may trigger a breakout or a hair shed. Unfortunately, this mechanism is so delicately balanced that hormonally vulnerable women may get the worst of both—enough testosterone for sex may be too much for hair.

This is not as grim as it sounds; when testosterone is unruly, there are a multitude of ways to restrain its misbehavior. In this chapter, I explain how to use currently available medications to keep testosterone in check. None were originally developed for this purpose; officially sanctioned research on drugs to counteract testosterone has been done exclusively for men, mainly for prostate problems and, to a limited degree, for male-pattern baldness. Keeping in mind the ancient Chinese principle that we are all a mixture of yin and yang, women can use several medications invented for other purposes when testosterone has not accepted its proper place in a female body.

Since oily skin, acne, unwanted facial and body hair, and alopecia are all caused by testosterone, they are treated with a similar approach. This also means that treating one of the conditions usually benefits the others when more than one is present. Of course, each has treatments unique to itself; these were covered in the chapters on the separate conditions.

AN OVERVIEW OF TREATMENT

Testosterone can be tamed in several ways; in many cases, these work best if combined. We can suppress its production so that blood levels go down; prevent its activation to DHT; and, most useful, block its ac-

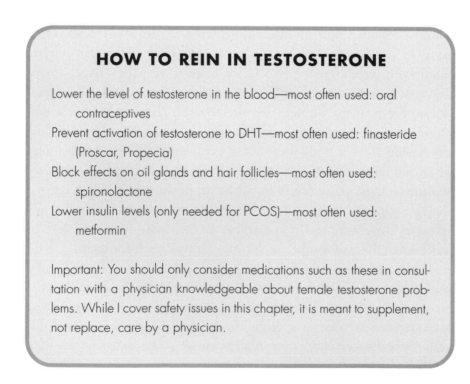

HOW TO REIN IN TESTOSTERONE

Lower the level of testosterone in the blood—most often used: oral contraceptives

Prevent activation of testosterone to DHT—most often used: finasteride (Proscar, Propecia)

Block effects on oil glands and hair follicles—most often used: spironolactone

Lower insulin levels (only needed for PCOS)—most often used: metformin

Important: You should only consider medications such as these in consultation with a physician knowledgeable about female testosterone problems. While I cover safety issues in this chapter, it is meant to supplement, not replace, care by a physician.

tions on oil glands and hair follicles. The sidebar on page 298 gives an overview; details follow in the remainder of this chapter.

Each of these treatments acts at a different stage of the journey testosterone makes through the body. First it is produced in the ovaries and adrenals. Next it travels through the bloodstream, from whence it enters tissues, including hair follicles and oil glands. There it is converted to DHT (dihydrotestosterone). Testosterone production can be suppressed in the ovaries by OCs or in the adrenals by dexamethasone. OCs also increase SHBG so that less testosterone escapes from the blood into tissues. Several medications block conversion to DHT, and others keep it from binding to receptors inside cells.

Based on the specifics of your problem, the treatment can be crafted that is most likely to be both effective and respectful of your hormonal vulnerabilities. Unfortunately, the majority of doctors are not familiar with many of these options. So to help you to be your own advocate, I provide you with detailed information in this chapter. Reading it will prepare you to work actively with your doctor to obtain the help to which you are entitled.

LOWERING TESTOSTERONE

If testosterone is doing bad things to your skin and hair, one logical step is to lower the level. The easiest and safest way to do this is with an oral contraceptive. The original Ortho Tri-Cyclen acne study, which I directed, showed that free testosterone was reduced by about half, which explains why this OC—as well as some others studied later—helps acne.

Its critical to choose the right pill to get this testosterone lowering benefit because some pills won't raise SHBG—the blood protein that keeps testosterone out of harm's way in the blood. Good choices are Ortho Tri-Cyclen, Ortho Cyclen, Desogen, Mircette, and Yasmin. Estrostep works also but is much more likely to cause inconvenient spotting. No studies have directly compared these different pills, but my experience suggests that they are about equal when used for treatment of androgenic disorders. The choice, then, depends on which is most likely to agree with you. Principles of choosing the right OC for your vulnerabilities are explained in chapter 4.

Many women are annoyed when an OC is suggested as the answer to a hormone problem because it seems like a brush-off. This reaction is not unreasonable because the pill is not a solution for all hormonal difficulties. Many of my patients tell me that they were prescribed an OC, such as Ortho Tri-Cyclen or Yasmin, by their gyn or family physician but felt it did not really help their problem, whether it was acne, hirsutism, or androgenic alopecia.

For mild cases the pill may be enough, but if oil glands and follicles are particularly vulnerable to testosterone, just lowering it by half, as the pill does, is not enough. To get a good result, it is usually necessary to also take a testosterone blocker. This combination works better than either alone.

If you are one of the women who cannot take an OC, the best approach is to use a testosterone blocker by itself. It will work almost as well as it does with the pill. It's essential to use another effective form of contraception, however, as explained in the next section.

When extra testosterone is coming from the adrenals, the pill is not likely to lower it by much. In this case, forms of cortisone can be taken to suppress the adrenal and thus lower testosterone. What works best and has the least likelihood of adverse effects is dexamethasone in a dose of 0.25 mg at bedtime. Doses higher than this risk significant weight gain and conspicuous stretch marks. Osteoporosis and high blood sugar are other possible dangers when these steroids are used in more than minimal doses. Careful use of very low doses can be safe but only with close monitoring.

BLOCKING TESTOSTERONE

I've already pointed out the total lack of interest on the part of the pharmaceutical industry in developing medications specifically for the benefit of women with androgen problems. Fortunately, several originally developed for men are also suitable for women, although there are possible side effects that I'll spell out as I discuss each medication.

Spironolactone This medication is the mainstay of antitestosterone treatment. Its role in blocking testosterone was unanticipated when it was introduced nearly fifty years ago as one of the first medications effective against high blood pressure. Unlike most antihypertensives, spiro acts on a blood pressure regulating hormone called aldosterone. This adrenal hormone causes the body to retain sodium and lose potassium—the opposite of what you want if you have high blood pressure. Spiro counteracts these harmful effects of aldosterone. It lowers pressure only slightly; it's main use is to prevent depletion of potassium by other blood pressure medications used at the same time. The effects on blood pressure and potassium are very slight in women with normal blood pressure who use it as a testosterone blocker.

The reason spiro helps hormonal skin and hair problems has nothing to do with its effect on aldosterone and blood pressure. The link is that testosterone and aldosterone are chemically similar, and so spiro blocks testosterone as well as aldosterone. This is a side effect if the drug is taken for blood pressure, but just what is wanted when it is used for acne, hirsutism, or androgenic alopecia. For men, of course, the antitestosterone effect is unwelcome, and so spiro is no longer used routinely for high blood pressure.

For women experiencing problems from testosterone, spiro has two beneficial actions: It lowers levels of the hormone, and it blocks its effects in hair follicles and oil glands. It is usually quite effective, though it works somewhat gradually. Like any medication, spiro has to be prescribed properly to work. When I see women who have tried it with no results, it is usually that the dose was too low, or they were not told what to expect. The sidebar on page 302 lists what you need to know to get a good result from spiro.

Testosterone blockers and pregnancy *It is essential to prevent pregnancy while you are taking any medication, including spironolactone, that blocks testosterone.* Since a male fetus needs testosterone to develop normally, there is reason to worry that any medication that interferes with this hormone will affect his development. That is theoretical; fetal injury has never been reported despite decades of use. Nonetheless, to be pregnant and worried that you may inadvertently have done something that could have harmed the baby is a torment to be avoided at all costs. The solution is to be scrupulous about contraception if you are taking spiro or any other medication affecting

HOW TO USE SPIRONOLACTONE TO GET RID OF UNWANTED HAIR, CLEAR ACNE, AND MAINTAIN A FULL HEAD OF HAIR ON YOUR SCALP

Be sure your dose is adequate. The old dose for blood pressure of 25 to 50 mg per day won't cut it for testosterone problems. Skin and hair need the full dose of 100 to 200 mg a day. Sometimes 75 mg a day will work, and it's worth a try if you experience side effects with higher doses.

Spiro works gradually. The minimum time needed to see a change depends on the condition, but is at least two to four months. Because skin and hair don't change overnight, the key to good results is hanging on long enough. Other testosterone blockers take just as long to work.

Improvement is usually slight at first but gets progressively better over ensuing months.

testosterone. There's good news, however: Spiro gets out of your system quickly and won't have any lingering effects on pregnancy health. I recommend stopping it about two months before trying to conceive, but this is being ultracautious—as is appropriate when the health of an unborn child is involved. Prior use of spiro will not affect the health of future pregnancies, nor will it impair fertility.

Spironolactone side effects Side effects can occur with spiro but are generally not serious, though they can be inconvenient or uncomfortable. Spiro has some diuretic (water pill) effect; a few women notice having to urinate more frequently, but most do not. Nonetheless, it does increase water loss and can cause very mild dehydration; symptoms are feeling tired, weak, or dizzy. This can be prevented simply by drinking enough water, usually 1 to 2 liters (quarters) per day is sufficient. Spiro causes sodium as well as water loss; many women like this effect because it decreases bloating. However if salt loss is excessive, you may feel wiped out. If you find yourself tired on spiro and also craving salt, your body is probably warning you that you need more sodium. All you need to do is add a little salt to your food so that it tastes right to you. However, if you have high blood pressure or problems with fluid retention, increasing your salt may not be a good idea.

The other common spiro side effect is shortening of the cycle so that periods come closer than every twenty-eight days, sometimes as often as every two weeks. As a general guide, so long as periods are at least twenty-four days apart, it is okay. Bleeding more frequently than this soon gets tiring, and so something needs to be done to regulate your cycle. Going on an OC will keep your cycle regulated if you are on spiro and also provides the necessary reliable contraception. As already discussed, the pill will further increase the effectiveness of your treatment by lowering your free testosterone. For these reasons, even if you are not sexually active, taking the pill with spiro is usually the best course.

If you cannot take the pill, you can still try spironolactone. You will need another form of contraception if you are sexually active, of course. You can start out and see what happens to your cycle. If periods don't come too close together, then nothing need be done. If they do, you can either try progesterone for twelve days each cycle to try to regulate things or try a lower dose of spiro. Sometimes if you simply stay on the spiro for a few more cycles, they will come back to normal.

Spironolactone safety You may be wondering, "If I take spiro for unwanted hair, what will happen to my blood pressure?" The answer is: very little. Spiro is quite weak as a blood pressure drug and so is no longer used for this purpose. It does have another use, however, an important one: extending the life of older people with heart or kidney failure. Recent research indicates that angiotensin, the active substance induced by aldosterone, has toxic effects on the heart and kidney. In heart and kidney failure, high levels of aldosterone, and therefore of angiotensin, compound the damage. Spiro protects these vital organs and has been found to prolong life in these critically ill individuals. Women in their hormonal years of thirty-five to fifty-five will not need spiro for their hearts or kidneys, but can be reassured to know that this medication is safe for these vital organs. I do want to emphasize this point because I am sometimes asked if taking spiro long-term will damage the kidneys. There is no basis for such a fear since any effect of spiro on these organs is protective. Another frequent fear is liver damage. Here too, one can be reassured. I have searched Medline, the database of the National Library of Medicine that summarizes nearly one billion medical articles, and found no convincing report that spiro can harm the liver.

If you cannot take spiro, or it has not helped you after an adequate trial, there are other options. While these have certain drawbacks, for some women, they work out very well.

Cyproterone acetate (CPA, Androcur) This is actually the oldest medication proven to help acne and hirsutism. Though spiro was introduced earlier, its use to treat androgenic conditions is more recent. Unlike spiro, CPA is not a diuretic and has no effect on blood pressure or the kidneys. Rather, it is a potent form of progesterone, which was also found to block testosterone. CPA is at least as effective as spironolactone, and for some women, it works when spiro doesn't. The main drawback is that while it has been widely used everywhere in the world for nearly forty years, it is not approved by the U.S. Food and Drug Administration. CPA is available in Canada and most other countries. Treatment with this medication should be monitored by a physician experienced with its use.

The reasons for nonapproval in the United States seem to be political and economic. CPA has been reported to cause breast cancer in beagle dogs, but this breed has a high risk of breast cancer anyway. Given that it has been in human use for decades without any evidence of causing breast cancer, this issue seems to have been satisfactorily resolved. An oral contraceptive called Diane-35 and a related one called Dianette contain CPA as the progestin. A report that this has a higher risk of blood clots than some other OCs received rather sensational media coverage in Canada a few years ago, but the government did not withdraw it. The risk is very small, but as with other OCs, it is not zero.

The other drawback of CPA, along with it not being available in the United States, is some tendency to cause low moods and weight gain. If you have a problem with depression and/or difficulty keeping your weight down, CPA is not the first choice. Spiro, in contrast, does not cause weight gain and, for many, has a mood-soothing effect. I don't want to overstate this; most women who take CPA feel fine on it and do not have abnormal weight gain.

CPA is usually used with an OC; Diane-35 is often used, but any nonandrogenic pill is equally suitable. The schedule is a bit unusual. You take the OC in the ordinary way, but take the CPA only on days one through eleven of each pill cycle. This is because CPA stays in the body for several days, so it will still be working for about ten days after you stop it. This regimen ensures that CPA will be out of your system in time for you to have a period during the last week of the pill cycle. CPA can also be taken daily and seems to be more effective this way. With daily use, you won't have a period, though you might have some spotting. There is no harm to taking it daily and not getting periods. CPA comes in 50 mg pills. The daily dose is 25 mg (half a tablet) or 50 mg.

Pregnancy safety is a nonissue with CPA because it is a powerful contraceptive. However, it might not prevent pregnancy if you take it erratically, so you must be sure you are not pregnant before starting CPA.

Bicalutamide (Casodex) This is the strongest testosterone blocker available—it blocks the hormone completely. Casodex was developed for treatment of prostate cancer because this tumor's growth is stimulated by testosterone, much as some breast cancer is stimulated by estrogen. An earlier drug, flutamide (Eulexin), is still available, but compared to bicalutamide is less effective and has more side effects.

The major problem with Casodex is a possible risk of serious liver injury. This is definitely a risk with flutamide, and the reason it should never be used, although occasionally I hear of a doctor still prescribing it. The risk is on the order of one per several thousand. Whether Casodex has a similar risk is not entirely clear; if so, the risk is thought to be less than with flutamide. It is said that liver problems do not occur in patients whose livers were clearly normal before treatment. This may be so, but a definitive study is lacking. Though Casodex can be effective when spiro and CPA have not been, the risk of liver problems must be taken seriously. If you decide to take this drug, your liver should be monitored with blood tests, and you should stop instantly if you have any symptoms, especially flu-like ones such as fatigue, aches and pains, or just blahs. These may precede the more specific signs of liver disease such as jaundice (turning yellow), dark urine, and light stools. If you have ever had liver disease such as hepatitis or even un-explained elevation of liver enzymes in your blood, Casodex is not for you. Effective contraception while on Casodex is a must.

Testosterone blockers that are unsafe Casodex and Eulexin are not the only testosterone blockers that can affect the liver. Ketoconazole (Nizoral) is an antifungal that lowers testosterone levels, but the risk of liver injury makes it unsuitable for treatment of androgen problems. It is available as a shampoo. This seems to be useful for oily scalp, but I doubt that it will do much for androgenic alopecia by itself.

5-alpha-reductase inhibitors (Propecia, Proscar, and Avodart) These medications were developed for treatment of prostate enlargement in men. They block the conversion of testosterone to its more active form, DHT (dihydrotestosterone), which makes the prostate bigger and hair follicles smaller.

Propecia and Proscar are the same drug (finasteride) but marketed under different brand names. Proscar ends up being cheaper, so I'll use that name. Avodart (dutasteride) is newer and more powerful; it lowers DHT by more than 90 percent, while Proscar lowers it by about 70 percent. However, it is not clear how much difference this makes in actual use.

Both drugs come with warnings that women should never take them. This is because of concerns about safety during pregnancy. There is a rare genetic disease, 5-alpha-reductase deficiency, in which males are born with improperly formed genitalia because lack of this enzyme results in inadequate DHT levels. Since Proscar/Propecia and Avodart also lower DHT, there is fear that they might affect the development of a male child. Needless to say, such an adverse effect would be extremely unfortunate and justifies the warnings attached to these drugs. However, there are no other specific risks for women who take these medications. Women can use them, despite the warnings, but *only if it is absolutely certain that they will not become pregnant while taking them.* The concern is even greater with Avodart because it stays in the body for up to six months after you stop taking it. Only women who are certain they will not have a pregnancy in the next several years can consider use of Avodart. Proscar/Propecia is out of the body faster and so is the only choice for women who want to keep open the possibility of a pregnancy within a few years.

Neither of these drugs is particularly effective by itself for female testosterone problems. They do not work at all for acne and only modestly for hirsutism. Men use them because they are the best option since most of the other alopecia medications are only suitable for women. Proscar and Avodart are mainly effective in combination with direct testosterone blockers such as spironolactone.

The most economical way to use a 5-alpha-reductase inhibitor is to get Proscar and take half a pill daily. (You'll need to get a pill cutter because the tablets are tiny and dense.) Propecia is exactly the same medicine, but tablets are 1 mg, yet cost as much as Proscar, which is 5 mg. Avodart costs about the same as Proscar, but comes in capsules, so it cannot be divided. Generic Proscar (finasteride) will be available soon and will be much cheaper.

WHAT HAPPENS TO SEX DRIVE WHEN TESTOSTERONE IS BLOCKED?

You may well be wondering: Blocking testosterone may help my skin and hair, but what about my sex drive? I don't want to do without that. Strange as it may seem, women's sex drive is only rarely affected by this form of treatment. Most do not notice any change at all. Some report feeling sexier because the improvements in skin and hair boost their confidence in their own attractiveness.

There are two reasons that testosterone blockers do not affect sex drive. First, they do not completely block all effects of testosterone in the body, and many women need only what amounts to a drop of testosterone to stay interested. For a vulnerable few, more testosterone is needed to keep the fires burning, and so blockers can be a problem. Second, the blockers don't seem to interfere with the action of testosterone in the brain, which is where we *really* experience sex. This may be because the blockers don't get into the brain or because testosterone exerts its brain effects as estradiol, which the blockers do not affect. (For a discussion of the paradox that testosterone acts in the brain by being converted to estrogen, see chapter 2.)

A very few women do notice a change in sexuality with antiandrogen treatment. Sometimes adjustments in the regimen will solve the problem. Bupropion can be tried as described in chapter 14. If that does not work, the only way to bring back sexual feelings may be to stop the antiandrogen. Of course it's a fundamentally unfair situation to have to choose between your appearance and your sex drive. With acne and hirsutism, nonhormonal treatments can be continued, even if they do not produce complete control. With hair loss, when antitestosterone treatment is needed, there is really no effective substitute. So far, all the women I've known who were faced with this choice have opted for hair over sex drive.

THE SECRET METHOD FOR KEEPING BOTH HAIR AND SEX DRIVE

Both appearance and sexuality are important aspects of life, and no one wants to be forced to give up one for the sake of the other. There is a final option, but it is not for everybody. This is to take both testosterone and a testosterone blocker together. With this combination, testosterone is counteracted in the skin and hair, where it is doing bad things for women, but still active in the brain, where it does good things. This is a complex treatment so needs to be prescribed by a physician experienced with these sorts of hormonal conditions. If you are considering this option, I recommend getting the alopecia under control with spiro before adding testosterone. If this induces hair loss despite the spiro, the testosterone usually should be discontinued.

ESTROGEN AND ALOPECIA

Alopecia is somewhat more complex hormonally than acne and hirsutism, which are always due to the action of testosterone. With alopecia, vulnerability to testosterone is usually the major predisposing factor, but, especially if the hair loss begins in the forties, decreasing estrogen levels also play a role. Without the nurturing effects of estrogen, hair grows slower and falls out quicker. Estrogen can be used to enhance hair recovery in a variety of ways. Prior to their early fifties, most women can use a hair-friendly OC as a safe form of estrogen. When taken for hair, the pill works best if taken continuously, that is, without the usual seven days of each cycle. Full instructions on how to do this are included in chapter 4. Use of estrogen, as well as a frank appraisal of the controversy, is discussed in Part VI.

PUTTING IT ALL TOGETHER

I've gone into detail in this chapter because treatment of hormonal skin and hair problems is somewhat elaborate and because information on these treatments is not readily available elsewhere. For most women, the combination of spironolactone and a nonandrogenic oral contraceptive works well. If this does not do it for you, then another, stronger testosterone blocker can be considered. Chances are high that you will get a good result—if you persevere. You'll need to work with your doctor, give the initial treatment a fair try, and be willing to try others if the first does not work out. It would be great if there were one pill that grew back hair for all women, but medicine is not there yet. Yet treatment for these conditions has advanced greatly in the past two decades. Those women who do persist are almost always glad that they did, since relief from acne; blemish-free, smooth skin; and abudant hair are life enhancing.

21.

The Hormone Problem That Affects Nearly Everything: Polycystic Ovary Syndrome (PCOS)

Although you or someone close to you has PCOS you probably never heard of it. The very name of the condition, which, as we shall see, is misleading, makes it sound arcane. Yet PCOS is far from obscure, affecting between 5 and 10 percent of women. Lack of awareness of PCOS among health professionals and lay public alike is particularly unfortunate considering that it affects eight to ten million women in the United States alone. Put another way, nearly one out of every ten women you know has it, quite possibly without being aware that she does. Even the name itself—polycystic ovary syndrome—is confusing, because the cysts are actually the least of the syndrome. A better name than polycystic ovary syndrome might be PHVS—poly-hormonal vulnerability syndrome—because the condition involves multiple sensitivities—to carbohydrate, to insulin, to testosterone, and to cholesterol and blood pressure problems.

If you are struggling to understand and cope with PCOS, it may seem hopelessly complex—it certainly did to me when I first began to study it twenty-five years ago. Part of the difficulty is that PCOS involves multiple hormones and body systems and has several variants. Publications on the subject often describe only a subset of the condition. Doctors too vary in their conception of PCOS; one consequence is that women with PCOS receive inconsistent advice from different doctors—each of whom has been taught a different definition.

I used to resist referring to this group of conditions as PCOS because the term is so misleading. We are stuck with it, however, and so I use it, though reluctantly. The biggest problem with this term is that the cysts themselves are of secondary importance in the condition. A more useful way to get a grasp on this condition, particularly how it affects you, is to break it down into five main features. There is variability within each of these features and in how many of them a particular woman has. Some women have partial PCOS. In this situation it's less important to decide whether to apply the label than to identify the features that are present and treat them. It's easy to get bogged down in semantics with PCOS. I try to avoid this and instead focus on working out the best treatment for the features that an individual woman has.

For a quick orientation, I've listed the five key features in the sidebar. I'll explain each in more detail as we go along.

THE FIVE MANIFESTATIONS OF PCOS

- Acne, unwanted facial and body hair, and loss of scalp hair—all caused by testosterone

- Ovarian problems, including irregular periods. Some, but not all, have difficulty becoming pregnant.

- Weight gain

- Abnormal metabolism, particularly insulin resistance, and, sometimes, increased risk of diabetes and heart attacks

- Depression—partly biochemical and partly due to the stress of coping with the condition.

PCOS is the ultimate hormonal vulnerability syndrome in which most of the important hormones get out of sync. *Fortunately, we now know enough to restore order to the jumbled biochemistry of PCOS.* Treatments are not perfect, but they can make a dramatic difference. To start to understand PCOS, let's look at the story of one of my patients.

PERIODS THAT NEVER CAME

Vanessa, an African American woman in her mid-thirties, came to see me because she had not menstruated at all during the past six years. Although she often felt premenstrual and fervently hoped that her period would come to relieve her bloating and fluid retention, it never did. And she was embarrassed by the gradually increasing amount of hair appearing on her upper lip and chin and even more by the forty pounds she'd gained over the previous three years. One doctor she had consulted told her not to worry about her cycle unless she was trying to get pregnant. Another told her she should lose weight but offered no advice on how to do so other than, "Push away from the table."

A friend told her it was probably stress. Vanessa's life did have some stresses—her work as a graphic designer for a magazine had strict deadlines, and she was having relationship problems. However, as she said, "Other women at the office are under stress too, but they get their periods." While searching the Internet, she'd found the excellent website of the Polycystic Ovary Syndrome Association (PCOSA), and thought she fit the description of the condition posted there. Her physical examination and tests confirmed that Vanessa did in fact have a mild form of this syndrome. An ultrasound done several years earlier did show the characteristic appearance of PCOS, but this had been overlooked.

Vanessa was not surprised when I told her that her irregular periods did matter; she'd known this intuitively, even though her doctor made light of it. She felt it to be obvious that not having periods indicated something amiss hormonally. In Vanessa's situation, her ovary made lots of estrogen but almost no progesterone, a situation which put her at risk for uterine cancer. Fortunately, taking birth control pills or progesterone itself would protect her against this.

When I asked Vanessa if she also wanted treatment for the increased hair growth, she was slightly surprised because she'd always been told that nothing could be done except electrolysis or a series of expensive laser treatments. I explained that several effective medical treatments exist, including a skin-friendly OC in combination with spironolactone and eflornithine (Vaniqa), a prescription cream that I helped develop.

Then we turned to Vanessa's difficulty with her weight. (Seemingly inexorable weight gain is one of the most distressing aspects of PCOS.) Vanessa knew that being overweight increased her risk of diabetes, a condition her father had and one that she was extremely anxious to avoid. Testing showed her to have normal blood sugars, but a somewhat elevated insulin level. Because high insulin causes the body to hold onto weight, I recommended a regimen to normalize her insulin: a low carbohydrate diet and metformin (Glucophage), a medication that can also help with weight loss and lessen the likelihood of later diabetes.

Vanessa had no specific plans for pregnancy but wanted it open as an option for the future. I explained that she would probably need medical help, but that she had a reasonably good chance of success.

Vanessa's story illustrates the difficulty women with PCOS often have in getting help, but also the positive effects treatment has on the condition. I'll give you the details in what follows.

THE PUZZLE OF PCOS

Women with PCOS gradually become aware that something is wrong. As skin breaks out, facial and body hair darken, periods fail to come on time, and weight goes up despite dieting, it's clear that something is amiss. The next step is a trip to the doctor, but too often, no diagnosis is provided or the label of PCOS is applied without much explanation of what it implies. Some consult additional doctors only to be given seemingly contradictory diagnoses. Frequently no treatment is suggested, other than oral contraceptives. (This is not entirely the doctor's fault; few receive any training in recognizing or treating this condition, an unfortunate state of affairs, considering that PCOS is the most common hormonal disorder affecting women prior to menopause.)

Many women with PCOS whom I see in my practice have become demoralized; to know something is wrong, but to be unable to get a straight answer, is profoundly discouraging. There may also be the sense, as so often with women's hormone problems, that the doctor does not really think it matters. This hormonal pessimism is not only sad, but also uncalled for. PCOS is complicated, but not so complicated that it cannot be understood. If you have PCOS, or think you might, you can work out what is happening to your body by using the list of five manifestations that I developed. This scheme will also prepare you to actively participate in selecting the best treatments for yourself and to be effective as your own advocate in inducing the health care system to respond to your needs.

In this chapter, I am assuming that you are reading it because you have PCOS or think you might. (It will be equally useful if someone important to you has it.) This assumption has to be qualified, however. Because PCOS has recently been in the media and on the Internet, I now see more and more women who've been told they have PCOS but actually do not. If you have a medical condition, you need to know that you do—but if you don't have it, it's just as important to know that you don't. All of the symptoms of PCOS, such as increased facial hair and irregular periods, can occur in women who do not have PCOS at all. Even if you do have PCOS, you may not have all the aspects.

WHY PCOS IS CONFUSING:
IT COMES DOWN TO SEMANTICS

I still remember the first patient I saw who had PCOS. Although she was only seventeen, she already had all five manifestations, including insulin resistance. Although I recognized that she had PCOS, I had not previously appreciated how extensive its effects can be. Unfortunately when I saw her, more than twenty years ago, we had no medications to lower insulin levels.

As I tried to understand the condition better, I found little help in gynecology or endocrinology textbooks; they mentioned PCOS but only in rather general terms. My next step was to review the world's medical literature on PCOS. I collected copies of all the medical journal articles I could find and ended up with a pile about a foot high, representing everything of any value that had been published on the condition. That was in the early eighties; now such a pile would be many feet tall; research interest in PCOS has fortunately blossomed. Each evening I would curl up on the couch in my living room, reading through the stack of articles, trying to make sense of them. As I read more, my confusion grew. Just when I was nearly convinced by one paper, another seemed to contradict it. Finally, by analyzing the details of the research methodology, I realized what was behind the apparent contradictions. It was not that the research was wrong, but that different researchers defined PCOS differently—they used the same term to apply to conditions that differed in manifestations or severity. Things became clear when I realized that the key to making sense of PCOS is recognizing that it is not one condition but many.

I've heard many debates between colleagues as to whether an individual woman has PCOS or not. One doctor might insist that a woman with regular periods cannot be diagnosed as having PCOS, another that there must be tiny cysts on ultrasound, another that testosterone must be elevated, and so on. Actually, though each of these is a general feature of PCOS, no single one is present in all affected women. As academic exercises, such debates are fine, but when the confusion is passed on to patients who are living with PCOS, it is demoralizing.

To me the question of whether a woman fits any particular arbitrary criteria for PCOS is really beside the point. What matters is which aspects of the condition she has and which she does not have. From this a treatment plan can be devised.

THE HEALTH CARE ESTABLISHMENT AND PCOS

When I lecture to doctors in training about PCOS, I begin by asking those in the audience to raise their hand if they think that PCOS is a major health issue for women. At most, one or two raise their hands. I then inform them of the statistic that PCOS affects 5 to 10 percent of women and go on to explain what it does to women's bodies and lives. At the end of my lecture when I take another poll, there is unanimity regarding the importance of PCOS in women's health. My point is this: Doctors will take an interest in PCOS, but they have to be taught about it. Most, however, are not taught. Internal medicine training tends to emphasize hospital care. Endocrinology specialty programs emphasizes diabetes, thyroid, and a variety of rare diseases. Generally little specific instruction is given about women's hormone problems. Gynecology is still primarily a surgical field, and residents are mainly concerned with learning to do deliveries and operations. These are all important matters—but so is PCOS.

If you have some or all of the appearance changes of PCOS—acne, unwanted hair, scalp hair loss—they will seem all too visible. Yet many doctors actually do not know how to detect them on physical examinations. My experience has been that obvious as acne, hirsutism, and alopecia are to the woman who has them, doctors need to be taught to recognize these changes. When I lecture to doctors about PCOS, I show examples of the skin and hair effects so that they will become familiar with them. I also place great emphasis on the risk of diabetes because for the medical establishment, diabetes is a real disease in a way that weight gain, acne, or hair loss are not. Once I have their attention, I try to get across the message that, while diabetes may be more serious than acne or hair loss, *all* effects should be treated. Any symptom that distresses the patient should be addressed.

It is still hard to convince doctors to apply a comprehensive approach to PCOS. A recent frustrating experience of my own illustrates this. While serving on the Reproductive Health Committee of the American Association of Clinical Endocrinologists (AACE), I worked with others on the committee to develop an official position paper about PCOS. The chair, however, decided that this should concern metabolic aspects only. During a conference call, I spoke up vehemently for presenting a more complete picture of the condition, including effects on skin and hair and on menstruation. I reminded them that women want help not only with the insulin resistance but also with the depressing effects on skin and hair and that their depression is often made worse when doctors turn a deaf ear. Finally, appealing to doctors' self-interests, I pointed out that a high proportion of PCOS patients are not satisfied with their medical care precisely because quality of life and appearance issues tend to be ignored. I'm glad to say that several others on the committee were responsive to this issue. Unfortunately, the chair was not. As I spoke out on the importance of the appearance changes for women's self-esteem, she interrupted me in a condescending tone and said that as chair she was exercising her authority to rule me out of order. Although I insisted on finishing what I had to say, she refused to allow the appearance effects to be further discussed.

The final statement was an excellent review of dysmetabolism in PCOS, but had very little to say about appearance and self-esteem. I find it sad, considering the excellent work done by many on the committee, that one person's narrow-mindedness resulted in loss of this opportunity to educate the medical profession about the needs of women with PCOS. It is also unfair to those on the committee who expended considerable time and effort to produce a document to guide doctors in treating PCOS, only for it to be weakened by the arrogance of one person.

There was another unfortunate consequence. At a press conference to announce the AACE position paper, the chairperson presented herself as a PCOS expert, despite her complete lack of interest in the quality of life issues created by the condition. The subsequent media coverage was disappointing, not surprising considering that the material presented was all highly technical with little mention of the concerns of PCOS women themselves. Thus an opportunity to raise public awareness of PCOS was lost.

This sorry affair typifies the situation faced by women with PCOS when they seek sympathetic care: There are excellent doctors out there who can really help you, but too many others do not take this condition seriously. There is no infallible system for finding the right doctor. All you can do is ask around. The individual is more important than the specific subspecialty; the best one for you may be an endocrinologist, a gynecologist, or a gynecologist-reproductive endocrinologist. Realistically, you may have to try several doctors before you get to the one who can help you.

WHAT YOU'LL FIND HERE THAT IS DIFFERENT

In the remainder of this chapter, I will provide complete state-of-the-art information on treatment of PCOS. To do so, I will draw upon research reports, including my own, but I will also rely upon what I think is equally important: my clinical experience, which has taught me much that textbooks leave out. (I know this because I edited one of the textbooks.) During the past more than twenty years in which PCOS has been one of my primary interests, I have seen more than 5,000 women with this or related conditions. So far as I have been able to determine, this is the largest experience of any physician in the world. This means that I have seen every possible form that PCOS can take. I've seen it in all ages and ethnic backgrounds and every possible combination of physical findings and lab results. Much of what I've learned has come from listening to my patients as they openly shared the intimate details of their condition. With a condition like PCOS, which affects so many aspects of a woman's life, emotions and experiences are just as important as the underlying biochemistry.

This experience has taught me the necessity of regarding each woman's PCOS as unique to her and developing a treatment plan based on her individual needs. In addition to providing detailed information to help you work out just how your PCOS is affecting you, I will cover every known treatment for *all* of the symptoms of PCOS: acne, unwanted hair, alopecia, irregular periods, weight gain, metabolism, and mood. If you have PCOS, this chapter will enable you to control it so that it doesn't control you. My approach is comprehensive because if you have PCOS, you want everything to get better, not just those parts in a particular doctor's specialty.

I pull no punches because to help your PCOS, you need to know as much about it as possible. I don't minimize the problems, but I don't exaggerate them either. My intent in this chapter is both to explain how you can undo the effects of PCOS and to restore your morale.

WHAT ABOUT THE CYSTS?

As I stated earlier, the very name "poly*cystic* ovary syndrome" is misleading because the cysts are not the key to the condition. The term originated long before the hormonal basis of the syndrome was understood. PCOS was first described in the 1930s by Doctors Irving Stein and Michael Leventhal in Chicago—hence an older name for the condition, Stein-Leventhal Syndrome. These gynecologists noticed during surgery that some women with increased hair and irregular periods had enlarged ovaries with a thickened outer layer, underneath which were many tiny cysts. They named the condition based on the appearance of the ovaries. Since in their day there was no practical means for measuring hormone levels, they were not able to recognize the variability of the condition or the fact that that similar hormone changes after occur with more normal-looking ovaries.

I don't ignore the cyst aspect of PCOS, but I downplay it because what affects a woman with the condition is not how her ovaries look but how they function—and the associated problems with weight and insulin. Confusion frequently arises because some women have all of the five defining aspects of PCOS, which I have outlined; yet on ultrasound, their ovaries do not look polycystic. The opposite situation is even more common: ovaries that look polycystic even though menstruation is normal and no features of PCOS are present. Often this is discovered by chance on an ultrasound done for pain or another reason. Most ultrasonographers are not particularly expert on the subtleties of PCOS and so their readings are not definitive. Overdiagnosis is particularly common with adolescents whose ovaries normally go through a phase with tiny cysts. The conclusion from all of this is that the ultrasound is not the way to diagnose PCOS. The five features are far more useful because they describe how the condition affects each individual.

The term *cyst* results in a lot of confusion because many think a cyst is a kind of tumor. In medicine the term simply means a mass that is filled with fluid. Cysts can form not only in the ovaries but also in skin, breasts, thyroid, even the brain. Cysts in different places have no relation to one another. The ordinary ovarian cysts that many women have at one time or another are different from the tiny ones in PCOS. The common cysts are usually enlargements of the follicles that develop normally each cycle. Generally only one cyst forms at a time. These typically cause pain or bleeding, or they may be picked up by chance on an ultrasound done for another reason. So long as they go away after one or two cycles, as they usually do, no treatment is needed. (Simple cysts must be distinguished from ovarian tumors, which may need surgery.) The multiple tiny cysts in PCOS don't go away by themselves. Sometimes women worry that the cysts of PCOS are tumors;

they are not. Although they often accompany hormone problems, the cysts of PCOS are harmless in themselves.

HOW TO FIGURE OUT YOUR PCOS

You can make use of the list of five manifestations I provided earlier in this chapter to analyze exactly how PCOS affects you. Many women with PCOS have only some of the symptoms. Treatment should be directed at what you do have, not at what you don't.

These different aspects are of course related to one another. PCOS involves multiple hormonal vulnerabilities in a chain reaction. These are reviewed in the next sidebar. I'll show how everything fits together as I go along.

It is possible to have some symptoms that can occur with PCOS, particularly the skin and hair changes, but not actually have PCOS. To help you avoid possible misdiagnosis, the sidebar on page 322 gives some guidelines for ruling out the diagnosis of PCOS.

TESTOSTERONE, SKIN, AND HAIR

If you have acne, increased facial and body hair, or are losing your scalp hair, it's pretty hard not to notice. Since these stare you in the face when you look in the mirror, they are usually what lead a woman to realize something is wrong with her hormones. This is why I put them first on my scheme of PCOS symptoms. As I've already discussed in the preceding chapters, these conditions are caused by the action of testosterone. Either the level is high, or the hair and skin are vulnerable to testosterone, or both—increased sensitivity to testosterone is often present with PCOS.

Women seem to have a harder time getting help for the skin and hair problems of PCOS than for the metabolic ones. This is a consequence of the tendency of doctors to focus on biochemistry over quality of life. The treatments I explained in the preceding chapters work well for women with PCOS; I suggest you refer back to those chapters for advice on treatment of the hair loss, increased facial and body hair, and acne that occur with PCOS. Later in this chapter I'll discuss metformin, possibly the best single medication for PCOS when insulin

MORE DETAILS ON THE FIVE MANIFESTATIONS OF PCOS

- **Testosterone causes oily skin, acne, increased facial and body hair, and even loss of hair from the scalp.** The specific changes depend on how your skin is vulnerable to this hormone.

- **Ovulation can be blocked by high-testosterone levels within the ovary.** When this happens, periods tend to be infrequent, but may be heavy when they do come. Not ovulating regularly makes it harder to get pregnant and increases the risk of uterine cancer. If fertility is one of your concerns, you will find information on getting pregnant with PCOS at the end of this chapter.

- **Weight is a major frustration.** It comes on easily but comes off with great difficulty, if at all. Extra weight tends to develop on the upper body and tummy. Hips and legs may be thin.

- **Dysmetabolism makes the body resistant to its own insulin.** Insulin goes up in compensation, but increases the risk of diabetes and heart attacks. Weight gain makes dysmetabolism worse.

- **Depression affects a high proportion of women with PCOS.** Though it is not listed in gynecology or endocrinology textbooks as a feature of the condition, many women with PCOS struggle with depression. The cause of the mood problem has not been adequately studied. It may be due to the frustration of trying to cope with the first four features on the list, or it may be a biochemical effect of the syndrome itself. I tend to think it is both. Whatever the explanation, what PCOS does to mood and well-being is just as important as what it does to the body.

YOU MAY NOT HAVE PCOS IF . . .

PCOS is not all or nothing—it's common to have partial PCOS.
Persistent acne, unwanted hair or alopecia can be signs of PCOS, but
frequently occurs in women without PCOS. PCOS is a *syndrome*—
you only have it if you have several of the symptoms.

PCOS is less likely if:

- You are of normal weight or no more than twenty-five pounds over-weight.
- Periods are regular.
- Testosterone is low or mid-normal.
- You have alopecia but no acne or hirsutism.
- Acne and/or hirsutism are mild.
- Your ultrasound showed normal ovaries.
- You have no family history of diabetes.

Although none of these criteria are absolute, if several of them fit, it's
reasonable to question the diagnosis of PCOS.

resistance is present. Here I'd just caution that, although studies have been published claiming that metformin helps reduce unwanted hair, this effect is very slight; to get a good result, you will also need a testosterone blocker.

For women whose testosterone is significantly elevated and for whom testosterone blockers are not adequate by themselves, there are other drugs such as leuprolide that can stop the ovary from making testosterone and its other hormones. This is a complicated treatment, more details are given in chapter 6 on PMS. I mention it here as an option if you have severe PCOS, and nothing else has worked. It will get your testosterone down no matter what.

IRREGULAR PERIODS AND ANOVULATION

Irregular menstruation was one of the defining signs of PCOS in the original report by doctors Stein and Leventhal. This is now thought to be caused by high-circulating insulin levels acting on the theca cells within the ovary to stimulate them to make more testosterone, which somehow acts inside the ovary to stop ovulation. The reverse situation seems to occur as well, though less commonly; high testosterone can induce the features of PCOS, including insulin resistance.

Some women with all the other symptoms of PCOS have regular cycles. This may be because the level of testosterone inside their ovaries is lower or because the ovulation mechanism within their ovaries is less vulnerable to testosterone. In general, when periods are normal, PCOS is milder. Weight is a big factor here. Being overweight tends to make PCOS worse and anovulation more likely. Some women with PCOS stop getting periods when they gain weight.

Regular ovulation (release of a mature egg cell) is necessary for pregnancy to occur and to maintain the health of the uterus. When ovulation does not occur this nonevent is referred to as anovulation. Since ovulation is followed either by pregnancy or a period, lack of periods indicate anovulation. In addition to making periods irregular, anovulation is significant for women in two ways. First, pregnancy cannot occur in any cycle that is anovulatory. (Treatments to help women with PCOS attain pregnancy are discussed at the end of this chapter.) Second, progesterone is not made during anovulatory cycles. Without monthly exposure to progesterone, the uterine lining tends to become thicker than normal. As a result when periods do come, they may feel as if you are having several at once: heavy, crampy, and uncomfortable. In between periods, there may oozing from the endometrium, which shows up as spotting or breakthrough bleeding.

Progesterone matures the cells of the endometrium and so protects them against turning cancerous. When the uterus is exposed to estrogen but not progesterone, as happens with anovulation, the risk of endometrial cancer is significantly increased. This form of cancer is almost 100 percent preventable; all that is needed is to provide the missing progesterone on a regular basis. As a general rule, if you have periods at least eight times per year, you are probably not at increased risk. This is something you should discuss with your gynecologist because interpreting menstrual patterns can be tricky.

For women with infrequent periods, there are several ways to replace the missing progesterone. For many, the simplest way is to use an OC; these provide excellent endometrial protection. If you have a contraindication to OC use or simply do not want to take one, oral progesterone is the alternative. Natural progesterone is available as Prometrium and is much less likely to induce PMS than the more commonly used synthetic Provera (MPA, or medroxyprogesterone acetate). The standard regimen of Promertrium for inducing periods is 100 mg in the morning and 200 mg near bedtime for at least twelve consecutive days each month. In some situations, every other month may be sufficient. A shorter course will often start off a period but may not provide full cancer protection—you need the full twelve days for that, even if bleeding starts earlier. MPA does protect the endometrium but can set off mood swings, so that many women end up hating it. A few, though, feel better with MPA than the natural form— hormonal vulnerability is highly individual. The standard dose of MPA is 5 mg once a day for twelve days. (Use of progesterone is also discussed in chapter 25, about hormone therapy for menopause.) The heavily promoted *progesterone creams do not provide adequate protection against endometrial cancer and should not be relied upon for this purpose.*

If you have an unusual bleeding pattern or other reason to be concerned about possible endometrial cancer, an ultrasound (US) and endometrial biopsy (EMB), both easy office procedures, are the next steps. Though the biopsy is uncomfortable, it is quick. Taking an NSAID, such as naproxen, two hours before can cut the pain. In general, hysteroscopy (using an instrument to look inside the uterus) or D&C are necessary only if the US or EMB give reason for concern.

I need to stress that the medical concern with infrequent periods is not the lack of bleeding in itself, but the hormonal disturbance that underlies it. In some situations not having periods need not cause worry, for example, if you take birth control pills continuously so as to avoid the inconvenience of menstruation.

CONTRACEPTION AND PCOS

When PCOS results in chronic anovulation, becoming pregnant is less likely, but not necessarily impossible. This is because most women with PCOS do ovulate at least occasionally and can become pregnant when they do. For this reason, having PCOS or irregular periods from any other cause, does not mean that contraception is unnecessary. The problem is that periods come *after* ovulation—your hormones give you no warning that ovulation is impending. You only find out afterward because you have a period—or are pregnant. Natural family-planning methods, such as checking cervical mucus, are not reliable if you have irregular cycles. The bottom line is this: Even if you have PCOS and infrequent periods, if you are sexually active and do not wish pregnancy, you will still need contraception.

Some PCOS treatments, such as metformin, glitazones, dexamethasone, and possibly spironolactone, may restore ovulation. So if you start one or more of these, you need to be alert to the increased possibility of pregnancy. Conversely, if you want to become pregnant, you need to be sure you are not taking anything, such as a testosterone blocker, that might pose a risk for the fetus. Although there is some reason to think antiandrogens can also restore ovulation, they are not a safe way to do so. (Testosterone blockers are discussed in detail in chapter 20.)

Many women who have not been able to become pregnant are understandably reluctant to use contraception. If you don't want to close the door on the possibility of pregnancy, just be sure to avoid any medications, such as antiandrogens, that might adversely affect the fetus.

WEIGHT PROBLEMS WITH PCOS

Seemingly inexorable weight gain can be the most frustrating part of PCOS. There is a double whammy here: PCOS predisposes to weight gain, and weight gain increases the effects of PCOS.

As the average American gets heavier, our culture gets more and more obsessed with thinness. A study showed that since the early days of *Playboy*, the models displayed in its pages have become progressively thinner. Women even more than men seem to have a preference for the ultraslender female figure. Fashion magazines have long shown models who are practically emaciated. Those in the *Sports Illustrated Swimsuit* issue seem to have scarcely any body fat at all. These media depictions give two misimpressions: first, that the only "normal" shape for a woman is very thin, and second, that only very thin women are attractive. It is my impression that women tend to be much more judgmental about their own shapes than men. While some men do prefer ultraslender figures, others are attracted to curvier ones. It is not necessary to look like a model to be appealing socially or even sexually.

I, of course, cannot do anything to change the unfortunate cultural atmosphere that makes almost all women feel that they are too fat. Even though there are now female celebrities who are voluptuous and a movement to empower "real women" or BBW (big, beautiful women), this has not gone mainstream. Women's reactions to getting weighed at the doctor's office suggest that most still fear they are too heavy.

It is sad that so many women are made to feel that their bodies are not right and even sadder that they are made to feel that their weight is entirely their own fault. This is clearly untrue; women with PCOS have particular difficulty losing weight because they are vulnerable to the fat-storing effect of insulin. PCOS really does make it easy to gain and hard to lose. Needless to say, no one chooses to become insulin resistant. So don't be taken in by the negative judgment of society that implies that being overweight is a kind of moral failing on your part.

Judgmental attitudes toward the obese are regrettably prevalent even in the health care establishment, as the following story exemplifies. A few months ago I was the program chairman for the PCOS Association's annual meeting. (This organization, founded by Christine DeZarn, does a wonderful job supporting and educating women with PCOS.) Unfortunately, one of the speakers—who'd been recommended but whom I'd never actually heard speak—took it upon herself to reproach her audience, telling them almost in so many words that they were too fat, eat too much, and are too lazy to exercise. Needless to say, her thoughtless remarks were devastating to many in the audience who'd come for help, only to be told it was all their fault.

I had to get up at the beginning of the next general session to apologize for the insensitivity of the speaker and reassure the audience that her views are not those of most PCOS experts.

I need to state clearly that there are some excellent nutritionists who do understand the problems of women living with PCOS. One is Martha McKittrick, R.D., who is nationally known in this area. Martha and I have worked together extensively, and she has greatly helped many of my patients. There are definitely good ones out there, but you may need to do some screening to find them. If you have been referred to a dietician, I suggest a phone call first to find out if she has had experience working with clients with PCOS and her attitude toward low carb. If she is unfamiliar with PCOS or disparaging toward carbohydrate reduction, I suggest continuing to look. Having run a program using an ultra-low-carbohydrate diet long before it became fashionable, I have no doubt that this approach can work even when others have failed. Low carb is not the answer for all nutritional problems, however, so a good dietitian will not recommend this approach for everybody.

Another caution: Nutrition is a popular subject these days, and there are some who bill themselves as experts who have no formal training at all. Be sure the person you consult is a registered dietitian (R.D.).

IS THERE ANYTHING THAT CAN HELP ME LOSE WEIGHT?

Though it's easy to feel helpless about your weight, there *are* things that can help. Since a fundamental cause of weight gain in PCOS is elevated insulin levels, it is important to implement strategies to get your insulin down. Metformin (met or Glucophage) is one medication that can help accomplish this. Met is not a miracle diet pill, but it does help move weight in the right direction. In several studies, people taking metformin for diabetes lost several pounds over the course of the year.

The greatest advance in nutritional treatment of PCOS is the low-carbohydrate diet. A small reduction in carb however will not make much difference; *to be effective for someone who is insulin resistant, a low-carb diet has to be not merely less carb but almost no carb.* Unfortunately, the term "low carb" has been coopted by the diet food industry as a marketing gimmick. To actually follow a reduced-carbohydrate diet, the consumer must tread warily because most claims on packaged foods are to some degree deceptive. Consider low-carb pasta, for example—this is an obvious contradiction in terms. Pastas so labeled are a few percent less in carb, but still more than 90 percent. To bill this as lower carb is misleading to say the least. The same is true of many other packaged foods. The only way to be sure is to read the fine print "Nutrition Facts," often placed inconspicuously on the side or back of the package.

Many women tell me that they tried a low-carb diet but that it did not work. Almost always they were not on a real low-carb diet but an ordinary one misleadingly labeled to take advantage of the low-carb fad. Several forms of authentic low-carb diets are explained in books such as *The Zone* and *The South Beach Diet*. The father of all of these is of course Atkins, now an industry by itself. Any one of these can give good results, if you can follow it. Given the complexity of nutrition and the multifarious ingredients hidden in many processed foods, it is difficult to know what you are actually eating. For this reason, I strongly recommend consulting a registered dietician (R.D.) for guidance in developing a low-carb regimen that will fit your lifestyle.

Let's consider the rationale for low carb and how this can be implemented in a realistic way. These diets aim to minimize insulin levels. We think of insulin as what keeps blood sugar down in people with diabetes, and it is. But did you ever think where the sugar goes when insulin lowers it? It goes right into the cells of the body. Insulin is basically a storage—read "weight gain"—hormone. It signals fat cells to store energy, which is advantageous during a famine, but not if you are trying to burn off extra pounds. To lose weight, you need to keep your insulin levels down. Proof of this is that people with insulin-requiring diabetes lose weight if they are not getting enough insulin. What I am suggesting is not dropping insulin to unmeasurable levels, as in juvenile diabetes, but reducing it from high levels to more normal ones. If you reduce calories but continue to take in lots of carbs, your insulin will fight you every inch of the way.

SLENDER PCOS

Some women with the skin and hair changes and irregular periods of PCOS do not have weight problems. This condition is referred to loosely as "slender PCOS." Since weight tends to make PCOS more manifest, those who are not overweight tend to have much milder symptoms. Only some slender women with PCOS have difficulty becoming pregnant and need medical help to ovulate.

Weight gain with PCOS tends to make the symptoms more pronounced, so if you are slender with the condition, controlling weight is still important. This is also an effective way to protect yourself against diabetes since it rarely develops in normal weight adults.

THE METABOLIC ROOT OF PCOS: INSULIN RESISTANCE

In characterizing PCOS, I've so far emphasized changes you can see. However, the metabolic effects you cannot see are just as important. I'll start out with insulin since, as I've already briefly noted, it is at the root of the first three features. I've mentioned both insulin resistance and high insulin levels and now need to explain the relationship between them.

Insulin was discovered by Frederick Banting and Charles Best as the missing factor in juvenile diabetes mellitus (DM). In juvenile, more properly termed type 1, diabetes the pancreas loses its ability to make insulin. As a result, blood sugar becomes extremely high. Yet, because the glucose cannot get into the cells where it is needed, the body wastes away. Insulin is lifesaving for children and adults with this type of diabetes, so there is a tendency to think of it as a good hormone. However, like other hormones, it can have both beneficial and harmful effects. Insulin promotes tissue growth by stimulating cells to take up glucose and amino acids (the basic constituents of proteins) from the blood. Unfortunately, this is not always beneficial, as we shall see.

To understand why high insulin is too much of a good thing, we need to look at the adult-onset form of diabetes. For a long time it was assumed that adult diabetes, like the childhood form, was due to lack of insulin. A great surprise occurred when it became possible to measure insulin because it was soon discovered that many adults with DM had levels of insulin that were actually *higher* than normal. It became clear that early in adult-type DM insulin levels are high; later on levels drop and blood sugar starts to climb. With the childhood form, on the other hand, insulin is low from the beginning. Both forms of diabetes involve high blood sugar, but what is happening with insulin is quite different. (Things can get a little more complicated because the juvenile-onset form due to insulin deficiency can occur in adults and the adult, insulin-resistant form in children, though neither situation is common. For this reason, the two forms have been renamed type 1, which is due to lack of insulin, and type 2, which is due to insulin resistance.)

DM2 usually develops in a characteristic pattern. First the body's ability to respond to insulin becomes impaired, and insulin levels go up to compensate. This insulin resistance can be caused by several factors, such as high levels of the hormone cortisol, but by far the most common reason is obesity. As a person's weight goes up, so does his or her insulin. Why being overweight interferes with the action of insulin is not entirely understood, though it is being aggressively researched.

THE NATURAL HISTORY OF INSULIN RESISTANCE

The pancreas compensates for insulin resistance (IR) by releasing extra insulin. This keeps blood glucose in check only temporarily because the pancreas eventually fatigues and cannot keep up with the body's need for more and more insulin. For a while, blood sugar is too high only after food intake and drops back to normal after two or three hours. Then, as the pancreas wears itself out, insulin drops below normal, and blood sugar stays elevated all the time. Usually it is at this point that the diagnosis of diabetes is made, but the metabolic abnormalities that led to it were already in place for a decade or more.

Diabetes is dreaded mainly because of its complications, which include vision loss, kidney failure, and cardiovascular disease. For a long time, the connection of these with the high blood-sugar level was doubted. (Sometimes scientists resist common sense.) Now however, we know beyond any doubt whatsoever that the main cause of the diabetes complications is the high glucose. Many large studies have shown that keeping glucose normal with aggressive treatment can delay, and may actually prevent, the complications. Effectiveness of treatment depends on how early it is started, which is why early detection of diabetes can be lifesaving. Many are not aware that some diabetes is preventable because the effective medications have been available only for a few years. The prognosis of diabetes is not nearly as gloomy as it was few years ago, especially if it is detected early.

DYSMETABOLIC SYNDROME

The insulin resistance that can culminate in DM2 is actually part of a cluster of metabolic abnormalities variously termed *syndrome X, dysmetabolic syndrome,* or simply, *metabolic syndrome.* Associated abnormalities include unfavorable cholesterol and high blood pressure. Unfairly, these major risk factors for heart attacks seem to go together in the same person. Obesity predisposes to this syndrome, which is present in some degree in as many as half of middle-aged Americans.

Though I recognized quite early that dysmetabolic syndrome in women manifests as PCOS, this obvious fact was ignored until quite recently because researchers concentrated on metabolism and did not inquire about the coexistent menstrual abnormalities and skin and hair changes. I suspect this results from an unconscious assumption that women's hormones are only for reproduction, so can be ignored when other aspects of bodily function are researched. It's now starting to be recognized that a woman's metabolism cannot be understood apart from her hormones, but research is still in a catch-up phase.

I mentioned earlier that insulin, while essential for life, can be harmful when levels are elevated. There is some evidence that excess insulin is involved in the development of coronary heart disease, the most prevalent cause of death in women. The theory is that the growth-promoting effects of insulin cause scars within arteries to grow thicker, eventually blocking vessels in the heart and causing myocardial infarction. Hence the extra amounts released by the pancreas to overcome insulin resistance and keep glucose normal comes at a price.

If you have PCOS and what you've been reading is starting to make you feel depressed, don't be; there are ways to remedy this metabolic calamity. First, you need to know if you have the dysmetabolic syndrome; many women with PCOS do, but some do not. To find out, you'll need to have the tests listed in the sidebar. If they show that you do have this syndrome, I strongly recommend that you get onto an active treatment program ASAP. Though this may mean taking several medications, the research results are unambiguous: If insulin, glucose, and LDL cholesterol are brought down to where they should be, people live years longer.

ACANTHOSIS NIGRICANS (ACN)

A clue to the presence of insulin resistance is a skin change called acanthosis nigricans, or ACN. This consists of darkening of the skin, thickening of skin fold markings, and, sometimes, skin tags. It affects intertriginous areas—places where skin rubs against skin. Most commonly affected are the back of the neck and underarms, but it can also appear around the groin and under the breasts. It is usually missed when a doctor does a physical because inspecting these areas is not part of the standard exam. Sometimes ACN is noticed by a family member who does not realize its significance. I've known mothers to suspect that their daughter's ACN was due to her not washing her neck, but the change is within the skin. If you notice skin darkening on your underarms or the other areas I've listed, you should be tested for dysmetabolism as itemized in the sidebar. Even if your insulin turns out to be normal, resistance tends to develop gradually, so you should be retested every year or two.

In the medical literature, cancer is given as one of the causes of ACN, but I am not convinced that this is correct because I have never seen a patient whose ACN turned out to be associated with cancer. I see no need to be concerned about this possibility unless ACN appears suddenly or there is another reason to suspect cancer. If in doubt, a checkup is warranted.

PCOS WITH NORMAL INSULIN LEVELS

I have emphasized high insulin as the metabolic root of PCOS, and in most cases it is. However, this is not the whole story because some women with PCOS have normal insulin levels, particularly those who are not overweight. Though some studies have shown slightly elevated

HOW TO CHECK FOR DYSMETABOLISM

Here are the main tests you need to detect abnormalities of the dysmetabolic syndrome.

Glucose tolerance test (GTT) With this test, you drink a slug of concentrated glucose to find out if your body handles it properly. Blood sugars are obtained at zero, one, two, and three hours. (Sometimes a five-hour test is ordered, but this is unnecessary and uncomfortable.) Fasting glucose over 100 mg/dL, or a two-hour value over 135 to 140, indicates glucose intolerance, which means that your sugars go higher than normal. Glucose intolerance is a sign of incipient diabetes and should be treated.

Fasting insulin This is a simple way to find out if you have insulin resistance. A level over 8 to 10 uU/mL indicates your insulin is too high and that you have insulin resistance. Upper normal limits printed on lab slips are usually up to 22 or 27, but these are far too high for health.

Hemoglobin A1c This sums up what your glucose levels have been in the past two to three months. It is useful to monitor diabetes but not sensitive enough to detect mild glucose elevations.

Lipid profile Women need the entire profile because hormones decide how much of your cholesterol is in the good (HDL) or bad (LDL) form. Your HDL should be 55 mg/dL or higher and LDL less than 100 mg/dL Triglycerides should be less than 150 mg/dL.

C-reactive protein Elevated levels suggest inflammation in the blood vessels. CRP usually improves with the same medications used to lower cholesterol.

Blood pressure This should be 135/85 or less, but if you have diabetes or insulin resistance, anything above 130/80 is too high.

insulin in slender women with PCOS, the elevation is too subtle to show up in standard clinical lab measurements and may not be significant. So long as normal weight is maintained, women with slender PCOS generally do not develop diabetes.

Even in women with PCOS who are overweight, insulin levels are occasionally normal. This is common in teenagers and women in their early twenties because insulin resistance seems to develop gradually with age. Sometimes older women with PCOS still have normal insulin, probably because they have a different form of the condition. It's hard to say much more about this variant because research has focused on those with IR.

Some day we will probably have a clear classification of PCOS into several specific types. Although we do not have such a scheme now, treatment can still be tailored to your individual situation. This is done by analyzing the extent to which you have each of the five manifestations and designing treatment accordingly. The take-home message is this: *All PCOS can be effectively treated, but there is no single treatment for all women with PCOS.*

TREATMENT OF DYSMETABOLISM IN PCOS

We now have excellent medical means of correcting dysmetabolism. Before I describe them, however, it is important to note that the most effective way to normalize all three abnormalities—high insulin, high glucose, and high LDL-cholesterol—is to lose weight. For someone who is significantly overweight, losing even twenty to thirty pounds will do wonders for their metabolism. Don't be discouraged about your weight loss efforts by the misconception that weight loss does not count unless you can get down to your supposed ideal weight. What is more important is the trend. So long as you are losing, however slowly, your metabolism will benefit.

No one's going to be shocked when I acknowledge that weight loss is difficult. For this reason, I suggest that if your insulin level, glucose, or lipids are unfavorable, you do not delay starting medication while working to get your weight down. Metformin can even help women with insulin resistance lose weight—a good reason to start this medication early. Cholesterol-lowering medications will not affect weight one way or the other, but does reduce the health consequences of being overweight. When you have lost enough weight to potentially help your metabolism, that is, twenty pounds or more, you can have another set of tests to see if you still need the medications. If, despite your efforts, the weight just will not come off, the medications will have given you a head start in lowering your insulin and cholesterol.

For those unable to lose weight, dysmetabolism tends to get worse over time. The very earliest stage of diabetes may be reversible with medication, but later ones are not. I am not spreading hormonal pessimism here; my message is that when unfavorable metabolism is recognized early, based on the presence of PCOS symptoms, there is the opportunity to start treatment when it will still be effective. Hence I do not suggest postponing medication more than three to six months if you want to try weight loss first.

Cholesterol is less sensitive to weight reduction or dietary change than insulin. Many with unfavorable cholesterol are not overweight at all. This is because most of the cholesterol circulating in our blood is not from food but is made in our livers. If LDL is quite elevated, medication will be necessary to bring it down.

NORMALIZING INSULIN LEVELS

Originally developed for diabetes, insulin sensitizers are even more effective when insulin is high, but diabetes has not yet set in. There are currently three insulin sensitizers available. Most often used to treat PCOS is metformin (met, Glucophage). This has been available in the United States for about ten years but was widely used in Europe for much longer. Metformin works by stopping the liver from massively dumping glucose into the bloodstream; as a result, there is less strain on the pancreas, and insulin levels drop toward normal.

Metformin is the first choice in treating insulin resistance because it can help with weight loss. Many also report that lowering insulin with metformin improves their mood and energy. Met is not quite a miracle drug because, while most feel good on it, some definitely do not. While chairing the PCOS Association conference last year I asked for a show of hands as to who thought met was a wonderful gift to women with PCOS and who thought it a disaster. The positives won, but there were plenty of dissenters. This is yet another illustration of the importance of considering individual vulnerabilities in designing treatment. The problem with metformin is that it causes upset stomach and/or diarrhea in some who try it. Often these go away in a couple of weeks, but for a few they persist. If you feel crampy and miserable on met, you'll be better off with a different medication.

The chance of GI upset with met can be lessened by going up to the full dose in gradual steps. Here's the best way to get started: Use the 500 mg size tablet and increase by one tablet every two to four weeks. Begin with one tablet after breakfast. The next step is to add a second tablet after supper. Then add a second tablet after breakfast, and, finally a second after supper. The final dose is 2000 mg—1000 mg after breakfast and 1000 mg after supper. There is also an extended-release form that is supposed to be easier on the stomach. I'm not convinced it makes much difference, but it's worth a try if the regular met is creating GI problems for you.

A dangerous side effect called lactic acidosis has been alleged to occur with met; in healthy people with normal kidneys, this happens, if at all, only during severe illness or as an interaction with X-ray dye or general anesthesia. If you are having either, be sure to notify the radiologist or anesthesiologist (they should ask you, but it's safest to be proactive) and stop the met five days before the procedure. Women with impaired kidney function should not take metformin, but kidney problems are extremely rare in combination with PCOS.

Two other insulin sensitizers are currently available: Actos (pioglitazone) and Avandia (rosiglitazone). Both belong to a family referred to as glitazones. The first drug in this class, Rezulin, worked well as an insulin sensitizer but was withdrawn because of rare but sometimes fatal liver reactions. A study on women with PCOS showed that Rezulin lowered insulin and often restored ovulation. There were several pregnancies among women who had not been able to become pregnant previously. (Although women in the study were asked to use contraception, some obviously did not.) Fortunately, none of the women in the study had a severe liver reaction; it was ended when the extent of the safety problems was recognized.

The two newer drugs of the glitazone family seem to be as effective as Rezulin for PCOS, but fortunately have little or no liver risk. They are definitely worth trying for PCOS, either as an alternative to met if side effects are too uncomfortable or if met does not bring insulin down completely. (The target for fasting insulin is 10 uU/mL or less.) Glitazones do have one significant drawback compared to metformin—they do not help with weight loss and may sometimes cause a slight gain. Many women, however, get good results without weight gain with either glitazone. Fluid retention can occur also, but I have not had complaints about this from women who have taken it for PCOS. One reason may be that it is often taken in combination with spironolactone, which helps prevent fluid buildup.

To keep track of whether the insulin sensitizer is helping you, it is useful to have fasting insulin and glucose done before you start and again after you have been on the medication for two or three months. While the ideal is to bring insulin to 10 uU/mL or less and glucose to below 100 mg/dL, any decrease is beneficial. If your insulin remains well above 10, it may be a good idea to add pioglitazone or rosiglitazone. Weight loss is always a good way to further reduce insulin levels.

LONG-TERM HEALTH MAINTENANCE FOR WOMEN WITH PCOS

If you look on the Internet or in recent publications about PCOS, you'll find a lot of scary talk about diabetes and heart disease. It's true that if you have PCOS and are overweight, you may have a higher risk of these conditions, but what is often unsaid is this: *Knowing you are at risk empowers you to do things that can greatly lessen the chance of developing diabetes or heart disease.* Because PCOS produces visible clues to the presence of risk factors, it gives the opportunity for very early intervention. For me, spending my professional life helping women with hormone problems, being able to actually prevent diabetes and heart attacks is a wonderful advance.

I have already stressed the importance of bringing down insulin and glucose levels if they are elevated. It's also important to bring down lipids. The meaning of lab results is outlined in the sidebar, but here I'll repeat that if your bad cholesterol (LDL) is over 100 mg/dL, it should be brought down with medication. One lipid lowering drug has been proven to be more effective than the others in reducing the risk of a fatal heart attack; this is atorvastatin (Lipitor). Rumors of liver problems circulate on the Internet, but these are extremely rare. The bottom line is that Lipitor increases life expectancy. Another medication, Crestor (rosuvastatin), may be more powerful than Lipitor, but because there is currently serious concern about its safety, I do not recommend it. Older lipid-lowering drugs are cheaper but probably less effective in preventing heart attacks. Lipid levels should be rechecked when you have been on atorvastatin for about three months.

A SYSTEM FOR DECREASING HEART DISEASE RISK WITH PCOS

- Get the basic tests listed in the previous sidebar on dysmetabolism

- Start an insulin sensitizer if:

  ○ Your fasting insulin is more than 10 uU/mL

      and/or

  ○ Your glucose is above 100 mg/dL fasting or 135 at two hours in the GTT

      and/or

  ○ You are thirty pounds or more overweight and have the other features of PCOS

- If your LDL is over 100 mg/dL, begin a lipid-lowering medication.

- Follow up with the lab to be sure treatment has brought your tests into the healthy range.

- Try to do aerobic exercise (jogging, cycling, swimming, or at least walking) for at least thirty minutes four times a week.

- Lose weight if possible, and remember *any* loss will improve your health.

- Take up a spiritual practice as described in chapter 28.

WHAT HAPPENS TO PCOS AFTER MENOPAUSE

A few years ago I was asked to lecture on PCOS and menopause for the PCOS Association annual meeting. I did not remember seeing anything written on this subject, and when I searched the National Library of Medicine database, I could find no publications of any substance. Even today, only a few studies have appeared. This oversight has occurred because PCOS tends to be categorized as a disorder of menstruation and fertility. Since by definition, menstrual abnormalities and infertility cannot happen after menopause, the later natural history of PCOS was ignored. In actuality, PCOS does not go away after menopause. The hair and skin problems continue; though acne usually gets milder, hirsutism and alopecia may get worse. With increasing age, risk of diabetes and cardiovascular disease rise.

If you have PCOS, it is just as important to receive treatment after menopause as before. This is especially true for the dysmetabolism, which should be addressed at as early an age as possible and will need lifelong monitoring. If you are in or approaching menopause, the preceding section on maintaining health will be particularly important.

It used to be assumed that testosterone rises after menopause. This is an example of the regrettable fallacy that a woman is somehow less female after the change. In actuality testosterone almost always goes down with age, not up; levels are usually quite low during perimenopause and menopause. The exception is an uncommon condition called thecal cell hyperplasia or hyperthecosis in which testosterone levels can become quite elevated. This condition seems to be the late stage of severe PCOS. After menopause, a testosterone level above about 75 ng/dL needs further evaluation. Causes include the already mentioned hyperthecosis and tumor of the ovary or adrenal. I have seen some women with hyperthecosis develop extremely high testosterone levels. If the source is clearly the ovaries, having them removed may be the best course. Removing the uterus at the same time can be considered if you are having any uterine problems such as bleeding. Not having a uterus also makes estrogen therapy easier and safer, but this is not by itself a reason for hysterectomy. Some of the issues regarding hysterectomy are discussed further in chapter 3.

I've discussed endometrial cancer earlier in this chapter. It often appears at or shortly after menopause. The only sign is unexpected bleeding; if this occurs an ultrasound and, usually, endometrial biopsy are necessary. Postmenopausal bleeding is often benign, but it must be checked out to be sure. (When bleeding occurs with hormone therapy, these tests are not always necessary, but you should check with your gynecologist.)

DEPRESSION AND PCOS

You may recall that I listed depression as a fifth feature of PCOS. I've deferred it until the end of the chapter, not because it is less important, but because I felt it would be most useful to treat those features unique to PCOS first.

Research on mood with PCOS is just beginning. My experience suggests that the causes are both psychological and biochemical. That coping with the multiple hormonal vulnerabilities of PCOS can be a significant strain for anybody is pretty obvious. Compounding the stress is the frustration so many women experience trying to get clear explanations and comprehensive treatment. To the extent that you feel depressed just to have PCOS, the essential first step is to learn about the condition and make sure all aspects are getting state-of-the-art treatment. Not only is it a relief to take action, but also many women notice that when their insulin resistance is treated, they feel better. This is hardly surprising because insulin is fundamental to the energy utilization system of the body; your energy will not be optimal if your body's response to insulin is sluggish. As skin and hair problems improve with treatment, some of the burden of the condition lessens and mood improves.

Weight also affects mood. Loss, even if only a few pounds, tends to improve well-being. Low-carb diets are mood-elevating—so long as the carb is really low—but this is one of those instances when you may feel worse before you get better. When carb intake is sharply reduced, major shifts in your metabolism have to occur, so you may feel wiped out for a few days, until your body shifts from its excess reliance on carbs to burning off extra fat. Once the changeover occurs, many feel much better on low-carb diets than they did before. Exercise helps restore sensitivity to insulin and is also a powerful mood elevator.

If you are confident that your PCOS is being competently cared for, but are still down in the dumps, you may want to consider treatment for depression. This usually means antidepressant medication but may mean counseling as well. The different ways to alleviate hormone-related mood problems are covered in chapter 6.

Some women are reluctant to take medicine for their depressed mood because they feel they should fight it mentally. I view this differently because I've seen how much antidepressants can help women with PCOS. It's not that such medications make it seem okay to have PCOS. Rather, they free up the energy that's otherwise drained away fighting low mood so that you can apply it to more productive purposes: school, work, homemaking, parenting, or simply enjoying life. So if your mood is adversely affecting your life, it's worth considering an antidepressant.

Counseling or talk therapy can be helpful. I absolutely am not implying that PCOS is caused by anything psychological, but simply that an outside perspective can make it seem less overwhelming. However, not all therapists understand how hormonal vulnerability, especially in the form of a complex condition like PCOS, affects the mind. It's critical to find someone who will not dismiss your physical problems as "all in your head" but will try to understand the organic factors. If you do not feel comfortable with a therapist or feel that she or he does not adequately recognize the medical issues you are facing, you may want to try someone else.

GETTING PREGNANT WITH PCOS

If your future plans don't include pregnancy, then what you need to know about PCOS has been covered in the main part of this chapter. If, however, you do want a child soon or simply want to know more about what is available to help with fertility, then read on.

While PCOS is one of the commonest reasons women need help becoming pregnant, the outlook is generally good—most women with PCOS will be able to have children. Sadly, many women with PCOS have told me that when they first consulted a doctor about their menstrual problems, they were told something like, "Don't worry that your periods are irregular; that's just you; and, oh, by the way, you'll never be able to get pregnant." A more insensitive comment can hardly be imagined. Fortunately, this prognosis is usually wrong. A nurse practitioner I worked with, who had five children, had been told in her teens that she would never be able to get pregnant. The moral of her story is not to take such discouraging advice at face value. For those women with PCOS who do need medical help, treatment has improved dramatically in recent years.

An important question is just how irregular your periods are. If they come most months or perhaps five to eight weeks apart, there is a good chance you'll be able to conceive without medical help, though it may take a little longer than usual. If you menstruate only a few times a year, the likelihood of spontaneous pregnancy is less, though it is not absolutely impossible. Some general guidelines for when to seek medical help are given in the sidebar. When in doubt, it is better to seek evaluation sooner than later. So as not to waste time, I recommend consulting a gynecologist specializing in infertility. These specialists are called reproductive endocrinologists and have undergone further training after completing their gynecology residency. The general level of expertise among fertility specialists is high.

Weight is an important factor affecting how readily a woman with PCOS can become pregnant. Both metformin and other methods of ovulation induction are more likely to be successful in women who are close to normal weight. This is just another example of the unfairness of PCOS: Weight gain is hard to control, yet it makes everything worse, including possibility of pregnancy. If you are trying to become pregnant with PCOS, weight loss is worth whatever struggle it takes, including ultra-low-carbohydrate diets.

THE SIMPLE WAY TO GET PREGNANT WITH PCOS

Fertility treatment was revolutionized with the development of pituitary hormone injections that stimulate the ovaries to release egg cells. This made in vitro fertilization (IVF) and related assisted reproductive technologies (ART) possible. These are wonderful inventions and have

GETTING PREGNANT WITH PCOS

- If you have definite PCOS, it is best to start on metformin before trying to become pregnant.

- If you are on a testosterone blocker such as spironolactone—and of course if you are on birth control pills—you'll need to stop these about two months before trying to conceive.

- The old recommendation to try for a year before seeking medical help for fertility is obsolete. If your are over thirty, have infrequent periods, or need to time pregnancy with career constraints, it's reasonable to utilize simple fertility treatments, such as metformin and clomiphene within a few months of starting to try.

- If your periods come very infrequently or if they are very light or very heavy, it's best to have a fertility evaluation as soon as you want to conceive.

- If you have PCOS and definitely want children, it is best to start trying as soon as you are ready since the odds do go down with age.

helped many couples have children who otherwise could not. Recent research has focused on the so-called male factor. Until recently, when the problem was the man's sperm, little could be done; now it is possible to extract sperm from the testis and insert them into the egg (ICSI, or intracytoplasmic sperm injection) so that even men with practically no sperm can fertilize a pregnancy.

The problem with these methods is that they are extremely expensive and also quite stressful, both physically and psychologically. I've seen some whose hormonal vulnerability seems to have been set off after they received the hormone injections required for IVF. These powerfully stimulate the ovary to a degree that seldom, if ever, occurs naturally. Most women do not have any permanent ill effects from this rigorous treatment, but if simpler, less expensive means work, so much the better.

Handling ova and sperm in the laboratory requires an extreme degree of skill, so not all centers achieve equally good results. Centers release statistics, but these can be misleading. Some, for example, turn away patients with a low chance of conceiving so as to make their figures look better. My remarks are not meant to disparage the field of ART. Many who work in this area are brilliant; it is one of the great advances of contemporary medicine. From the consumer point of view, however, it can be difficult physically, psychologically, and financially. Fortunately, a second revolution is beginning.

Largely unheralded, this second revolution consists of treatments, such as metformin, that do not stimulate the ovary directly but correct the hormonal dysfunctions responsible for anovulation. When physical problems such as scarred tubes are present, IVF remains the best approach and will probably continue to be. For most women with PCOS, however, the problem is that insulin acts within the ovary to increase testosterone and thereby blocks ovulation. By lowering insulin, metformin can restore ovulation in women with PCOS. If metformin does not work by itself, pioglitazone or rosiglitazone can be added. Research is less complete on using the latter two for restoring ovulation, but it is clear that they often work. Metformin also reduces miscarriage risk, which is slightly higher for women with PCOS.

Not all fertility specialists offer these medical approaches for restoring ovulation. However, if your regular doctor or gynecologist will prescribe them, you can try them for six to twelve months before going on to consider ART. If your periods do not regularize on the medication, this would be a reason to consider other methods sooner. In any case I suggest no more than a six-month trial of insulin sensitizers before starting to consider ART in addition to the metformin, especially if you are more than thirty-five years old.

I've been able to give only a very brief overview of ways medicine can help women with PCOS get pregnant. Technology in this area is advancing very rapidly, so if you have not become pregnant despite trying, getting specialized medical advice early is the best course.

SOME FINAL THOUGHTS ON PCOS

If your condition seems impossibly complicated, don't let yourself become discouraged; it's hard for everyone at first, doctors included.

With some study, however, PCOS becomes understandable. My list of five manifestations seems simple (at least I hope it does) but is really a distillation of two decades of studying and treating the condition. It is what I use to individualize treatment of each patient I see—you can use it too as a tool for hormonal self-understanding. You will, of course, need a physician who is both knowledgeable and willing to listen. Not all physicians have these traits, but some do, so don't give up if the first you see is unhelpful. As with other forms of hormonal vulnerability, learning to be your own advocate is the key.

PART VI

Menopause: Straight Talk on the Tough Questions

22.

The Great HT Scare:
What They Didn't Tell You
About All Those Studies

When the Women's Health Initiative reported in July 2002 that hormone replacement therapy increases the risks of breast cancer, heart disease, and stroke, it made headlines all over the world. The cover of one national news magazine even proclaimed "the end of the era of estrogen." Tens of millions of women who were taking estrogen stopped it immediately. Over the next few months, something strange happened, something that never made headlines: Many women who had stopped their estrogen started taking it again. Not everyone, of course, but a large number. It's not that these women were oblivious to the risks that had been reported—this would hardly be possible considering all the front-page coverage. Rather, despite their fears, they had decided that they could not do without estrogen. Upon abruptly stopping their hormone replacement, they had come up against their body's vulnerability to the hormonal changes of menopause.

Not everyone restarted. Some felt fine without estrogen and realized that they probably did not need it in the first place. They were the lucky minority. Of those who resumed because they needed estrogen to feel well and function, some did so at the cost of ongoing anxiety that they might be damaging their health. Yet another group felt miserable off estrogen but were afraid to go back on. Except for those who felt perfectly well off estrogen, few felt entirely confident with the course they had chosen.

Women whose menopausal transitions are uncomfortable are between a rock and a hard place. Or so it seems. Actually, the media coverage was misleading in the extreme. To be fair to the press, reporters are not epidemiologists trained to analyze complex studies. It did not help that those in charge of the study—who did have such training—played for the headlines and left out the nuances. It's taken more than two years for a clearer picture to emerge. More complete results have been published, and outside experts have had a chance to review the data, giving us a much clearer idea of what the risks really are. I will share some of the findings of this more nuanced analysis with you. While what I present in this chapter are my opinions, they are based not only on many years of treating women for menopause and conducting research on hormone therapy, but also on presentations at specialized conferences and informal discussions with other menopause experts. I think most physicians and scientists who are informed about the study would agree with the views I will present to you here, though obviously controversy remains.

You are probably familiar with the technical terms and acronyms used in discussions of hormones and menopause, but in case some are new to you, I've provided definitions in the sidebar on pages 352 and 353.

A general sense of fear now surrounds the entire subject of menopause, and until this is addressed, it is hard to focus on specific issues. For this reason, I'll start with the WHI study and the risks it reported. I'll then talk about what happens to a woman's body during menopause and give you the necessary background to help you make your decisions about menopause treatment.

HORMONE THERAPY: THE POSSIBLE RISKS

In a nutshell, the Women's Health Initiative found several possible health risks with hormone therapy and a possible fourth. These are breast cancer, heart attack, stroke, and possibly Alzheimer's. (A fifth risk, blood clots in leg veins, was known previously. This risk is extremely small and can be minimized by using patch estrogen as described in chapter 26.) These are all very serious diseases; no one wants to take a chance on any of them. Yet to make an informed personal decision regarding HT for menopause, it is necessary to look beyond the headlines to the actual data. To clarify the findings, I need to go into some detail regarding the design of the study.

Like most studies, WHI had several "arms"—groups of patients who received different treatments. The largest arm received Prempro, a combination of the horse-source estrogen, Premarin, and the synthetic progestin, Provera. This arm was the first to be discontinued because of adverse effects. While both the initial medical journal reports and the public media tended to refer to WHI as a study of estrogen, it was actually a study of estrogen *and* progestin in combination. Any risk found could be due to either or both hormones. This is extremely important because, as we shall see, *it was not estrogen but the progestin that caused an apparent increase in breast cancer risk.* There is a certain irony in this because the progestin is taken for the sole purpose of preventing another form of cancer, that of the lining of the uterus.

A second arm consisted of women who'd had hysterectomies and therefore had no need for the progestin. They received Premarin alone in the same dose as those in the Prempro arm. A third arm received placebo—inactive pills made to look like the active ones. It is to this untreated group that comparisons were made.

In writing this book, I've tried to avoid dry statistics, which too often miss the human impact of a condition. With HT, however, the main story can be told only with numbers, but I've done my best to select those that are truly informative for women who must decide about HT. The following sidebar shows some of the reported adverse effects in terms of a statistic called *hazard ratio* (HR). This is a decimal fraction that can easily be converted to a percent. An HR of 1.3, for example, indicates that the rate of events in that group was 130 percent of that in the comparison control group. Even this is somewhat confusing because it means the risk was 30 percent higher, not 130 percent higher. Let's say there were two groups of 100; those in one group received a drug and those in the other did not. A hazard ratio of 1.3

MENOPAUSE TERMINOLOGY

Menopause is defined technically as the cessation of menstruation. More generally, it refers to all the physical and mental effects produced by the decline in estrogen as the ovaries slow down.

Perimenopause is a recent term that refers to the life stage during which the physical and mental effects of waning estrogen have begun, but periods are still occurring. Perimenopause may precede actual menopause by several years. The distinction between perimenopause and menopause is somewhat artificial—the same symptoms occur in both phases—and so for convenience I often refer to this time of a woman's life as perimenopause/menopause.

Hormone replacement therapy (HRT) or hormone therapy (HT) refer to use of estrogen and a form of progesterone when the ovary's production of them has decreased at perimenopause/menopause. Recently the term hormone therapy has been favored. ET or ERT refer to therapy with estrogen alone, as is appropriate for women who have had a hysterectomy.

Estrogen is the main female hormone, as discussed in chapter 2. There are three kinds of estrogen in the human body; the main form made by the ovaries prior to menopause is estradiol. The other forms—estrone and estriol—are discussed later in this chapter. It is estrogen that relieves the symptoms of menopause (see sidebar on page 364). The forms of estrogen most commonly prescribed for menopause are estradiol, the natural human hormone, and conjugated equine estrogens (CEE Premarin), which come from pregnant mares.

Progesterone is made by the ovary every month following ovulation. It prepares the uterus for pregnancy or for menstruation. Natural progesterone is available by prescription, as Prometrium. **Progestin** is the term applied to the many synthetic forms of progesterone as used in oral contraceptives or in various HT formulations. MPA (medroxyprogesterone acetate, Provera) is the synthetic currently most commonly prescribed. Its many problems, including a possible role in breast cancer, are described in several chapters in this section. It is combined with Premarin in Prempro. The sole reason for including progesterone or a progestin in HT is to prevent cancer of the endometrium.

Endometrium is the medical term for the lining of the uterus. It is shed monthly during normal cycles. When exposed to estrogen but not progesterone, overgrowth of the endometrium—and even cancer—can occur. For this reason, women who have not had a hysterectomy usually need a form of progesterone if they are taking estrogen. Women who have had a hysterectomy do not need progesterone.

Women's Health Initiative (WHI) is the formal name for the menopause study that made all the headlines. It was organized by the National Institute of Health and followed more than 16,000 women on Prempro and nearly 11,000 on Premarin alone. The value of the study was its large size; some of its limitations are discussed later in this chapter.

would mean that one group had ten events and the other thirteen. Presumably three of the thirteen cases were due to the drug. Note also that an increased risk of 30 percent does not mean that 30 percent of those who took the medication had the adverse event, but 30 percent more than in the group that did not receive the medication.

I've picked the 30 percent example because this is the approximate increase in breast cancer risk found in one arm of WHI. The sidebar on page 354 gives more specifics.

WHI HAZARD RATIOS

	Prempro	Premarin only
Invasive breast cancer	1.24	0.77
Heart attacks	1.24	0.91
Stroke	1.44	1.39

One of the most important findings, not well publicized, is that *breast cancer risk was only higher after four or more years of treatment.* This risk peaked at five years and seemed to fall after six or more years. Furthermore, the increased risk of breast cancer at four years was seen only in those who'd used HT prior to study entry, so actually more than four years of exposure were involved. Some interpret this pattern of increase-followed-by-decrease to mean that Prempro increased the growth of existing tumors rather than creating new ones. Another possible interpretation is that only a few are susceptible to breast cancer as a result of using HT. This suggests that if a woman has been on HT for six years without developing breast cancer, there is no further risk from the HT per se. The data supporting this is limited, however. It needs to be pointed out that the risk of breast cancer is present for all women—unfortunately about 12 percent of women will eventually develop this disease, even if they never use HT. I am not trying to be gloomy, but to make clear that even if you are not on any hormones, you still need regular breast exams and mammography.

A critical fact was hidden in plain sight in the WHI data and barely mentioned in media reports. If you look at the sidebar above you'll notice that the risk of breast cancer for those on Premarin alone was actually less than for those women not on hormones at all. Since then, additional studies have confirmed that it is progestins, not estrogens, that are the major risk factor with HT. Suppressing this finding was more than inaccurate journalism; it betrayed women by failing to inform them that by taking the least progestin possible, they might reduce the risk of breast cancer and heart disease from HT.

These data, despite many remaining questions, have two very clear implications for women considering HT. First, trying it for up to four years will not increase your risk of breast cancer. Second, if you have had a hysterectomy, you can take estrogen without any increase in breast cancer risk because you don't need a progestin.

A question of great importance for women is whether different forms of estrogen and progestin, specifically those that are natural for human females, would create the same risk. My own view is that it is common sense to proceed on the assumption that natural forms—estradiol and progesterone itself—are the safest. I must stress that this supposition has not been tested in any large-scale study. Though reasonable, it is based as much on hope as science.

CORONARY HEART DISEASE (CHD)

The biggest surprise of WHI was the finding of a small increase in risk of heart attacks in the Prempro group—about 28 percent overall. This was surprising because extensive research in monkeys and some in humans had suggested a protective effect. It is important to be aware that the increased risk was found only in women who were more than ten years postmenopause. (The risk of death from a heart attack was increased by 10 percent, but this was not statistically significant. There were not many heart attacks, and nearly all, fortunately, were nonfatal.) Another study, the Heart and Estrogen-Progestin Replacement Study (HERS) trial found that in women who had already had one heart attack, Premarin and Provera increased the risk of another. With estrogen alone, in the WHI study, there was actually a suggestion of a slight *decrease* in heart attack risk.

How can we make sense of all this seemingly contradictory data? The most reasonable interpretation, the one most experts believe is correct, is that for women with healthy blood vessels, estrogen may delay atherosclerosis. Once the vessels are scarred and narrowed, however, it is too late for estrogen to help. Age, too, may make the arteries less able to open up in response to estrogen. The increased risk when estrogen is started later may be due to its tendency to cause clots. So it is still plausible that estrogen, if started early enough, is cardioprotective. Enough uncertainty remains, however, that no one is recommending estrogen for cardiac prevention. Indeed, using estrogen for this purpose is unnecessary. Statins (Lipitor and related drugs) and aspirin work just as well. In fact, when statins are combined with HT, there is no increase in cardiac risk.

I must emphasize again that WHI mainly studied women in their sixties and seventies; in general risks for women in their forties and early fifties are far lower. For women with premature menopause—before forty or forty-five—estrogen clearly does have health-protective effects.

Even experts on biostatistics and epidemiology become confused by the immense amount of data accumulated in WHI. After wrestling with the numbers, patients and physicians alike want to know what it means for them. The sidebar distills the WHI findings down to a few clear guidelines.

HORMONE THERAPY, HEART DISEASE, AND YOU

If you have had a heart attack or other evidence of coronary heart disease, you should not use HT.

If you are under fifty-five, with no evidence of heart disease, HT is unlikely to increase your risk.

Use of proven treatments to decrease heart disease risk—statins (Lipitor, Zocor, Pravachol, and others), aspirin, blood pressure control, or insulin sensitizers if indicated—is the best way to protect your heart and blood vessels, whether or not you use HT. With statins, HT does not increase heart disease risk.

Improved diet (mainly less saturated fat and red meat) and regular exercise are good ideas, too.

SOME IMPORTANT THINGS TO KNOW ABOUT WHI

WHI was an immense effort involving many scientists and 161,809 women in an effort to determine health effects of HT and also of a low-fat diet. (Most of the women were in the dietary part; those in the hormone part numbered just over 26,000.) Such an enormous effort and expense will probably not be duplicated in the foreseeable future. Given this, it is disappointing that so many questions remain. The dilemma now facing women is self-evident: What does this study mean for me, and how can I apply it for decisions regarding my own health?

Most women considering HT are in their late forties to mid-fifties. For women at this point in life, the major limitation of the study is that the average age of women starting was sixty-three. Also, those whose menopause was causing them significant discomfort were excluded because it was felt that too many would drop out. Despite this, more than 40 percent discontinued participation before the study ended. For these reasons, it is far from clear that the risks found in WHI apply to women in the younger age range at which estrogen is usually first considered.

The media coverage of the WHI results consistently emphasized possible harmful effects and underplayed or ignored the reassuring ones, such as the discovery that estrogen by itself does not increase breast cancer risk. This was not entirely the fault of journalists—the initial publications and accompanying commentary in medical journals were similarly unbalanced. To keep matters in perspective, it's important to remember that the great majority of women who use HT never develop breast cancer or premature cardiovascular disease; for them HT is safe. The real questions are these: How do I determine the risk for me as an individual, and how much can I minimize the risks for myself? In the section that follows, I'll consider these practical implications of WHI.

THE CASE FOR ESTROGEN

Ironically, presenting the positive side of estrogen fell not to medical experts, nor to self-styled consumer advocates, but to an actress, Suzanne Somers, in her book *The Sexy Years*. As one of my patients who decided to try estrogen after reading the book told me, "She's in her mid-fifties, she's using estrogen, and she looks fabulous." Indeed, as Ms. Somers tells us loud and clear in her book, she enjoys sex and everything else in her life. *The Sexy Years* has done much to balance the debate on estrogen by eloquently proclaiming how it can enhance a woman's life. I do need to add some cautions, however. While I agree that the most natural forms of hormones should be used, the oral compounded estrogens recommended in *The Sexy Years* do not quite live up to their billing as "bioidentical." There are better ways to mimic your own body's way of supplying estrogen and progesterone; I'll tell you exactly how to do this in chapter 26. Also, in her enthusiasm, Ms. Somers tends to pass too lightly over the safety issues and does not seem informed about some important research findings, such as those I have summarized in this chapter.

Like many doctors, I am bemused that many women seem to trust an actress's advice more than those who, like myself, have spent our professional lives working with women's hormonal issues. There are two ways we can react to this: with annoyance or—my own choice—by reflecting on why Ms. Somers struck a chord with so many women. I can think of at least two reasons. First, instead of rehashing statistical minutiae, she responded to the natural desire to feel and look good. She also sets an example for women of her age of being actively involved in life. This includes being sexy, but goes beyond it. The book recognizes that sexuality is representative of many important aspects of a woman's life: continuing health and vitality, delight in life's many pleasures, confidence in one's own attractiveness. Suzanne Somers sets a wonderful example of how life can be active and fulfilling, despite the hormonal vulnerabilities of menopause. (I must state that all I know about Ms. Somers is what she chooses to reveal publicly in *The Sexy Years;* I have no specific knowledge of her case and would not discuss it if I did.)

I do want to emphasize that the decisions that Ms. Somers made for herself would not necessarily be those that are right for all women. In the first chapter, she describes the shock of discovering—from an ultrasound, as it did not show up on mammogram—that she had breast cancer and the difficulty of making decisions about treatment. She opted for surgery, but no chemo and no tamoxifen (an estrogen blocker that intensifies menopausal symptoms). She also decided to continue with her hormone replacement.

Now it is clear that Ms. Somers assembled all the information available and thought through her decision with great care. What cannot be known at this point is what the final outcome will be—whether her cancer will come back. I hope you have not, and will not, be faced with a diagnosis of breast cancer. If you do, reading how Ms. Somers made her decision will be helpful, but you should most assume that the decision that was right for her will necessarily be the right one for you. Although she emphasizes the virtues of bioidentical hormones, it has not been proven that these will not have some of the hazards of the synthetics. Only time will tell if her cancer will recur, although we are all hoping that it will not. In considering hormone therapy, you will need to make your own decision, not simply follow that made by someone else.

WHICH SIDE AM I ON?

When the subject of estrogen therapy comes up among nonmedical people, I am often asked bluntly if I am for it or against it. My answer is that I am neither—or both. I am for estrogen for some women and against it for others. The question is the wrong one. HT is not a political issue on which one must take sides. It is a complex health issue that needs information, not opinion. The media likes controversy and so often treats scientific issues as if they were political ones. The standard way to write a health care story is to quote an expert willing to say that a treatment is good, then find another to declare that it does not work or is dangerous. It's not hard to do this because scientists, like other people, like to air their pet opinions. To the journalist, this is balanced reporting; to the reader, who must use the information to make vital decisions about her health, it is at best confusing and at worse demoralizing.

In the HT debate both sides want what is healthiest for women; they disagree on just what that is. Given the complexity of the issues, many tend to base their position on the aspect of the conundrum that is most familiar to them. Those who consider themselves activists or advocates for women define their role as warning women of possible dangers. Doctors who prescribe hormone replacement are hoping to maintain the well-being and health of their menopausal patients. The gynecologist or endocrinologist hears daily the discomfort and disabilities that menopause produces. Women experiencing a difficult menopause get our attention more than those who have an easy time, for the simple reason that people come to doctors because they don't feel well.

Within medicine, there are two major camps in the HT debate. On one side are the epidemiologists, the specialists in statistics who run the huge studies. These scientists are great at crunching numbers but never actually meet the women who participate in their research projects. They spend their time looking at computer printouts that describe populations, not individuals. On the other side are many gynecologists, endocrinologists, and others who actually provide health care to individual women. All of us have seen how HT can help hormonally vulnerable women who are trying to keep things together through the biochemical turbulence of menopause. Listening to women whose well-being has been restored by HT shows us the positive side. (Of course, clinicians do not all agree. The cardiologist or breast surgeon who spends his or her days with people with heart disease or breast cancer tends to focus on these possible risks. The generalist may simply want to avoid the issue and not prescribe estrogen at all because he or she is too busy caring for a wide variety of problems to be able to deal with the intricacies of the HT studies.)

As with most bitter controversies, the truth lies between the extremes. We needed the epidemiologists to pinpoint the risks, and we cannot argue with their powerful techniques—though we can point out places where their results have been widely misinterpreted. Clinicians, however, are also right that some women feel terrible without HT.

The only resolution is to recognize that each woman's estrogen decision is an individual one. Most articles and books on menopause are slanted one way or the other. This one is not. It neither discounts the risks nor exaggerates them. My goal is not to persuade women to take or not take estrogen. Rather, it is to put together the information you need to make the decision that is right for you.

Some suspect that doctors have improper motives in trying to persuade women to use HT or are manipulated into it by pharmaceutical industry sales reps. In my experience, the influence of pharmaceutical industry marketing is exaggerated. The days when the industry offered expensive perks are largely over. Most doctors want to do the right thing for their patients—which is not to say mistakes are never made. Aggressive marketing will not sell drugs that doctors perceive as bad for their patients. Thus Evista (raloxifene), a menopause drug that turned out to make symptoms worse, never did well financially for its manufacturer despite heavy marketing. Of course, doctors are influenced to some degree by marketing, as are consumers. But we are a skeptical bunch, and we are well aware that drug reps will put a positive slant on what they tell us. To view HT as a sinister plot of the pharmaceutical industry is unhelpful for what is really important: sorting out the pros and cons about HT so that you can make the best decision for yourself.

WHAT YOU REALLY NEED TO KNOW ABOUT HT

In this and the next chapters, I'll cover HT risks in detail, based on the most accurate, up-to-date research. I'll explain alternatives that can help women feel well during the menopausal years without taking HT. But I'll also pass along the experiences of women in my practice who felt that for them estrogen was life enhancing. I'll also emphasize crucial facts about HT risk that you may not have read elsewhere, facts that have been kept almost secret such as the following:

- All studies have consistently shown that *there is no increased risk of breast cancer with less than four years of estrogen.*
- *For women in their late forties or early fifties who are just entering menopause, the risk of heart attacks is not increased.* The heart attack risk reported by the WHI study only applies to women ten or more years after menopause. Active measures can greatly reduce heart attack risk, whether or not a woman is using HT. However, women with heart disease should not take estrogen.
- Even though the headlines were about estrogen, the study showed that *most of the risks reported, except stroke, were not*

due to estrogen but to the synthetic form of progesterone that was taken with it. How you can apply the latest research to make HT safer is spelled out in chapter 26.

- Anxiety about estrogen can affect quality of life. If HT stops you from being awakened by night sweats, but you wake up anyway because of worry, you are not better off. No matter how bad your symptoms are, if the idea of taking estrogen terrifies you, it is probably not for you.

23.

What Menopause and Perimenopause Feel Like

Menopause is not just the end of menstruation. No woman had ever told me that she was to sorry stop getting periods. What makes menopause so challenging are the subtle bodily changes that occur as the ovaries gradually lose the ability to make hormones. For most women, the ovary begins to slow down by their mid- to late-forties. Periods may still be regular, but for those women vulnerable to loss of estrogen, symptoms begin. Perimenopause can be quite difficult because, as has only recently been recognized, hormone swings during this phase can be wider than at any other stage of a woman's life, even puberty. Women are often particularly frustrated by the less publicized symptoms of these shifts, such as hair loss, mood swings, and general aches and pains because doctors often dismiss them as merely psychological.

I've listed the main symptoms that can emerge in this phase of a woman's life in the sidebar on page 364, but keep in mind that almost any change in how you feel, even if you can't put a name to it, can be due to perimenopause or menopause. So if you are in your forties, or even your late thirties, and have many of the symptoms I've listed, or just have started to feel different, declining estrogen levels may be the reason. If your periods have gotten lighter or closer together, this is further evidence that your ovaries are putting out less estrogen. Please remember, however, that nearly every symptom in the list can have other causes that may need to be ruled out. Not all that flashes is menopause.

ARE YOU IN PERIMENOPAUSE/MENOPAUSE?

The symptoms of the change are listed below. If you have stopped menstruating and have these symptoms, you are in menopause. If you have these same symptoms, but still get periods, you are probably in perimenopause. The effects of tiring ovaries can begin years before periods stop.

Here are clues to perimenopause.

Age over forty-four—But it can begin years earlier or later.
Periods lighter—They may also be closer together or less frequent.
Hot flashes or night sweats—Yes, they can start when you are still having periods.
Restless sleep
Mood swings—even if you had them before, these probably feel different.
Hair loss, sometimes quite rapid
Mild but definite discomforts:
    Body not feeling right
    Discomfort when touched
    Pain when combing hair
    Aching muscles or joints
Mild problems with memory
Slower thinking
Less lubrication with sex

If you have four or more of these symptoms, it may be that your ovaries are making less estrogen. Look in chapters 25 and 26 for ways to relieve its discomforts.

THE CLASSIC SYMPTOMS: HOT FLASHES AND NIGHT SWEATS

With respect to temperature control, our pet dogs and cats are much better off than we are, neither needing to put on, nor take off, their coats. The human temperature regulating system works efficiently only within a narrow range. When the room or outdoor temperature is too hot, more blood flows through the skin so as to bring heat from the core of the body to the skin where it can be released into the atmosphere. Sweating often accompanies this shift in blood flow and compounds the discomfort.

The hypothalamus, the part of the brain that regulates our internal environment, acts as a thermostat to keep our body temperature within the narrow range needed for comfort and health. For reasons we do not understand, the drop in estrogen at menopause alters the setting on the internal thermostat so that the body thinks it should be cooler. This means that temperatures that were previously comfortable now feel too hot. Hot flashes (also called flushes) tend to come on abruptly: You feel comfortable, then all of a sudden your hypothalamus decides to cool you off and sends signals to increase skin blood flow and initiate sweating. Actually, the body temperature is normal before a hot flash; the problem is a malfunctioning internal thermostat. Unfortunately, our bodies lack dials that can be twisted to reset the hypothalamus.

A typical hot flash begins with a sensation of warmth in the chest that then travels up to the face and head. There is flushing, which is particularly noticeable in fair-skinned people, and sweat may drip down the face or soak clothes. Stress tends to set off hot flashes, which is not surprising because the same part of the brain, the hypothalamus, controls many of the body's responses to threatening situations. Hot flashes, when severe, can be quite distracting and force stopping of activity; this can be quite a problem when it happens at a critical moment.

A night sweat is simply a hot flash that occurs during sleep. The discomfort usually wakes you up, and the sweating often soaks the sheets, further adding to the misery by inducing a chill. Some women have told me that the sheets get so wet that they have to change them in the middle of the night; needless to say this is conducive neither to a good night's rest nor a happy husband. Night sweats may begin before daytime hot flashes and become noticeable.

Some women have a generalized feeling of being too warm, rather than sudden flashes or sweats. Though less embarrassing, these milder forms of temperature imbalance are still uncomfortable. Prior to menopause, women usually feel cold more than men; afterward this reverses itself. Arguments about whether to open the bedroom window continue, but this time it is the woman who wants them open and the man who wants them closed.

Hot flashes and night sweats are the sort of symptoms that don't sound so bad—until they happen to you. A common bit of advice for dealing with flashes is to wear clothing in layers that can be put on or taken off as one's temperature sensitivity changes. This is perfectly sensible, but most women I see for menopause-related symptoms have already figured it out for themselves. Furthermore, it is not always convenient or practical. Estrogen, in adequate doses, completely stops flashes and sweats. There are other treatments too, which are discussed in chapter 25.

NOT ALL THAT FLASHES IS MENOPAUSE

In recent years, I've heard women who are not even remotely close to menopause age express concern that they are having hot flashes. Actually flushing can occur at any age, but before menopause hormones are not likely to be the culprit. These other kinds of flushing tend to be infrequent, while the flashes of menopause can occur ten times a day, or more in women who are very vulnerable to low estrogen levels.

In my experience, flushing unrelated to menopause is particularly common in northern climates during fall and spring, when temperatures are at their most variable. To go from 20°F degree weather, as we are having in New York City as I write this, to a 74°F degree interior is a thermal stress that our bodies were not designed to withstand. In summer, the opposite occurs; we move from sweaty outdoor weather to excessively chilly indoor air conditioning. The flushing does not necessarily occur at the exact time of the temperature change, however. These flushes are uncomfortable but not a sign of anything dangerous. The only answer is to dress flexibly, for example, to take off winter coats and sweaters as soon as you enter an overheated interior and to bring a sweater for indoor use in summer if you are sensitive to air conditioning.

Another common trigger for flushing is sudden embarrassment. In this case it is called blushing; the cause is usually obvious.

There are rare diseases that manifest as flushing such as pheochromocytoma, a tumor that releases adrenalin or related hormones. However, these are exceedingly rare and generally have much more severe symptoms. This condition can easily be ruled out by a blood test called metanephrine, but it is rarely necessary.

THE VAGINA: WHAT HAPPENS TO IT INSIDE AND OUT

In many traditional cultures, it was assumed that women should stop being sexual after menopause. Of course many women did stay interested, but they may have felt ashamed of their still vigorous sexuality, and husbands tended to fulfill their needs elsewhere. This oppressive situation has greatly improved; one of the unheralded changes of modern culture is appreciation of the charms of mature women. Our culture is criticized for its youth emphasis, but is starting to offer more and more examples of women, like Suzanne Somers, whose glamour extends well beyond their fifties. Women reasonably expect sex to be part of their lives so long as they are healthy enough to enjoy it. Though bodies have changed—the fifty-five-year-old of our time is likely to be in far better shape than the fifty-five-year-old of earlier generations—what we expect of our bodies has changed even more. Yet our bodies do impose limitations on sexual expression. Estrogen is needed to maintain a woman's sexual areas, and its decline in midlife may interfere with physical intimacy, even when interest is undiminished. For intercourse to continue to be comfortable during perimenopause and menopause may require some accommodations.

Estrogen has profound effects on vaginal tissues. Before puberty, a little girl's vagina is very small, with the mucosal lining dry and thin. As puberty progresses, the vaginal lining grows in size, thickens, and starts to secrete mucus for lubrication. Pubertal changes are not irreversible because estrogen is needed to maintain the vagina in a functional state. When estrogen begins to decline, the earliest change, which may be evident while periods are still coming, is a slight decrease in moisture. Full arousal produces lubrication but less than previously. At first, use of a lubricant such as K-Y or Astroglide will usually maintain comfort during intercourse. (Sexual lubricants are discussed in chapter 14.) Later this may not be enough because as estrogen drops further, the vaginal lining becomes thinner and less resilient. What used to feel good may now simply make you sore. Not only the vagina, but also the surrounding tissues in the pelvis bear the impact of the erect penis during intercourse. No other internal structure in the body is subject to the same degree of mechanical stress as the female reproductive system.

One reason that coital pain (dysparunia) is not more common among women in their late forties and fifties is that men's erections at this age are less rigid than in earlier decades. Hence the stress to the vagina and surrounding structures is less. With the advent of erection-enhancing drugs such as Viagra, the vagina must cope with harder knocks during intercourse.

As women go into their sixties, estrogen levels fall further, and the vaginal mucosa becomes so thin as to be almost translucent. Less obvious but just as important, it shrinks so that the vagina becomes much narrower. After many years, intercourse may not be possible at all, though this is far from invariable. This will not occur during the hormonal years of thirty-five to fifty-five, which are the subject of this book. The important point is that when it comes to sex, the principle of use it or lose it definitely applies; regular intercourse can limit later vaginal shrinkage.

Comfort is obviously critical for pleasure. It's hard to stay interested in having sex if it hurts. When thin and dry, the vagina can suffer abrasions or tears during intercourse. If sex has started being painful, a pelvic exam is essential to determine the cause. If you notice bleeding after sex, you should have this checked by your gynecologist promptly.

MOOD AND MENOPAUSE

Some women breeze through menopause feeling perfectly fine. Women who are less fortunate in their relationship with their own hormones must endure greater challenges from waning estrogen levels. When friends boast of being untroubled by menopausal changes, those more vulnerable can get caught up in self-blame, as if their difficulty coping is a character weakness. Rest assured this is not the case. The miseries of perimenopause or menopause are due to hormones, not neurosis or wimpiness.

Prominent among the effects of waning estrogen is lowering of mood. Depression, like the other symptoms, can begin before or after periods stop. Early on in the perimenopause phase, because estrogen levels are unstable, mood may fluctuate unpredictably. Later, as estrogen sinks to consistently low levels, an overall dull feeling takes over from the previous more volatile mood swings. Depression due to the hormonal vulnerability of menopause has more or less the same symptoms as depression due to other causes. If you find your zest for life has evaporated as your hormones change, I urge you to take action sooner rather than later so that you do not sink into a permanent slump. Everyone knows women in their late fifties or older who seem to find their lives without pleasure or interest. (Men can lose interest in life, of course, and it can result from low testosterone, but this is uncommon as a cause of male depression.) After many years, the depression precipitated by lack of estrogen becomes habitual and it is far harder to pull oneself out. For this reason, and because depression takes the meaning out of life, I think that it should be treated promptly, lest depression become a way of life.

I am often asked: Why didn't my mother or grandmother have such a hard time with menopause? One answer is that she may have, but believed, very likely correctly, that it would do no good to complain. While women's ailments are not always taken seriously, even now, things were far worse in earlier generations. One teaching was that if symptoms of menopause lasted more than one year, they were psychosomatic; this is refused by the fact that the symptoms resolve completely with estrogen. The other reason menopause seems harder now is that for many women, the late forties and early fifties are years of peak demands. Children are likely to be in their teens and demand close supervision, for which they are not always appreciative. The troubles adolescents can get themselves into are worse than in the past, making parental anxiety more pervasive. Careers tend to blossom at this stage of life, and so responsibilities rise at work as well as at home.

Whatever challenges arise during this phase of life, hormones don't make them any easier.

IS IT DEPRESSION, OR IS IT MY HORMONES?

Although women know better, many in the medical profession doubt a connection between hormones and low mood. Because hormonal depression has similar symptoms to other kinds, its reality is often doubted. To many doctors, irritability, tearfulness, discouragement, and lack of energy simply mean depression, and hormones are not considered as a factor. Yet it usually is possible to recognize when hormones are involved, though it comes down to experience and even intuition on the part of an experienced physician because tests rarely tell the whole story. FSH, the standard blood test for menopause, only turns positive late in the process. Though estradiol is clearly involved in the mood changes of perimenopause, it fluctuates so widely that a single measurement gives only limited information. What's really important is how your hormones are interacting with neurons in your brain, something we can only infer.

I am not succumbing to hormonal pessimism here. Quite the contrary, I am urging that test results not be an excuse to ignore hormones as a cause of mood changes. Once identified, hormonal depression is highly treatable, either with HT or with the measures explained in chapter 25. I've seen countless women's moods quickly turn cheerful when they got help for their menopause.

The sidebar on page 371 itemizes the important clues that suggest mood change is due to hormones.

These guidelines assume that there are no significant life events that might be affecting you. If you've had a relationship end, lost a job, had a child become seriously ill, or experienced another unhappy life event, your mood and energy will certainly be affected. On the other hand, hormones can make events like these even harder to endure. My view is that any time a woman is depressed, hormones should be considered as a contributing factor. When sad life events come together with hormonal changes, treatment for the hormonal component will not in itself solve the problem, but it may free up energy to help you deal with the external causes.

IS FALLING ESTROGEN PULLING YOUR MOOD DOWN WITH IT?

PMS is the more likely cause if you are under forty, have normal cycles without any recent change, and your mood swings occur at the same time every cycle, usually the week before menstruation.

Perimenopause as a cause of low mood and/or decreased energy is likely if:

You are over forty.

Your periods are unchanged or have gotten slightly lighter and/or closer together.

Mood and energy fluctuate throughout your cycle, not just premenstrually.

You have more difficulty sleeping throughout your cycle.

You are having symptoms associated with low estrogen, such as:

Hot flashes and/or night sweats

Decrease in vaginal moisture and lubrication

Menopause is the probable cause of low mood and/or decreased energy if:

Periods are infrequent or have stopped.

You have other menopausal symptoms, such as flashes or sweats.

Your mood problems began at about the same as periods changed or stopped.

You were not depressed before—or depression that was mild has taken a turn for the worse.

TREATMENTS FOR LOW MOOD: HORMONES VERSUS ANTIDEPRESSANTS

A basic principle of therapeutics is to treat the underlying cause, not just the symptom. In this sense, if low mood is due to estrogen changes, then giving estrogen is the logical approach. Hormone replacement with a patch and natural progesterone allows individual dose adjustment so as to give you a steady supply of estrogen at the blood level at which your body feels best.

Paradoxical as it may seem, taking estrogen is effective for mood swings due to estrogen. This is because of the principle I have emphasized throughout this book: Women's hormone problems are due not so much to the hormones themselves as to their fluctuations. When estrogen is supplemented at perimenopause, blood levels become more consistent and are less likely to set off the hormonal alarm system. It is striking how often a modest dose of estrogen will help soothe even severe mood swings at this phase of life. Later on, when perimenopause has progressed to menopause, estrogen fluctuates less, but levels are much lower. Supplementation helps this as well. So estrogen can help in both perimenopause and menopause, but for somewhat different reasons.

If you can't take estrogen or prefer not too, antidepressants are a reasonable alternative. I've covered the ins and outs of this class of medications in detail in chapter 6 on treatment of PMS. Certainly, if you have a reason not to use estrogen or simply are apprehensive about it, trying an antidepressant first is a valid option. However, if this kind of medication does not do it for you, it's reasonable to reconsider at least a trial of estrogen. Keep in mind what I've already explained: If you are in your late forties or early fifties, there is no increased risk from being on estrogen for at least the first four years.

Psychotherapy is a usual treatment for mood problems, but studies have shown that for depression not clearly caused by disturbing life events, medication generally works better. If you are feeling overwhelmed and would like an outside perspective, then counseling may be a useful adjunct. Psychotherapy cannot make you invulnerable to your hormones, so you will still need medical help with the biochemical factors.

DOES MENOPAUSE *REALLY* CAUSE DEPRESSION?

In an earlier era, doctors assumed that the symptoms of menopause were psychological—since the function of women is to have children, they must be universally depressed at the loss of this ability. All of us mourn our youth to some degree—though few would want to relive it—and there is a natural sadness at getting older. But this does not necessarily translate into physical symptoms. One obvious flaw in this psychological theory of menopause is that it does not explain why hot flashes do not occur at other times.

The standard textbook on gynecological endocrinology, Clinical *Gynecological Endocrinology and Infertility* by Leon Speroff and Marc A. Fritz, says this about depression and menopause (pages 643 to 645):

> . . . many of the problems reported at menopause are due to life events. Thus, there are problems encountered in the early perimenopause that are seen frequently, but their causal relation with estrogen is unlikely. These problems include fatigue, nervousness, headaches, insomnia, depression, irritability, joint and muscle pain, dizziness, and palpitations.

The authors go on to a conclusion that is rather confusing or, perhaps, merely confused:

> The perimenopausal transition, therefore, is not a cause of clinical depression; however, labile emotions do seem to be improved in many women administered hormonal therapy.

In other words, the low estrogen of perimenopause does not cause depression, but many women feel less depressed when they take estrogen! This is a blatant contradiction. I've quoted this textbook, which in most respects is excellent, because I think it well reflects the current muddled thinking in the medical establishment regarding menopause and well-being. On the one hand is a dogma that perimenopause or menopause does not cause depression; on the other is the obvious fact that mood difficulties are common at this time of life and usually get better with a little estrogen. Here are some of the comments made by some of my patients after they have gone on HT for mood problems: "Now I feel myself again." Or "I no longer cry at the slightest frustration." Or "My husband and children tell me there is a huge difference; I no longer snap at them all the time." (This is not to say that husbands and children never deserve to be snapped at; even so, losing one's cool rarely results in improved relationships.)

Another argument sometimes advanced to buttress the claim that low estrogen does not affect quality of life is the finding in the WHI study that women did not feel better on HT. Actually, this is not surprising because *women were admitted to the WHI study only if they were not having troublesome menopausal symptoms in the first place.* Of course, treatment won't reduce symptoms that don't exist! This detail was somehow left out of the press coverage.

Now, I am certainly not suggesting that estrogen is the solution to all women's midlife problems. Nor do I think that every woman should take it during her change. My point is that estrogen does have significant benefits for women whose perimenopause/menopause years are grueling ones. This is a major reason that doctors who treat women are more positive about estrogen than the epidemiologists who spend their days pouring over computer printouts: We see the immense difference it makes in many women's lives. I've emphasized estrogen in discussing midlife mood problems because it is often the most direct solution. However, there are many ways to help the symptoms of menopause besides estrogen; I enumerate them in chapter 25.

TWO CAUTIONS

Because some symptoms of depression, such as low energy, can be due to physical illness, it is vital that you have a medical checkup before attributing them to depression or hormonal changes.

In this book, I mostly discuss mild or moderate mood problems, those that can be coped with, though they sap energy and may tax relationships. However, *if your depression is so severe that you are in real despair, you should seek professional help without delay.*

MENOPAUSE AND THE MIND

Many women in perimenopause-menopause notice that their thinking has been affected, that it takes a little longer to remember a name or find a word, or that their mind just works more slowly. Lapses in attention seem more frequent, and many describe sometimes forgetting what they had just started to do. Many secretly fear they may be in the early phase of Alzheimer's. This is never the case because Alzheimer's and related diseases don't begin this early.

The changes in thinking that occur during perimenopause/menopause are not extreme. No one goes out and forgets where she lives or the names of her children or any of the other terrible things that happen to some of the elderly. It may take a second longer to remember a name, but it still comes. Nonetheless, when memory seems slow, it's easy to feel that you are losing your mental edge and fear that it will get worse. Information recall is critical in modern working life. It's vital in sales, in which remembering a customer's name and personal details is expected; or information technology, in which the details of software quirks must be remembered; or teaching, in which one does not want to lose one's train of thought in front of a class. To feel confident about almost any work requires mental sharpness. At home, as women are well aware, multitasking is the name of the game, especially since children's schedules nowadays can be busier than those of adults'.

Research confirms that cognitive function is affected by estrogen deficiency. (An excellent book on this subject is *Menopause and the Mind,* by Claire Warga, Ph.D.) Some studies, though not all, have shown that estrogen replacement produces slight improvements in memory, especially verbal recall. It is not surprising that estrogen has such an effect, since women overall perform better in tests involving verbal ability. Recent studies suggest that small doses of testosterone, such as those used to treat sexual dysfunction, may also help cognitive function at menopause. This is not surprising either, since testosterone seems to play a role in facilitating certain other aspects of mental function, especially spatial relations.

My own experience helping women deal with the hormonal tumult of perimenopause/menopause indicates that changes in thinking are real, but small in magnitude. Competence is not affected, though confidence may be. After going on estrogen, most women who noticed slower thinking report that it returns to normal. Men as well as women have significant brain levels of estrogen, so its role may not be entirely different in the two sexes. Another theory about the effect of low estrogen on brain function is that it is a result of sleep disturbance. There is no doubt that even mild sleep deprivation lowers mental acvity. How much the effects of menopause on cognitive function are due directly to lack of estrogen and how much to impaired sleep is a moot point, since estrogen solves the problem. Sleeping pills are not a substitute because by sedating the brain, they tend to dull thinking.

There is another reason for apparent memory difficulties that has nothing to do with hormones: Women in their forties and fifties typically have more to remember because their responsibilities are greater, and the consequences of forgetting potentially more serious. College students forget things all the time but usually are rather blasé about it. All they really have to remember is when their classes are and the dates of exams and papers. I remember one patient, a research scientist, who worried because after reading through a pile of scientific papers, she could not remember all the details. This is a consequence not of hormonal or brain dysfunction, but of being human.

ESTROGEN AND DEMENTIA

Anyone who has seen a relative or friend deteriorate from Alzheimer's or a related condition knows how terrible it is. The thought of ending up physically alive but with the mind gone is horrifying. The overall medical term for conditions in which memory and thinking progressively decline is dementia. Alzheimer's is the most common form, but dementia can occur from other causes, for example, from multiple tiny strokes.

The role of estrogen in maintenance of cognitive function is not fully resolved. Since Alzheimer's is about three times as common in women, it is plausible that estrogen is involved. But this could go either way. It might be the decline in estrogen at menopause that predisposes women to dementia, or it might be that higher levels over a

lifetime increase risk. These two hypotheses have very different implications for what estrogen therapy might do regarding dementia risk.

The WHI reported an increased risk of dementia with estrogen;
however, this was not Alzheimer's but vascular in nature. This means
that the mental changes were caused by blockages in the arteries supplying blood to the brain. It is likely that this is due to the increase in
clotting caused by estrogen, particularly oral forms such as the Prempro used in the study. The average age of the women diagnosed with
dementia was seventy-five, so one cannot assume a similar effect in
younger women.

Several earlier studies have shown a protective effect of estrogen
therapy against later dementia. There is no benefit, however, in those
with a gene predisposing to Alzheimer's, nor for those starting less
than ten years before symptoms appear, probably because the condition is already present in subtle form.

How do we put together this seemingly conflicting data regarding
estrogen and risk of later cognitive decline? What seems most likely is
that estrogen is protective if started early, while the brain is in good
shape with good blood circulation. Once dementia has set in, estrogen
may make matters worse, perhaps by causing clots in brain arteries.
This is analogous to the story with cardiovascular disease, for which
early estrogen may be protective to the healthy heart but not to one in
which coronary disease has already started.

In the short term, thinking is improved with estrogen. Although the
studies report only small effects, women frequently tell me that estrogen has made a major difference in their mental sharpness. Not that
they could not meet demands before, but they become more secure
about their memory when on estrogen.

The bottom line: If started in the forties or early fifties, estrogen
seems to be good for the brain.

DYSESTHESIA: WEIRD SENSATIONS AND PAIN

The word I have used to title this section, dysesthesia, is not a common
one, but I think it is useful because it describes a common group of
menopause symptoms that are otherwise hard to put into words. *Dys-*
means not normal, and *-esthesia* refers to sensation, as in *anesthesia*, a

drug that stops all sensations. It is also the root of *aesthetic,* which refers to the pleasing quality of beautiful things. Dysesthetic sensations are uncomfortable but not quite like ordinary pain. They are disturbing out of proportion to the pain associated with them. Remember hitting your "funny bone" as a child, or perhaps, rubbing velvet? These are dysesthetic sensations. I've already told the story of one woman whose husband thought she was a little crazy when she told him it hurt when she combed her hair. Some find that previously trivial sensations like this or clothes rubbing against their bodies become quite disturbing. Dysesthesia is a common symptom of menopause but one which, because it sounds strange when described, is often not taken seriously by physicians. To say, "My body just does not feel right," or "I don't like to be touched," sounds neurotic, but is actually due to hormones. As I overheard one woman say to another during a recent train ride, "Hormones do crazy things."

Sexual touching can be dysesthetic in the absence of arousal or when too much pressure is applied. The sexual tissues are actually quite delicate, and pleasure may depend on your partner rubbing in just the right way, neither too soft nor too hard. One cause of loss of sexual interest at menopause is a change in the character of genital sensation from erotic to dysesthetic.

Dysesthesia quickly resolves with estrogen treatment. I have not found anything else that works, although the problem sometimes gradually goes away by itself.

OTHER DISCOMFORTS OF MENOPAUSE

Sleep disturbance I've already mentioned that insomnia is extremely common in perimenopause or menopause. Studies have shown sleep at this phase of life to be shallower than ideal, even in women without any subjective sense of sleeping poorly. Recently, it's been recognized that sleep deprivation is a major factor in low-grade depression. Many studies, some of which were done on doctors in training, show that mental acuity, alertness, and coordination suffer when sleep is inadequate. In the terrible days of the Soviet Union, the KGB found that simply by not letting a person sleep, he or she would eventually confess to anything, even though it meant execution. Having spent many thirty-six-hour-plus intervals without sleep during internship and residency, I recall only too clearly what a totally miserable feeling this is. Thinking is erratic, the body feels uncomfortable all over, and minor problems seem overwhelming. While I am not entirely convinced that sleep deprivation is the entire story of menopausal depression, it is certainly a contributing factor.

Joint and muscle pain Many women whom I see for menopause express concern that they may have arthritis because of pain in the arms and legs. Careful physical examination invariably shows that their joints are quite healthy; the pain is actually in the muscles. Because muscle pain is common and does not produce any changes on physical exam, it is often dismissed as unimportant. Like any constant low-grade pain, muscle aches can impair concentration, mood, and sleep.

A similar condition, fibromyalgia, is particularly common in women but usually begins before estrogen levels have begun to fall. Fibromyalgia is diffuse muscle pain; the cause is still not understood. It is frequently associated with chronic fatigue, and both are thought to be related to inadequate sleep. In order for muscles and joints to recover from the mechanical strains of a normal day, the body must go completely slack during sleep. When sleep is not deep enough, the muscles and joints are not able to fully heal during the night and so feel stiff and sore during the day. This is a vicious circle because the pain prevents sleep from being deep enough to allow the muscles to recover. Shallow sleep leads to pain, which leads to shallow sleep, and so on.

Restoration of normal sleep can greatly help muscular pain, whether due to fibromyalgia or to declining estrogen. Conversely, good pain relief can improve sleep, further decreasing pain. Menopausal muscle pain can be treated in various ways. NSAIDs such as naproxen or the cox-2 inhibitor Celebrex (celecoxib) may help. (The current issues regarding these classes of medications are discussed in chapter 7 on female pain.) Very warm baths (but not so hot they burn or make you dizzy!) and massage help. So does exercise, but this is a case where you may feel little worse before you feel better.

Estrogen replacement usually relieves muscle pain to the degree it is due to menopause. Sleeping medications may help, but because of their addiction potential, they are not a good long-term solution.

Women with muscle discomfort sometimes worry that it is due to osteoporosis, but this is virtually never the case. Osteoporosis causes pain only when there are fractures, which occur only after years of bone loss.

HORMONAL OPTIMISM

Once when a teenage patient was describing her symptoms to me, she suddenly stopped and said, "I'm sorry to complain so much." I was amused and pointed out to her that if a person has no complaints at all, she would not come to see a doctor. My treatment of menopause in this chapter is directed at what women complain to me about. In this sense, what I have written so far is not a balanced picture. For this reason, I need to state quite clearly that, despite the challenges imposed by hormones, *for most women, the years around perimenopause and menopause are at least as good as any others in their lives.* I focus on what can go wrong because this is my function as a physician. Hormonal pessimism is no more justified at perimenopause/menopause than at any other phase of life. It is true that maintaining well-being often requires some extra effort when hormones are changing, but the effort is small in proportion to the likely reward.

24.

Menopause: The Decision

TWO WOMEN AND THEIR MENOPAUSES

Let's set aside statistics for a moment and look at the experiences of two women as they went through the menopause transition. Sandra and Ellen worked together as partners in a natural foods catering business. Although both were about the same age, Sandra developed menopausal symptoms first. She'd read many things about the change, mostly from an alternative viewpoint and decided that she would use soy and herbs and avoid hormone therapy (HT), which she felt to be unnatural. Ellen had read less about it, but assumed she'd do the same things when her change came.

Sandra came for consultation because she was having hot flashes, despite the soy, and wondered what else she could do, making it clear that HT was not an option on the table. Although Sandra was already well informed about natural remedies, I was able to help by giving her some advice on how to fine-tune her regimen. I explained that to get the benefit of soy, she needed to use actual tofu or fresh soy milk, because most of the prepared capsule forms do not have adequate amounts of the healthy isoflavones and proteins. She had also been using evening primrose oil, but I told her that black cohosh is more likely to be effective. A few months earlier she'd begun taking pyridoxine—vitamin B_6—which she thought helped a little. However, her dose was too high—200 mg daily, which can cause nerve damage—so I suggested that it would be prudent to cut back to 100 mg per day. Sandra was taking adequate calcium and vitamin D but needed a monitoring program to be sure her bones were getting the same protection that prescription medications provide.

We also discussed meditation, something Sandra had tried a few times but had not stuck with. In my experience, regular practice is needed to get real benefit. Meditation does not necessarily stop hot flashes, but it can make them less disruptive to one's equilibrium.

At her follow-up visit four months later, Sandra reported that her hot flashes were much less bothersome. They had not gone away but, she told me, "I can live with them. I'd rather put up with feeling a little hot and sweaty than take estrogen. And I think the meditation is starting to help, now that I do it nearly every day."

About a year later, Sandra's partner Ellen came to me for her menopause. She'd been having night sweats for several months and each morning woke up feeling clammy and exhausted. She said, "I came to you because of what you did for Sandra. We both work with natural foods, and I want to go the natural route also. I've started to eat tofu with her every day and am taking the same herbs and vitamins, but they do not seem to be working for me. Maybe I'm not doing it right."

Ellen and I reviewed her regimen, which she had based on Sandra's. I suggested she add l-phenylalanine because she was also having mood problems, and Valerian to help her sleep. These made some difference, but not enough for Ellen. "I'm afraid Sandra won't approve, but I'm thinking that maybe I should try estrogen. When we prepare the food, I'm the one who spends most of the time in the kitchen; it's too uncomfortable having hot flashes while I lean over the stove—especially if I start to drip sweat. Plus, I still wake up at night soaked."

Ellen worried that she was deserting her principles and wondered why what worked for Sandra had not worked for her. I pointed out that she'd given the alternative treatment a very thorough try and ought not to feel she had failed. Her body simply had a different pattern of vulnerabilities than Sandra's and needed a different approach. We worked out a plan using natural progesterone and an estrogen patch. This form of estrogen is derived entirely from plant sources and releases estrogen in a way similar to that of the ovary. She had not wanted Premarin, the preparation made from horses, and I reassured her that the only hormones I prescribe are those made entirely from soy and yams. I also explained that no study has ever shown an increased risk of breast cancer from less than four years of estrogen.

At her next visit Ellen was smiling and reported that her symptoms had nearly gone, that she could sleep through the night, and that her mood was more stable. "But," she said, "I hope that eventually I will be able to get off hormones and go back to soy and herbs." We agreed that we'd reassess her need for estrogen at her follow-up visits every six months.

Sandra and Ellen both had a preference for natural treatments, yet Ellen ended up taking hormones while Sandra did not. Both had similar concerns and on the face of it the same problem: menopause. But their bodies responded differently. Possibly Ellen's ovaries were making less estrogen than Sandra's were, but clearly her body was more vulnerable to estrogen deprivation.

Who made the right decision, Sandra or Ellen? I think both did. HT is a very complex issue for women now, and each woman must decide for herself. Both using estrogen and not using it can be valid decisions.

DECIDING ABOUT YOUR MENOPAUSE

Women have been going through menopause since the human species began; only recently has it been thought of as a medical problem. This has led some critics of modern medicine to suggest that current widespread treatment of menopause is mainly motivated by the marketing efforts of the pharmaceutical industry. Without doubt, this industry has been more than happy to sell hormone replacement preparations. It was aided in this goal by the recent and unfortunate misconception that all women should use HT, rather than just those who are hormonally vulnerable. The rationale for this extensive overtreatment was based on animal and human studies that we now know to have been inadequate. However, in my experience, the main reason that women choose to take HT is not marketing but simply that they do not feel well without it. Some insist that menopausal symptoms are really culturally induced, but this theory does not get you through the night if you keep waking up in a cold sweat.

You may be wondering, how did women in the past make it through the change without treatment? One reason is that they were given no choice. Women's problems were not taken seriously, especially when they were "over the hill," as was then thought to happen at about age forty. Menopause-related complaints were often dismissed as psychosomatic, perhaps due to the dubious "empty nest syndrome"—the assumption that a woman without children at home must feel worthless. Hormonal pessimism, the assumption that having a woman's body means not feeling well a lot of the time, was accepted unquestioningly, not only by doctors but also by women themselves.

Many did not even consider complaining—and those who did were usually not listened to. Now, however, a fifty-year-old woman is likely to be working at a demanding job; if she has children, they are likely to be in their teens and need considerable supervision as they navigate the perils of today's world. She does not have the luxury, if that is the word, of retiring from active life while waiting for her menopausal symptoms to go away. For today's perimenopausal woman, a night without sleep due to night sweats may precede a day of sales calls or critical business meetings where dozing off is not an option. Women's bodies have not changed, but what is expected of them has.

The estrogen decision-making process begins with your answer to a single question: Do you feel well enough without estrogen? If the answer is yes, there is no reason to take it. If on the other hand, your symptoms are making life as much a burden as a joy, estrogen becomes at least a consideration. It comes down, once again, to hormonal vulnerability. Some women breeze through menopause and do not need to consider estrogen. Others have mild symptoms but are able to tough it out. Still others, whose symptoms are more severe, decide, often reluctantly, that they need estrogen to function.

To help you think through whether there is any reason to consider HT, I've provided a self-assessment quiz as a sidebar on page 385. There are three steps in this HT self-assessment. First is to use the quiz to determine how many symptoms you are having and how much they are disrupting your life. Second is to consider if there might be other causes for your symptoms. Because there are so many possibilities, you'll need your doctor's input for this. Third is to weigh the pros and cons of HT for you as an individual. For this, you can use the HT

MENOPAUSE: ASSESSING YOURS

Beside each of the symptoms in this list, write a number between 0 and 3, with 0 being not at all and three being most severe:

Hot flashes that interrupt your activity or make you embarrassingly sweaty. _____

Night sweats that interfere with sleep so that you are not refreshed in the morning. _____

Slowed down thinking, difficulty concentrating, or decreased memory that interfere with work or other activities. _____

Excessive effort needed to keep up with work and home demands. _____

Greater vulnerability to stress. _____

New appearance of mood swings or depression not related to any life event. _____

Loss of energy. _____

Muscle and joint discomfort to the extent that your body almost never feels comfortable. _____

Skin sensitivity so that being touched or combing your hair are uncomfortable. _____

Vaginal dryness or discomfort that take the pleasure out of sex. _____

If your total score is less than 10, you may be in perimenopause or menopause, but symptoms are tolerable—unless you scored a 3 in one or more categories. A score of 10 to 20 or higher indicates definite discomfort, which may or may not be something that you can live with. If your score is higher than 20, menopause is significantly impairing your quality of life and finding relief should be a priority for you.

balance sheet provided on page 387. When you've come to a tentative conclusion, you'll be ready for the next two chapters, which give full details on alternative remedies as well as hormone therapy.

Part of the self-assessment is to consider if there might be other explanations for your symptoms besides menopause. You probably won't sleep well if you are anxious or stressed, whatever is happening with your hormones. Sleep deprivation from worry, pain, or any other cause can make your mind less efficient and your body less comfortable. It's not always easy during perimenopause to figure out which discomforts are due to hormones and which to stress or other factors. One important clue is the onset of the symptom. If you have many of those I've listed in the sidebar, they began at about the same time, and you are in your forties or beyond, there's a good chance that falling estrogen is at least part of the problem. On the other hand, if you've suffered from fatigue or mood swings for many years, perimenopause won't be the whole story—though, it may be part of it.

Once you've done your symptom self-assessment, the next step is to think through whether the advantages of HT will be worth the possible problems. Many women whose bodies are highly vulnerable to the hormonal roller coaster of perimenopause/menopause do discover that their lives are dramatically better with HT. As the stories of Sandra and Ellen illustrate, each woman must make her up her mind for herself. To help you weigh the multiple factors regarding HT, I've itemized them in the sidebar on page 387.

The most important thing to keep in mind as you weigh these assets and liabilities is that whichever decision you make, you are not signing a contract that commits you for the rest of your life. You can change your mind at any point, based on new medical information or simply because you've rethought your situation. A good idea is to plan a reassessment about every six months. Remember that if you are in your forties or early fifties, the risks are small to nonexistent. In a sense, you have a free trial period. You can see whether the actual benefits to you are sufficient to be worth any slight risk or if they are not. I do encourage you to think through any change in your regimen carefully so that you do not go on and off repeatedly. Starting and stopping HT is not necessarily harmful to your body but does confuse it.

HT: THE BALANCE SHEET

Assets:

Restored well-being

Skin more resilient, fewer wrinkles

Hair less likely to thin

Skin, muscles, joints more comfortable

Hot flashes and night sweats go away

Vaginal tissues moister and more flexible for comfortable sex

Bones kept strong

Arteries kept open for better blood flow

Better mood

Quicker memory

Faster thinking

No increased breast cancer risk in the first four years of use.

Liabilities:

Nagging worries about safety

Chance of periods or spotting

Sometimes nausea and breast discomfort (but not if dose is properly individualized)

Not the only way to protect bones

Breast cancer risk increase of 0.8 per 1,000 women per year, after four or more years (Only if both estrogen *and* progestin are used.) No increase if you've had a hysterectomy and need estrogen only.

Stroke and heart attack risk each increase by 0.6 per 1,000 women per year

(Heart attack risk not increased if you take estrogen alone or use a statin to control cholesterol. Daily aspirin may help reduce risk of stroke.)

WHEN MENOPAUSE COMES EARLY

The safety issues with HT concern its use after normal menopause age. In the WHI study, the average age when women started was sixty-three. The obvious implication is that the findings in the study cannot be applied simplistically to younger women in perimenopause or menopause. I've already indicated that the risk is probably very small for women in their early fifties or younger. It's important to realize than neither WHI nor any other large-scale study considered women with early menopause. Here, there is no controversy among medical experts—*when menopause is premature, estrogen reduces health risks, including heart disease and osteoporosis.*

According to textbook definitions, menopause is abnormally early when it occurs before age forty. However, given that the average age of menopause is about fifty-one, even when the change occurs in the mid-forties, it can be considered premature. Since it's normal for a woman's body to have full estrogen levels until her early fifties, taking estrogen if you have early menopause is more natural than not taking it.

25.

How to Feel Good Without Estrogen: Alternative Treatments

My view is that before trying estrogen, it usually makes sense to first consider the alternatives. (There are a few situations, such as right after total hysterectomy or premature menopause, in which starting estrogen promptly is probably best.) Perhaps the greatest change in health care over the past two decades is the explosion in availability of botanical and other alternative healing modalities. While I think that this is overall a good thing, I do have some reservations, as I'll explain.

SOME THOUGHTS REGARDING ALTERNATIVE MEDICINE

I first became interested in alternative medicine as a result of my study of Asian spirituality. From medical school I have been aware, as are a surprising number of other physicians, that Western scientific medicine, despite its marvelous accomplishments, has significant limitations. The public thinks so too, as shown by the enthusiasm with which alternative healing techniques have been taken up. Some physicians are distressed by this trend, but I think doctors must reflect on why so many people are not fully satisfied with orthodox medicine. Not all the criticisms of establishment medicine are fair, but some are;

by being open to other approaches, we can enhance our ability to heal.

In my efforts to consider everything that might help women with hormone problems, I've studied several forms of alternative healing, particularly botanical medicine and meditation. During the twenty years I have practiced and taught meditation, I have come to appreciate the power of spiritual practices to stabilize mind and body, not only against external stresses, but also internal ones such as hormonal shifts. For about a decade I've been prescribing plant- or herb-based remedies, such as soy and vitex, with good results. I've come to avoid prescribing animal source preparations, such as Premarin, since there is virtually always a better option.

Yet, there is another side to alternative healing that is less positive. In my practice, I often see women who have been subjected to treatments that are ineffective, or even harmful, carried out by self-styled healers whose knowledge of the conditions they purport to treat is minimal. Even alternative practitioners who are sincere may not be aware of the limitations of their method. An example is the use of acupuncture for alopecia; some women I see have lost valuable months being poked by needles before finally realizing that nothing was happening. This is not to say that acupuncture never works, but I have rarely seen it work for hormonal skin and hair problems.

In some areas, for example thyroid conditions, some alternative practices have caused real harm. I've seen some women placed on excessive doses of the powerful hormones made by this gland; the result can be nervousness, decreased concentration, hair loss, thinning of bone, even heart problems. Since alternative medicine is largely unregulated, you are on your own with respect to safety and effectiveness. Alternative medicine magazines are not reliable because, like other consumer magazines, they see their function as helping their advertisers sell products. This does not mean that the products are necessarily bad, but it does mean that much of what you read about them is not objective. Similarly, sales personnel in health food stores are there to sell; they lack real training in nutrition and have no qualifications to make diagnoses.

It is far from my intent to discredit alternative medicine across the board, but simply to warn that not everything alternative can be trusted. The basic problem is incomplete information. This is gradually being remedied as some excellent scientists devote themselves to research in this field.

A final admonition before I move on to the positive aspects: *Just because something is a vitamin or supplement does not guarantee that it is safe—they can have risks just as prescription medications can. Decisions about alternative therapies should be made with the same care as those regarding conventional medical ones.*

BOTANICAL MEDICINE FOR MENOPAUSE

Menopause is one of the conditions for which alternative and nutritional treatments have an important place. Though the number of supplements now available is overwhelming, I felt it would be most helpful to limit what I cover here to those few for which there is evidence of effectiveness and safety.

Black cohosh This is the most widely used herb for relief of menopausal symptoms. The most familiar brand is Remifemin. Evening primrose oil has been used as well. Although there was much enthusiasm for these a decade ago, controlled studies have not demonstrated any reduction of symptoms. Nonetheless, some women report that black cohosh helps them, so it is reasonable to try, if hot flashes are mild. If you don't have a clear benefit within about a month, there is no point in continuing. The cost of such preparations can be considerable, and they are not covered by insurance.

Soy Considerable evidence supports the effectiveness of soy as a treatment for menopause. Several studies reported reduction of hot flashes, as well as reduction of elevated cholesterol levels. In monkey studies, soy has inhibited development of cardiovascular disease. Yet the effectiveness and even safety of soy are debated. My reading of the evidence has led me to conclude that soy is beneficial. Most persuasive is the dramatically lower incidence of breast, endometrial, and prostate cancer in countries with very high dietary soy intake, such as Japan, Singapore, China, and Australia. In fact, the highest life expectancy in the entire world is in Okinawa, where soy consumption is extremely high. This Japanese protection against heart disease and breast cancer cannot be attributed to better genes because it is lost with change to a more Western, meat-intensive diet. The better health of Japanese on their traditional high soy diet makes it hard to argue that this food is anything but beneficial.

Soy has two important kinds of active ingredients. The isoflavones are phytoestrogens; that is, they have slight estrogen-like effects. However, they also partially block estrogen, which could account for a protective effect against cancer. It is the isoflavones that help menopausal symptoms. Also beneficial for health are special proteins that lower cholesterol.

Most research, although not all, has confirmed beneficial effects of soy preparations on menopause symptoms and on cholesterol. The limitation of most of the studies is that they used isolates of various soy ingredients, assuming that these will have the same effects as whole soy. As with fruits and vegetables generally, to get the health benefits of soy you need to eat the complete food, not simply pop it in capsule form. Soy extracts lack the cholesterol-lowering proteins and may not contain adequate amounts of isoflavones. Use of supplements can be a cop-out—the hope that one can gain the benefits of a healthy diet just by swallowing a pill. Processed forms of soy may also lack the healthy ingredients.

If you want to try soy as a way of controlling menopausal symptoms, you will need to use the real thing. About one cup a day of tofu or two cups of soy milk should be enough. I suggest soy milk should be the fresh form sold in milk cartons, but the powdered forms are an alternative. If you do not like the taste and texture of tofu, addition of seasoned sauces can help as can mixing with other foods in a stir fry. Soy can also be blended in fruit smoothies.

It is not clear that soy will work for everyone. The long-term health benefits seem to be due to an isoflavone metabolite called equol, but not all humans convert the soy isoflavone daidzein to equol; those who do not may not benefit. Overall, however, soy is the most effective botanical for control of menopausal hot flashes. The quality of protein in soy is high, so it can be a good substitute for less healthy protein sources, such as red meat—which, among other things, increases the risk of breast and colon cancer.

Lots of scare talk has dissuaded many women from using soy. In evaluating this, keep in mind that the antisoy forces have some hidden agendas. First, not only the meat producers, but also other segments of the food and restaurant industries have a vested interest in meat consumption. There is also a subtle cultural prejudice against any trend toward vegetarianism. Many recall our mothers insisting that meat was necessary for us to grow. The health food industry also has a stake in the antisoy propaganda because it is a vegetable-based food that they do not control or profit from. Yet, a balanced look at the evidence shows that soy is one of the healthiest foods a woman can eat.

DONG QUAI: THE WORLD'S OLDEST MENOPAUSE REMEDY

Herbal preparations for female problems have been used for thousands of years. One still still widely used is dong quai, an herb consumed by millions of Chinese women to "nurture yin." As with many such traditional botanicals, it is difficult to translate its effects into the concepts of Western medicine.

Dong quai is available in expensive capsules at health food stores and quite inexpensive dried root in Chinese herbal pharmacies and groceries. My preference would be for the latter because the raw form is less likely to be adulterated.

Though dong quai itself does not have estrogenic effects in women, one cannot assume that preparations are unadulterated. I know of one woman who took a powder allegedly made of ground up pearls—believed by many Chinese women to give a clear, pearl-like complexion. (Tiny pearls are also put in the eyes to make them brighter; this I definitely do not recommend!) After taking the pearl powder, she began to have spotting. The only plausible explanation is that the preparation was spiked with estrogen. Sadly, one cannot be sure of avoiding estrogen, if one uses Chinese herbal preparations. There are many other examples of such adulteration, sometimes with dangerous substances; for example, a probably effective prostate cancer medicine was banned by the FDA after it was found to contain rat poison. With Chinese medications, one does not know what one is getting. Japanese herbal products (kempo) are prepared to high standards but are not readily available in the United States. I do think the Chinese botanical medicine tradition has much to offer, but we will not be able to use it with confidence until manufacturing is effectively regulated. The same is true of Indian Ayurvedic preparations.

Vitex (chasteberry) is definitely helpful for PMS, especially breast discomfort. Since PMS is also set off by hormonal swings, Vitex is worth a try for menopausal symptoms. Vitamin E may have some slight benefit for flashes and sweats. Safety issues with E are covered in chapter 6.

MONITORING WHILE ON ALTERNATIVE MENOPAUSE TREATMENTS

With the possible exception of soy, none of the herbs that have been tried for relief of menopausal symptoms will protect bone. Soy does seem to be good for bones but is less potent than estrogen or recently developed bone-conserving medications. For this reason, if you opt for the no-hormone route, you will still need to have your bones monitored with the DXA test. (Maintaining bone health is covered in chapter 27.

Alternative and hormonal treatments are not mutually incompatible. Soy, for example, can be supplemented with a low dose of estrogen. Nor does estrogen have to be forever. Alternative treatments tend to work slowly; if symptoms are so severe as to disrupt your life, you might consider using estrogen until things are back in order, and then seeing if the natural approaches will maintain the benefit.

NONHORMONAL MEDICATIONS FOR MENOPAUSE

A number of medications have been reported to diminish hot flashes and night sweats. Some women get a good result with them, so they are worth a try if your hot flashes are disruptive and you do not want, or cannot take, estrogen. None is an ideal solution because, for some women, their side effects can be worse than the flashes they are supposed to control.

Effexor (venlafaxine) is an antidepressant that can help hot flashes, according to well-designed studies. The problem with Effexor is that it can produce what psychopharmacologists refer to as "activation"—a delicate way of saying that it makes some people feel extremely hyper.

It's worth a try because some women feel fine on it and have fewer flashes, but if you dislike its mental effects, it is probably not worth it. The dose is 37.5 to 75 mg daily. Other antidepressants that have been studied to see if they help flashes include Prozac (fluoxetine) and Paxil (paroxetine), but I have been less impressed with these, and Paxil in particular can cause weight gain. A variety of other drugs have been tried, including Neurontin (gabapentin), which does not seem very effective, and clonidine, which causes drowsiness. The latter might be tried at bedtime, but you need to be cautious about getting up suddenly because dizziness may also be a problem. Given that hot flashes are triggered by events in the central nervous system, the failure to find a more satisfactory CNS-active drug to control hot flashes is disappointing. Nonetheless, Effexor or other antidepressants do work for some women.

26

If You've Decided to Try Estrogen: Choosing the Best Preparation for You

If you want to try hormone therapy for perimenopause/menopause, you will need to pick a specific preparation. Some are clearly better than others, but standard sources rarely give the whole story. Because women need more than banal generalities about estrogen and progesterone, I will tell it like it is, even revealing inside information that most doctors don't know. In doing so, I will spill the beans on why some of the most popular hormone preparations are among the worst. First, I'll go over the general principles then, at the end of the chapter, you will find a practical guide to reducing estrogen risks as well as a quick reference guide that reveals names and tells tales about all the popular forms of HT.

ORAL CONTRACEPTIVES AND MENOPAUSE

It's hard to tell exactly when perimenopause is far enough along that pregnancy is no longer possible. For this reason, unless you can be completely certain that your ovaries have shut down, it's safest to continue to use contraception. It's rare, but women in their fifties do sometimes get pregnant. You probably don't need contraception if you haven't had periods for several months, are experiencing hot flashes, and have an FSH over 20—but check with your gyn to be sure. (FSH goes up when the ovary runs out of egg cells.)

Birth control pills are a convenient way to get both HT and contraception at the same time. However, standard pills provide estrogen for only twenty-one days out of each twenty-eight day cycle, not all the time as HT regimens do. Once you are in perimenopause/menopause, your ovaries will no longer make enough estrogen to keep you comfortable through the inactive pill week. One solution is to use the OC Mircette (generic, Kariva), which has active pills for twenty-six days out of twenty-eight days. The other option is to apply an estrogen patch during the last seven days of each pill cycle. Climara is convenient because each patch lasts for a week. Women in their late forties or even very early fifties can use the same OCs as any other women. (At the end of chapter 4, you'll find a guide to picking the best pill for your body.) OCs often soothe moods when used at perimenopause because the ovary no longer has to strain to make enough estrogen. If you are vulnerable to mood swings on OCs, you can get equally good symptom relief with an individually customized hormone regimen using an estrogen patch and natural progesterone.

Though it was once thought that the pill should be stopped by the time a woman reaches thirty-five, it is now recognized that the main pill risks after this age are confined to smokers. If you do not smoke and have no specific contraindications, you can remain on the pill until your early fifties. There is no exact cutoff, but I suggest considering changing to HT around the time you reach fifty stretch though you can it out a little longer. If you are taking an OC, you may not know when you go through menopause because the hormones in the pill prevent symptoms and keep periods coming. For this reason, if you are in your mid-forties or older when you go off the pill, you should be prepared for the possibility of menopause symptoms appearing suddenly. Options for controlling symptoms are the same as when perimenopause/menopause declare themselves under other circumstances.

PILLS, PATCHES, GELS, AND RINGS

Estrogen comes in several different forms: pills, patches, gels, and vaginal rings. Implants and injections were once used but are now obsolete. Having done research on all the main forms, I have come to consider the patch to be best for most women. The advantages of patch estrogen are listed in the sidebar on this page.

For the reasons listed in the sidebar, the patch is actually the most bioidentical form of estrogen. The second most natural is estradiol gel. Estradiol in pill form (Estrace and generics) comes in only third because much is converted to another estrogen—estrone—as it travels through the liver. Most of the other oral forms, including the notorious Premarin, contain forms of estrogen that otherwise never occur in the human body. Estradiol gels have been used by European women for decades but have only recently been introduced into the United States. When I did research on Estrogel more than ten years ago, most of the women in the study liked it. Since then, however, patches have improved to the point where I regard them as the first choice over gels,

---

WHY PATCHES ARE THE BEST WAY TO TAKE ESTROGEN

All contain estradiol, the most natural estrogen, derived from yam and soy.

Blood levels are much smoother than with pills, avoiding the ups and downs that can set off hormonal vulnerability.

Release of the hormone into the blood more closely mimics that of the ovary.

Passes through the liver gradually, not all at once as happens with oral estrogen.

Less estradiol ends up as estrone, a less desirable estrogen.

More accurate dosing than with gels.

which are less convenient to apply and produce less consistent blood levels. On the other hand, if you get significant skin irritation from the patch, the gel is a good alternative.

Another way to get even release of estradiol is the Femring vaginal ring. This is inserted into the upper vagina like a diaphragm (though it does not provide contraception) and releases estrogen for three months. It offers less flexibility in dosing than the patch, but requires less attention. Discomfort is rarely a problem, yet not all women like the idea of using a device that stays in the vagina. From a medical point-of-view, there is nothing wrong with getting estrogen through the vagina, however.

ESTROGEN IN PILL FORM

While pills are not ideal, they are still a viable choice if patches or gels don't work out for you, or you simply don't like the idea of putting something on your skin. I can think of no reason to use anything other than estradiol, since the other forms are not natural to the human body and have no advantages. Orally effective estradiol has been available only for about twenty years because it requires a technology known as micronization, which produces pills able to disintegrate in the stomach. Without micronization, estradiol or progesterone will pass through your stomach and intestines without being completely absorbed. The first brand of micronized estradiol to be developed was Estrace. I still recommend this over generic, if you can afford it, because proper manufacturing is necessary for the hormone to get into your body.

Estradiol does not stay in the blood for very long. Though the manufacturer recommends taking the entire dose at once, you can get a better result with the same amount of estradiol by dividing it into two or, if you can remember, three doses. (The total daily amount stays the same. For example, if you have been taking a 2 mg Estrace tablet once a day, dividing your dose would mean taking 1 mg twice a day.) Especially if you are hormonally vulnerable, you are likely to feel better with the smoother levels you get with a divided dose. For those who have alopecia, the daily estrogen dips that occur with any oral form are potentially bad for your hair follicles, so the patch is definitely the best bet.

I've saved the worst estrogen for last. For reasons that I cannot fathom, the oldest estrogen is still the most widely prescribed. This is Premarin or conjugated equine estrogens (CEE), a.k.a. horse estrogen. My negative view of this preparation is not simply because I am a vegetarian. CEE is, to my mind, an irrational preparation because it contains forms of estrogen that otherwise do not occur in the human body. To be fair, there is no proof that Premarin is bad for women—though it was the estrogen used in the WHI study—but there is also no proof that it is as safe as more natural forms. Given the lack of research comparing Premarin to estradiol, it seems to me plain common sense to go with the natural form. (Actually, research was done in an effort to find special health advantages from using CEE instead of estradiol, but it never panned out.) The argument many doctors use to justify prescribing Premarin is that it has been around for decades and works in controlling symptoms. To me this is a nonargument. There are plenty of drugs that are properly forgotten when better ones come along.

NATURAL AND BIOIDENTICAL ESTROGEN
AND PROGESTERONE

Suzanne Somers's popular book, *The Sexy Years*, advocates the use of hormones that are "bioidentical." This term implies estrogen and progesterone that are identical to those normally made by the human ovary. If bioidentical is defined this way, I agree that the natural forms of the hormones are the best ones to use. Unfortunately, various forms of estrogen are promoted by compounding pharmacies as "natural" or "bioidentical" that are not. We need to look critically when something is billed as *natural* or *bioidentical* because use of these terms is entirely unregulated. (There are rules about what can be labeled "organic," but this applies to foods, not medications or supplements.) In my view transdermal estrogen, although it employs advanced technology, is far more natural in how it affects the body than is possible with any oral preparation.

Compounding pharmacies prepare medications on their own premises. The implication that such preparations are somehow more natural is misleading because the ingredients are actually bought in bulk from chemical companies. Some women have been misled into thinking that the only way to avoid horse or other nonhuman estrogen is to buy a compounded preparation. This is totally untrue; all patches, as well as oral estradiol, are bioidentical and derived solely from plant sources. As I have already emphasized, transdermal estrogen more closely mimics nature than pills; all oral forms, including those compounded by a pharmacy, have the same problems of wavering blood levels and excessive effects on the liver.

An example of the sort of preparation that is billed as bioidentical, but should be avoided, is what is commonly called "TriEs," a mixture of all three forms of human estrogens. A usual claim implied in promoting TriEs is that one of its ingredients, estriol, can protect against breast cancer. This is based on a theory that was already on its way out when I was in medical school. More recent research suggests that estriol may actually *increase* breast cancer risk. TriEs does include estradiol, but it also contains estrone, a form of estrogen that is made in fat tissue and sometimes predominates after menopause. This is generally considered less desirable than estradiol.

A further problem with compounded preparations, especially creams and gels, is that they may not contain accurate amounts of hormones—it is actually very difficult to get the exact concentration of hormone into a topical; adequate quality control is very expensive. Furthermore, compounding pharmacies in the United States do not test their products to be sure the concentration is identical from batch to batch, or even within different areas of the same tube of cream or gel. (Pharmacy standards are much better regulated in Germany, which leads the world in assuring safety of alternative preparations.) Perhaps the biggest worry with compounded preparations is that they are never tested in actual use by women, so their safety and effectiveness can only be guessed at.

I hope I have made it clear that compounded does not equal bioidentical. *I do agree with the principle that HT should be as natural as possible. However my view, based on years of doing research on several forms of estrogen, is that transdermal forms are the most bioidentical.*

ESTROGEN FOR A YOUTHFUL VAGINA

Different parts of a woman's body need different amounts of estrogen. Bones need the least and the hair, usually, the most. The vaginal tissues are somewhere in between. Some women whose hot flashes and other bodily discomforts are adequately relieved by a moderate dose of patch or oral estrogen still find that their vaginal tissues are drier than is comfortable. When this happens, there is no need to expose the entire body to a higher level because estrogen can be applied directly into the vagina. Several forms are available: Estrace (estradiol) cream; Estring, a small ring of plastic-like material that is impregnated with estradiol, and Vagifem; a small tablet designed for easy vaginal insertion. The cream's advantage is an added moisturizing and lubricating effect; its disadvantages are inconvenience and slight messiness. Premarin comes in cream form as well but has no particular advantage over estradiol. The ring lasts for about three months; discomfort is unusual. (Note that Estring and Femring, mentioned earlier, are somewhat different. Estring supplies estrogen for the vagina, while Femring provides a larger amount for whole body estrogen replacement.) The Vagifem tablet is more convenient than the cream, but if the vagina is very thin and dry—as can happen when menopause occurred some years previously—insertion can be uncomfortable at first. A solution is to start with the cream, then if you prefer, you can switch to the tablets or ring some weeks later— after tissues have become moister and more resilient. Many women tell me that they are happy with the cream, however.

The ring and Vagifem have fixed doses. Estrace cream comes with a soft plastic applicator that allows it to be inserted much like a tampon. Although the smallest marking on the applicator is 1 gm, half this amount two or three times a week is usually adequate. If you are very dry or sore, you can start with 1 gm daily for the first two to four weeks, then cut back. Most notice improvement within a couple of weeks, but it may take a little longer if you've been estrogen deficient for several years.

Intravaginal estrogen by itself will not always restore the resiliency of pelvic tissues sufficiently for comfortable sex. It supplements, rather than replaces, patch or oral estrogen. Since intravaginal estrogen is sometimes absorbed enough to affect the uterine lining; unless you have had a hysterectomy, you'll probably need a form of progesterone as well.

Doctors do not always think to mention supplementing oral or patch estrogen with intravaginal forms, so don't be reluctant to suggest it for yourself, if dryness is a problem.

WHAT ABOUT PROGESTERONE?

If the lining of the uterus (endometrium) is continually exposed to estrogen but not progesterone, its cells can grow out of control; this in turn can lead to cancer. This sometimes happens during perimenopause or menopause when the ovary is still making estrogen but cannot make progesterone. (Another possible cause of progesterone deficiency is PCOS, covered in chapter 21.) In the early days of menopausal hormone replacement, estrogen was given alone—until it was finally recognized that this put women at risk for endometrial cancer. This is not as grim as it sounds because endometrial cancer is almost completely preventable by providing its natural adversary, progesterone. For this reason, a form of progesterone is included in all HT regimens, unless a woman has had her uterus removed, in which case progesterone is not necessary. All you need to do is to take natural or synthetic progesterone for at least twelve days in a row, every one or two months. OCs work too because they provide more than ample progestin to prevent overgrowth of the uterine lining.

Taking progesterone as part of menopausal HT may mean having to put up with periods, though they are usually light. Most typically these start about two days after you finish the medication, but they can begin earlier, while you are still taking it. When this happens, you still need to finish out the twelve days to get the cancer protection. If you are on a very low dose of estrogen, you may not have noticeable bleeding after finishing the progesterone. This is nothing to worry about; what is important is that your uterus be exposed to the anticancer effect of progesterone, not that you bleed.

Many women are placed on so-called continuous-combined regimens in which both estrogen and progestin are taken every day. The idea is to get the protective effect without having periods. This sounds good, but in reality about 70 percent of women on this type of regimen spot on and off for months. The bleeding tends to be quite light, but still gets tiresome. There is an even more important reason to take only the minimum amount of progestin needed for endometrial protection: In the WHI study, it was the daily use of Provera that seemed to increase breast cancer risk, not estrogen. Given these findings, it seems prudent to take progesterone, whether natural or synthetic, only intermittently for twelve days every month or every other month. It may seem paradoxical that progesterone decreases the risk of one form of cancer, that of the endometrium, only to possibly increase the risk of another, that of the breast. The reason is that the breast and uterus are hormonally vulnerable in different ways.

WHEN PROGESTERONE IS UNNECESSARY

The only established use for progesterone as part of HT is endometrial cancer protection. If you have had a hysterectomy, you have no uterus and so cannot get endometrial cancer. Yet some women whose uterus has been removed are still given progesterone.

You may have read that after menopause women should have their estrogen and progesterone "balanced." Sometimes a progesterone blood level is obtained and declared to be low. This borders on deception because after menopause, the ovary never makes progesterone, and so all women's levels are unmeasurable. Some practitioners urge giving progesterone after menopause and checking blood levels. This is bizarre. There is no normal level for progesterone after menopause except zero. If you have gone through a hysterectomy, one of the benefits is that HT is simpler and safer because you do not need progesterone. There is absolutely no evidence that taking progesterone has any benefit other than endometrial cancer protection, and so I do not recommend it for women who've had a hysterectomy. As I have emphasized, for those women who do have their uterus, only the minimum amount of progesterone needed to protect against endometrial cancer should be used.

ESTROGEN-PROGESTIN COMBINATIONS

A variety of combination preparations put estrogen and a progestin together in one pill or patch. These are designed for the average woman, and they work well—if you're average. On the other hand, if you are hormonally vulnerable, you will probably do better with separate estrogen and progesterone. Although it is slightly less convenient to use two preparations, this allows the dose of each to be separately matched to your body's needs. For this reason, I rarely prescribe the combinations. I've found that with more flexible forms I can virtually always work out a regimen that restores well-being, even for women whose hormonal disposition is very delicately tuned.

If you have been using a fixed combination and feel perfectly fine, there is no arguing with success, and it is quite reasonable to take the attitude of "if it ain't broke, don't fix it." However, if your symptoms are mostly gone but still sneak up on you from time to time, you might feel even better using a regimen customized for your body. With most of the fixed combinations, you take progestin every day; I've already explained why I don't think this is a good idea.

IF YOU TRIED ESTROGEN, BUT IT DIDN'T HELP OR MADE YOU WORSE

It takes about a month to start to experience the benefits of estrogen therapy. Some effects take a bit longer, especially the recovery of vaginal tissues. If you are not starting to feel better after a month, you may need a higher dose. However, if symptoms are starting to improve, it's reasonable to wait a little longer.

In my practice, I see women who've become discouraged about HT, which they started in the hopes of feeling better, only to discover that it made them feel worse. These women are hormonally vulnerable and need to be on exactly the right dose to feel well. The same amount will have very different effects on a forty-six-year-old woman who is just transitioning into perimenopause and a fifty-four-year-old woman who has had very low levels for several years.

If you are in perimenopause or just recently stopped menstruating, you can usually start on an intermediate dose of estrogen right away without discomfort. This would be a 0.0375 or 0.05 patch. On the other hand, if your estrogen has been very low for several years, its essential to begin HT gradually, so your body can get used to it gradually. The symptoms produced by a too sudden estrogen jump are breast tenderness and nausea—milder versions of what happens in early pregnancy, when levels zoom up even faster. Later in pregnancy these symptoms go away because the body has become acclimated to higher estrogen levels. Estrogen levels rise at puberty too, but so slowly as not to cause symptoms.

The solution is to mimic the way estrogen rises gradually during puberty by starting on a very small dose and increasing in small steps. How low to start and how quickly to go up depends on how long your estrogen has been low and on your own degree of vulnerability. The sidebar gives a method I developed that enables even the most hormonally vulnerable woman to start estrogen comfortably. This method brings your dose up gradually while minimizing the chance of setbacks, such as sore breasts. While breast tenderness is not a sign of impending cancer, it still hurts.

I don't want to make starting estrogen sound complicated or difficult. For most women, getting on HT goes smoothly. Many times, the schedule I have given can be done a little faster. This book is for women who are hormonally vulnerable, however, so I felt I needed to give a method that will work even if you've previously had difficulties taking estrogen. This gentle way of starting estrogen is outlined in the sidebar on page 407.

PROGESTERONE PROBLEMS

I've already given you the good news about progesterone, which is that taking it can prevent a common form of female cancer. The bad news is that it can bring on PMS-like feelings. Since the main point of HT is to make you feel better, it's more than frustrating if it has the opposite effect. This is mostly a problem with the synthetic progestin Provera, one of the least woman-friendly drugs in existence, which might even be called "PMS in a pill." If you feel out of sorts on this or another synthetic form of progesterone, changing to the natural form usually solves the problem. (Natural progesterone is available by prescription as Prometrium. Compounding pharmacies market their own versions, but these tend to be less reliable and costlier.) There are some hints that Provera may not be good for the heart or breasts; even if you feel okay on it, you may want to switch to Prometrium.

A few women are particularly vulnerable to progesterone and so

THE GENTLEST WAY TO START ESTROGEN

Patches are best because they avoid the swings that occur with pills and also permit fine-tuning your dose.

Start with the Menostar patch, which is the lowest dose available.

The next dose steps are: 0.025, 0.0375, and 0.05. Increase your dose at four week intervals, but more slowly if you develop either morning nausea or breast tenderness. You can go up faster, at two week intervals, if you are not having any side effects whatsoever.

If you do have nausea or breast discomfort:

If mild, stay at your present dose until the discomfort goes away. This sometimes takes a few weeks.

If severe, cut the dose to the previous level. If this does not help, it may be best to stop for a month or so. Vitex (see chapter 6) may help.

Once you are at 0.05, hold for at least two months to see if your symptoms are controlled.

Dose can be further increased to 0.075 or 0.1, if absolutely needed to control symptoms.

If you cannot use the patch, you can use micronized estradiol tablets. The steps are half of a 0.5 mg tablet once a day, then twice a day, then a whole 0.5 mg tablet twice a day. If this does not control your symptoms, you can work up to 1 mg twice a day.

Micronized progesterone (Prometrium) should be taken for at least twelve days on alternate months. You can start when you have been on estrogen for two or three months.

It's essential to work out your individual plan with your doctor. There may be other factors in your situation that would require a different approach.

have mood problems even with the natural form; this is not surprising when one remembers that this hormone can play a role in PMS. Here I have to give just the sort of advice I try my best to avoid: to try to tough it out for those twelve days every other month. Remember, by taking progesterone you are protecting yourself against a form of cancer. If the mood changes are just too much to bear, there are two options. One is to start an antidepressant from a week before you start the progesterone until you are finished—this is an adaptation of a proven PMS treatment. The last resort is to take estrogen only but with very careful monitoring of your endometrium. If you begin to spot, a common event when estrogen is taken alone, try stopping for about five days to let the bleeding run its course and then resume. Bleeding can be a sign of endometrial overgrowth and so needs to be checked out by your gyn.

I do need to emphasize that estrogen by itself is only for those few women who are extremely vulnerable to any form of progesterone. *If you are on HT and have your uterus, but don't take regular progesterone for at least twelve days every other month, it is vital that you be monitored closely by your gynecologist to be sure you are not developing endometrial hyperplasia, which can be a precursor to endometrial cancer.* This can be done by endometrial biopsy, an office procedure. Fortunately, the biopsy can detect abnormalities before they turn into cancer.

WHAT YOUR DOCTOR SHOULD NOT TELL YOU ABOUT MENOPAUSE

Ever since Dr. Katharina Dalton advocated progesterone for PMS, it has been promoted on and off as the wonder hormone for all female ills. The present fad for progesterone cream was kicked off by a book entitled *What Your Doctor May Not Tell You About Menopause* by Dr. John R. Lee and Virginia Hopkins. Building on the popularity of Dr. Lee's book, the alternative health establishment has been marketing progesterone creams relentlessly. Significantly, not a single mainstream menopause expert thinks that progesterone cream is effective in treating anything. Fortunately, its popularity seems to be waning as more and more women discover that it does not help them.

Nor can it be assumed that progesterone cream is innocuous. I've already explained that the WHI study suggests that it was the synthetic progesterone, that increased breast cancer and heart attack risk. While we hope that natural progesterone will not have this risk, this remains to be proven. A second problem with progesterone creams is erratic blood levels. Since progesterone swings are involved in PMS, the creams may actually aggravate hormonal vulnerability for some women. Third, *progesterone in cream form does do not protect against endometrial cancer because too little is absorbed.*

If you are wondering why you have heard such wonderful things about progesterone creams, let me share an experience that will give you insight into how unbalanced coverage in the alternative health media can be. About a year ago, I was interviewed by a writer at *Alternative Medicine* magazine for a story about progesterone creams. I explained my concerns, just as I have to you in this chapter. It was clear that the reporter understood these safety issues because she asked many questions about them. However, when the article appeared, there was no mention whatsoever that progesterone creams may not be effective or even safe. It was a pure promotion piece. Since the alternative medicine establishment is not always up front about problems with its treatments, we cannot place automatic reliance on its claims. Conventional medicine is far from perfect, but drug problems do eventually get out into the open.

HOW MUCH ESTROGEN SHOULD I TAKE AND FOR HOW LONG?

Current official recommendations are to take as low a dose as possible for as short a time as possible. This sounds reasonable but is really too vague to be helpful. The old teaching was that most women can stop HT after a year or two without their symptoms reemerging. No doubt this is true for some women, but for those who are vulnerable to low estrogen, symptoms can be troublesome for a decade or more after menopause. A good approach is to try tapering your dose after one to two years to see if you will feel comfortable on less. If you start to feel bad, then you'll need to made a decision as to whether to go back to your previous, higher dose.

The following sidebar gives a guide to the various doses and their effects.

ESTROGEN DOSING—WHAT THOSE STRANGE NUMBERS MEAN

It's not enough to pick the right kind of estrogen; to get a good result without side effects you need to be on the right amount. Estrogen doses are confusing; they vary between different preparations, and some are rather odd-looking decimal fractions. In this sidebar, I give a general idea of the effect of each dose.

The first number is the dose for the patch, which is the number of milligrams that are absorbed into your body during each twenty-four hour day. Doses for pills seem higher, but that is because not all is absorbed; I've given the equivalent doses for oral estradiol and Premarin in parenthesis. Keep in mind that your response may differ from the averages I've given here.

0.014—(Available only as Menostar.) The lowest dose available. Mainly for osteoporosis prevention but can help mild symptoms.

The following doses are available as Vivelle Dot, Climara, Alora, Esclim, and others. (Not all sizes are available in all brands.)

0.025—Reduces symptoms for a few women, but by no means all. (Estradiol 0.5 mg; Premarin 0.3 mg).

0.0375—The next step up, but still too low if symptoms are severe.

0.05—A high proportion of women get adequate relief at this level. (Estradiol 1 mg; Premarin 0.625 mg.)

0.075 and 0.1—These are the highest dose patches. They usually control even severe symptoms, such as those that occur after removal of the ovaries. These doses are sometimes needed to control alopecia. (Estradiol 1.5 and 2.0 mg; Premarin 0.9 and 1.25 mg).

The best plan is to start on a low dose, then work up at one month intervals as in the sidebar on page 407. There is no best dose for all women, but there is a best dose for each individual.

Because accurate patch manufacture is complex, I do not recommend generic estradiol patches at this time.

PATCH PROBLEMS

Throughout this book I have presented alternatives whenever possible, based on the obvious fact that women's bodies are not all alike. While the patch is the best form of estrogen for most women, a few do have problems with it.

Very mild skin irritation is common but can be minimized by switching sides each time you change the patch. Be sure not to put it on any area of skin that is irritated. The slight redness you may notice just after you pull off the old patch generally resolves quite quickly. If it persists, 2.5 percent hydrocortisone cream can be applied; once is usually enough. Some women notice a dark ring around the edge where the adhesive has oozed out and lint has stuck to it. This comes off easily with cotton soaked in a little rubbing alcohol.

A few women find that the patch does not stick well to their skin. If one brand of patch does not stick well, another can be tried. If the patch comes loose, try pressing it back on. If it still will not stick, you'll need to apply a new patch.

I've seen a few women who were using the patch correctly but did not get symptom relief. Blood tests showed that the estradiol was not being absorbed. Why this happens has not been studied; I assume something is different about the chemistry of their skin surface, though it looks perfectly normal. If the patch does not seem to be working, despite an adequate dose, measuring your estradiol, preferably on the second day of a patch, can determine if you are having an absorption problem.

WHAT NOT TO DO ABOUT MENOPAUSE: EILEEN'S STORY

Some unscrupulous practitioners capitalize on the fears engendered by the WHI study to lure patients with nonstandard treatments that they claim are "holistic" or "bioidentical," but may actually be quite bizarre. The pitfalls facing women today as they try to negotiate their health care are illustrated by the story of Eileen, one of my patients.

Eileen had hot flashes, night sweats, and vaginal dryness, all of which she recognized as due to menopause. But there was more: Eileen could not sleep, felt anxious much of the time, had lost her sex drive, had aches and pains, and thought her memory was slower than before. She had thoroughly researched HT and made a decision to try it in the hope of getting relief from symptoms that had gotten progressively more severe. A few months earlier, she had consulted her regular gynecologist, who recommended Prempro. Eileen quite sensibly did not want either the horse estrogen or the synthetic progestin continued in this preparation. Hoping for a more natural approach, she next went to a doctor who claimed to be "holistic" and prescribed a bevy of hormones in cream form that could be obtained only from a nearby compounding pharmacy. Eileen showed me these creams, each packaged in a plastic syringe, supposedly to help her measure the dose, though the syringes were too large to permit accurate measurement of the small amounts she was supposed to use. The hormones claimed to be present in the various creams included estradiol, estrone, estriol, progesterone, and testosterone. After trying the creams for three days, Eileen had to stop. As she told me, "I felt absolutely awful on them." Worst of all was an intense headache, "like my brain was in a vice." When she returned to the holistic doctor for help, she was told haughtily that no other woman had ever reacted that way and was summarily dropped as a patient. No less rigid than some conventional doctors, the holistic one had refused to consider that Eileen might react differently to the hormones that she had prescribed—in short, that she was hormonally vulnerable.

The main reason Eileen felt so bad was that the hormones were given in greatly excessive amounts, particularly for a woman whose estrogen levels had been extremely low for several years. Though Eileen's hormonal vulnerability was not extreme, this ill-conceived regimen was too much for her. Understandably apprehensive about trying hormones again, she believed, correctly, that without estrogen she would continue to feel terrible.

I am baffled that any doctor could suppose that abruptly starting a menopausal woman on a mixture of just about every possible female hormone, plus one male hormone, could be considered natural—yet, that is how the regimen was presented to Eileen. The doctor who prescribed it was holistic in name only. She clearly did not consider the whole person in her treatment approach. Nor is Eileen's story unique. Almost every week I see women whose menopausal discomforts could have been relieved by a carefully individualized dose of estradiol, but who were placed on other forms of estrogen with poor results.

Eileen's story had a happy ending. She started the patch using the slow-but-sure regimen I detailed in the earlier sidebar on page 407. Although she did not feel much better on the starting dose, once she reached 0.05, she felt fine. As she put it, "I'm myself again." As so often, the solution was not to use exotic and untested hormone preparations, but to use standard ones properly.

When women are given hormones misrepresented as bioidentical and end up feeling worse, their confidence is shaken, as Eileen's was. Worse, doctors sometimes respond with annoyance toward patients who do not react to medication as expected. This can lead women to fear that they are a little crazy, when all they are is hormonally vulnerable. What enabled Eileen to finally get effective treatment was a trait that is all too necessary in dealing with the health care system today: perseverance. It shouldn't take true grit to get the help you need, but in reality it often does. Eileen had seen both a conventional gynecologist and a "holistic" doctor who supposedly specialized in bioidentical hormone treatment. Yet, both failed to give her an estrogen regimen that suited her needs. If this is happening to you, my first advice is: Don't give up and don't ever forget that you have a right to treatment tailored to your individual vulnerabilities. If you are not getting what you need, summon up your determination as Eileen did, refuse treatments you don't want, and keep looking until you find the doctor who can help you.

ESTROGEN: HOW TO MINIMIZE THE RISKS

Although it is clear that the risks of HT can be dramatically reduced, critical information on how to do this has not gotten out to women who need it. It is as if we were warned that driving is dangerous without being told to wear seat belts. I've outlined the hormonal equivalent of wearing a seat belt in the following sidebar. Much of this advice is dull—have regular checkups including pap, breast exam, and mammogram; minimize saturated fat; cut down alcohol—but the evidence is clear that these do cut risks for breast cancer, heart attack, and stroke.

MENOPAUSAL HORMONE THERAPY—REDUCING THE RISKS

Breast cancer risk increases only after four to five years of HT; after that, carefully assess your need for continued treatment.

The breast cancer risk with HT is due to the progestin, not estrogen. Use natural progesterone but take only the minimum needed to protect against endometrial cancer.

Alcohol intake of two or more drinks per day increases breast cancer risk as much as HT. Minimize alcohol intake.

High saturated fat intake is also a breast cancer risk factor. Cut down on saturated fat as much as you can.

Have a breast checkup at least yearly, including physical exam, mammogram, and ultrasound.

Breast self-exam is a good idea too.

Be sure your blood pressure meets the new guideline of 125/80 or less.

Be sure your LDL-cholesterol (the bad kind) is 100 mg/dL or less.

To lower stroke risk, take a baby aspirin (81 mg) daily, unless it irritates your stomach.

If you are overweight, especially with a family history of diabetes, get tested to see if you have high blood sugar and insulin resistance; get treatment if you do.

Even if you are not on HT, following these guidelines will help you stay healthy.

A QUICK GUIDE TO THE BEST—AND WORST—ESTROGENS AND PROGESTINS

The Best   As I explained earlier in this chapter, patches are usually the best way to take estrogen.

Vivelle Dot is the smallest patch and, for this reason, the most popular. Alora is older; it works fine but is much larger. Both are changed every three and a half days, but if you are paying for it yourself, you can stretch each out to four days. Climara is larger than Vivelle Dot and lasts seven days instead of three and a half. This is actually a disadvantage because skin irritation is more common. Nor does it save money because one Climara patch costs about twice as much as one of the three and a half day patches. It is the only patch that currently comes in a 0.06 mg dose, which is just right for some women.

Esclim is an oddity. Because it is thick and opaque, Esclim is the ugliest patch, but the one that will stick if none of the others do.

Estraderm was the first patch to be introduced. It is not actually a patch but a sack with an alcoholic solution of estradiol. It is awkward to use, irritating to skin and inconsistent in absorption; for all these reasons, Estraderm, though still available, is awkward to use and obsolete.

Menostar is a very low-dose patch intended for osteoporosis prevention. It will not relieve severe symptoms but may take the edge off mild ones. An advantage is that you do not need to take a progestin with it.

Two patches combine estradiol with a progestin, making them slightly more convenient. Combipatch uses norethindrone acetate and Climara Pro levonorgestrel. Both have slight testosterone-like activity, but not nearly enough to boost libido. These should be avoided if you have acne, unwanted hair, or loss of scalp hair. As explained earlier, I think it is better to take natural progesterone for twelve days on alternate months, rather than a daily synthetic.

Gels have been used in Europe for more than a decade and are very popular there. I did some of the early research on Estragel, and many of the women who used it during the studies were very happy with it. The other, Estrasorb, is packaged for use at a single dose, equivalent to a 0.05 mg patch. Because dosing with gels is less consistent from day to day, I recommend them only if patches are too irritating, or keep falling off.

The Best Estrogen in Pill Form If you want to use oral estrogen, micronized estradiol (Estrace, Gynodiol, and generics) is the only form that is identical to human estrogen. For this reason, it is the only pill I have included in the "Best" section. Estradiol is removed quickly from the blood, so to be fully effective it should be divided into two or three times a day doses (see page 399), not the once a day regimen recommended by the manufacturer.

Progesterone Here the best choice is Prometrium, currently the only prescription form of natural progesterone. Prometrium is formulated with peanut oil, so if you are allergic to peanuts it is not for you. Only in this circumstance do I recommend getting progesterone from a compounding pharmacy, but if you do so, be sure to tell them of your allergies. Other prescription forms of natural progesterone may be introduced in the future.

Some women find that oral progesterone makes them drowsy, so it is best to take it at bedtime. If this does not solve the problem, an alternative is using 4 percent progesterone vaginal gel (Prochieve), also for twelve days every other month.

Combination Pills These are convenient because you simply take the same pill every day, but they do not allow for individualizing doses. They also expose you unnecessarily to synthetic progestin every day. Femhrt is basically a scaled-down version of the birth control pill LoEstrin 1/20. Some studies suggest a more favorable effect on bone than some other HT regimens possibly because it has slight testosterone-like effect. Bleeding rates may be lower than with some of the other fixed combination pills. This preparation is fine if it works out for you, but if you are hormonally vulnerable, you'll probably do better on estradiol and natural progesterone. Activella uses estradiol but is not as potent for controlling symptoms.

The Worst Estrogens Premarin (CEE or conjugated equine estrogens). If there is ever an award for the worst pharmaceutical product for women, this one would at least tie for first place. The only close contender is Provera, the synthetic progesterone, which comes as a combination with Premarin in Prempro and Premphase. Oddly these are the most popular of all HT preparations, for the not very good reason that doctors are used to prescribing them.

Premarin to give it its due, does work to stop symptoms, and if you have been on it for many years with good results, there is no urgent reason to change. Even in this situation, I would suggest Cenestin, which has exactly the same ingredients but is derived entirely from soy and yam instead of horses.

Estropipate (Ogen) is an old alternative to Premarin but not much used now. It has no advantages. Esterified estrogens are contained in Estratest and Estratest H.S.; reasons to avoid any oral form of testosterone are explained in chapter 14.

Progestins As already mentioned, Provera ties with Premarin as one of the worst pharmaceutical preparations intended for women because of its propensity to induce mood swings. Fortunately, natural progesterone is readily available as Prometrium.

Combinations Prempro and Premphase combine the worst forms of estrogen and progestin. Bleeding is common with Prempro, which was the preparation used in WHI. I see no reason to choose either of these for HT.

27.

Planning for Your Bones' Future: Preventing Osteoporosis

Many women give more attention to planning for their financial future than their bones' future. Even though osteoporosis has been extensively publicized, many women put off thinking about it. The standard statistic that broken bones cause more deaths after seventy than breast cancer leaves out something just as important: the loss of comfort and mobility that result from fractures. Too many women still have their later years bedeviled by painful bone problems including curvature of the spine, which can make it impossible to find a comfortable position for sleeping and even constrict breathing. For this reason, I emphasize how taking good care of your bones now can result in a more active and involved life into your seventies and beyond. In a sense, osteoporosis is a form of hormonal vulnerability—inability of the bones to hold up their strength after menopause. During the hormonal years of thirty-five to fifty-five, symptomatic osteoporosis is virtually unknown. (There are rare bone diseases that can occur in this age, but they are not related to female hormones.) Since these years are when women tend to start thinking about hormones, it is a good time to get in the habit of taking calcium and vitamin D.

It's easy to procrastinate on bone protection because bone seems as solid and unchanging as a rock. In actuality, however, bone is a very dynamic organ whose structural elements are continually being broken down and built back up. For strength to be maintained, deposition of new bone must keep pace with removal of old. When bone is resorbed faster than it can reform, it progressively weakens. The main role of estrogen is to slow the breakdown of existing bone. Calcium is also essential because it is the raw material that gives bone its strength. Poor calcium intake harms bone in two ways: Not only is there not enough to keep existing bone in shape, but also the body has to borrow calcium from bone for other purposes when not enough can be absorbed from diet. If the borrowing is short term and the body repays its calcium debt to bone, there are no problems. But if not enough new calcium can be absorbed from food, the calcium debt mounts up, and bone gets thinner and weaker.

During childhood, and especially adolescence, bone is built up to its maximum strength. Nutrition is critical during this phase because if bone formation is suboptimal in these early years, it will be thin ever after, making it more vulnerable after menopause when calcium starts to dribble away. Ideally, calcium supplements should be started by age ten or twelve, but this rarely happens because we think of bones as not needing attention until later in life. Assuming no underlying disorder is present, bone loss in adult women is quite slow until menopause, when it greatly accelerates due to loss of the bone-conserving effect of estrogen. The consequences of menopausal bone loss depend on the state of your bones going into the change—the less you have, the less you can afford to lose. Those with fairly dense bones are less likely to have later fractures.

There are definite ethnic differences in vulnerability to osteoporosis, but all groups should take calcium and vitamin D as well as have their bones checked regularly. Black women have the lowest risk. Caucasian women are generally at high risk, especially if they are slender and/or fair-skinned. Asian women have more delicate bones than Caucasians but somewhat less risk of fracture.

A period of low estrogen, for example if periods were stopped for a while because of thinness or extreme exercise, can increase the risk of later osteoporosis. On the other hand, obesity and PCOS are associated with stronger bones. Both smoking and drinking increase the risk of osteoporosis and fracture.

MINDING YOUR BONES

The state of your bones can easily be determined by the simple DXA test. (The full name of this test is dual-energy X-ray absorptiometry. Despite the name, the amount of X-ray exposure is slight.) A blood chemistry profile can screen for other causes of bone loss, such as overactivity of the parathyroid gland. In some cases, more extensive testing is necessary.

Though DXA results are given in printouts that are quite elaborate and confusing, interpretation is usually fairly easy. The critical number is the T-score, which compares your bone density to that of healthy young adults. Ideally, the T-score should be above −1. A T-score between −1 and −2.5 is considered osteopenia, while −2.5 or lower is osteoporosis. (In case your algebra is a little rusty, negative numbers run in the opposite direction, so that −3 is less than −2.) Treatment to prevent further loss should be considered if the T-score is below −1. If your T-score is near or below −2.5, treatment is imperative.

Response to treatment is also monitored using the DXA test. Since bones change slowly, there is no reason to repeat the DXA scan at a shorter intervals than one year. Blood tests for osteoporosis are not very helpful except for research.

TREATMENTS FOR OSTEOPENIA AND OSTEOPOROSIS

It's very important to realize that *once menopause is reached, bone density never improves without treatment*—just waiting to see what will happen is a bad idea. As I write this, I am about to leave for the hospital to visit an eighty-nine-year-old friend who fell two days ago and fractured her hip. She always refused any preventive measure for her bones because of her fear of side effects. Fortunately, she was successfully operated on and will soon be walking again. But she would have been spared much pain and worry had she accepted medical help to maintain her bones.

Calcium supplements and exercise can slow loss but do not completely prevent it. To arrest, or even reverse, progressive weakening of bone, there are three sorts of treatment. That in longest use is estrogen. Even a very low dose, such as that in the Menostar patch, will inhibit bone loss. Not all women's bones respond to minidoses of estrogen, however; sometimes higher doses are needed if estrogen is the primary treatment.

The current view is that estrogen should not be used for bone loss unless it is also needed for symptom control. (It is possible that the very low dose forms of estrogen, such as Menostar, will not have any of the safety issues found in the WHI study, but long term safety data is pending.) At this time, the primary treatment for osteopenia or osteoporosis is the class of drugs known as bisphosphonates. Two have been available for several years now—Actonel (risedronate) and Fosamax (alendronate); another Boniva (ibandronate) has just been released. Bisphosphonates can restore lost bone to some degree. Nonetheless, since osteopenia is progressive, sooner is better than later as far as treatment is concerned. Fosamax and Actonel are available in convenient once a week forms; Boniva needs to be taken only once a month. There is concern that any bisphosphonate can get stuck in the esophagus and cause problems, and so the instructions inform you to swallow the pill with a whole glass of water and to remain upright for at least a half an hour. (You don't have to stand; sitting counts as upright.) There are no definite differences in either side effects or effectiveness between the different drugs in this class.

Another bone treatment, one that has never really caught on, is Evista (raloxifene), an altered form of estrogen that has a protective effect against breast cancer. The main drawback of Evista is that it frequently makes menopausal symptoms worse. If symptoms are no problem at all for you, Evista may be a good option, particularly if you are apprehensive about breast cancer.

Another recent development in osteoporosis treatment is Forteo (teriparatide). This is a form of parathyroid hormone, which is involved in normal regulation of bone metabolism. At this time, it is mainly reserved for osteoporosis with severe pain. Since it must be taken by injection and long term safety is unclear, it is not likely to be an option for many women under sixty.

Though bone metabolism is a complex subject, in practice treatment of osteopenia or mild osteoporosis without fractures is fairly simple for both patient and physician.

THE BEST FORMS OF CALCIUM AND VITAMIN D

Low calcium intake is commonly a contributing factor to bone loss, especially since health considerations have led many to limit their dairy intake. This is a wise move, but there is no other readily alternative source of calcium. Vitamin D is necessary for calcium to actually get into the blood, but our food does not supply enough. The human body can make its own D, but only with lots of sun exposure—not a good idea if you want to maintain healthy skin. Realistically, then, the only way to get enough calcium and vitamin D is to take supplements.

BONING UP: THE BUSY WOMAN'S GUIDE TO MAINTAINING BONE HEALTH

Have a DXA (bone density test) before you turn fifty.

If your density is low, have a chemistry profile and TSH (thyroid test) to rule out hormonal conditions that can cause abnormal bone loss.

Take calcium citrate with vitamin D, one 600 mg tablet at each of two main meals. This is recommended for all women, not just those approaching menopause.

If your T-score is much lower than −1.0, either begin treatment or have another DXA in a year.

If you want estrogen for symptom control, this is usually adequate treatment for a low T-score.

If you do not want estrogen, take the once a week Actonel or Fosamax. Monthly Boniva may be a good alternative, but there is less experience with it because it is newer.

If a single drug does not give an adequate result, estrogen can be combined with either Actonel or Fosamax.

Raloxifene is an additional option but is mainly for women not having significant menopausal discomforts.

Stay in shape with weight-bearing exercise, but remember that this by itself will not prevent bone loss.

Many forms of calcium are available. Calcium carbonate is widely sold but not always easily absorbed, and some preparations may be contaminated with lead. In my view, calcium citrate (Caltrate, Citracal, and others) is clearly the best. Choose one with vitamin D and your requirement for this vitamin will also be met, so long as you also take a daily multiple. (The official requirement for D is stated as 400 U per day. Mature women actually need 800 U per day.) Calcium requirements are 1000 mg per day prior to menopause and for postmenopausal women on estrogen. For postmenopausal women not on estrogen, the daily requirement is 1500 mg. Since all women get some calcium in the diet, supplement doses can be somewhat less. A simple way that provides enough calcium for all women is to take two 600 mg calcium citrate with Vitamin D tablets a day—one with each of two meals.

I've put all this together in the sidebar. Remember, preventing bone loss is simple and painless, dealing with fractures is not.

PART VII

Hormones and the Soul

28.

Hormones and Spiritual Healing

HORMONAL VULNERABILITY AS SPIRITUAL CRISIS

We think of soul and spirit as helping us overcome the limitations imposed by our bodies. Yet spirit and body are mutually dependant. Better to acknowledge the degree to which the body affects the soul, as the Buddha and the Chinese sage Laozi did.

Hormonal vulnerability, because it seems so limiting, creates crises that are both physical and spiritual. Yet, others rarely accept hormonal disruptions as a justification for temporary impairment. It is acceptable to call in sick for the flu, but not for PMS. Since hormone problems tend to be recurrent, they create dread that even when you feel good, it is only temporary. There is guilt too because their very elusiveness makes one wonder if they are real or all in the head. To help you pin down what your hormones may be doing to you spiritually, I've listed some effects in the following sidebar.

HORMONAL VULNERABILITY: ADVERSE EFFECTS ON MIND AND SPIRIT

Loss of hope

A feeling that the good part of life is over

Forcing oneself to go through the motions

Shame

Feeling like a complete failure—as a woman, worker, wife, mother

Guilt

Helplessness—exacerbated by doctors who offer no help or comfort

Anxiety over future

Loss of pleasure

Meaninglessness

A psychologist or psychiatrist might say that what I have listed as spiritual effects are just symptoms of depression. This ignores the fact that depression itself is a state of spiritual crisis. But more to the point, to apply the label of depression is to ignore the cause—hormonal vulnerability. Time and time again I've seen the supposed "depression" lift when the underlying hormone problems—PMS, acne, hair loss, menopause, or insulin resistance, to name a few—were solved.

Let's admit that hormones can affect everything, including the spirit, despite the fact that no endocrinology textbook mentions the soul as a target organ for hormone action. This omission does not mean that spiritual healing cannot help hormonal vulnerability. On the contrary, spiritual healing is particularly valuable in coping with the elusive, but very real, effects of hormones on mind and body.

I am sure that if you have read this far, you know that I believe in using all the resources of scientific medicine to correct hormone problems. But I recognize that this is not always enough. Even when treatment works perfectly, something else may remain: the sense of vulnerability, a certain apprehension that the problem will return or another arise. Such uneasiness, however, is part of the human condition. Those who are hormonally vulnerable are particularly aware that the human body is neither completely reliable nor indestructible. It is just when we are up against these physical limits that spirituality is needed. Also, since treatment of hormonal conditions tends to work gradually—indeed, it is often better this way—it is important to enhance your coping skills while you are waiting for treatment to work. Medications help many things, but more is needed to meet life's challenges than pills.

SELF-CARE

Americans tend to be hard on our bodies. We treat ourselves harshly—working long hours relieved, if that is the word, by strenuous exercise. Like the rest of our bodies, our hormones are not allowed much rest; instead they must fluctuate practically nonstop to compensate for the extra demands placed on the body. Many take physical limits as challenges to be overcome rather than as warning messages. We have lost sight of what the ancients well knew. Laozi wrote 2,500 years ago that our difficulties come from having a body. In place of pressing against limits he taught cultivating a sense of what can actually be accomplished at each moment. In India, Shakyamuni, the historical Buddha, taught a middle way between overindulgence and extreme asceticism. To those of his followers who wanted to practice self-mortification, he pointed out that one cannot develop spiritually without attending to the needs of the body. These lessons are of great value to moderns who tend to forget that at certain moments in life, quiet reflection is better than nonstop activity. With prayer, meditation, and other states of quiet receptivity, we can better develop our sense of when and how to act. Sometimes the first step in solving a problem is to simply be with it for a while. Women tend to be much better at this than men and so are ideally suited to cultivate this natural ability for their own healing.

SPIRITUAL HEALING METHODS FOR THE HORMONALLY VULNERABLE

If I omitted a discussion of meditation and prayer, this book would not fully reflect my own approach to healing, which definitely embraces the spirit as well as the body. There is now no lack of books about spirituality, but with this information overload, the basics sometimes get obscured. In this chapter, I'll pass on some of the easy-to-use, practical methods that I've learned from my own experience studying meditation both here at home, and in China, Japan, and Thailand. I've refined these methods in workshops I've conducted for health care professionals and for women with PCOS.

Women who share hormonal vulnerabilities will not necessarily hold identical beliefs about religion and spirituality. Recognizing a spiritual principle in the universe can take many forms. For that reason, I discuss prayer and meditation in general terms, rather than from the viewpoint of any specific religion. I've drawn more heavily upon Buddhism and other Eastern philosophies for the simple reason that they've inspired my own practice over more than twenty-five years. But the techniques should be equally comfortable for followers of all religions, and even agnostics.

In the United States, prayer has become politicized of late, which I regard as unfortunate because it is a particularly intimate act, connecting to one's deepest emotions and beliefs. There is nothing wrong with expressing these publicly but nothing wrong with keeping them private, either. My view toward prayer is not an obligation but a way of enhancing one's sense of harmony with the infinite universe in which we find ourselves.

As has been emphasized throughout this book, hormones and emotions are intimately intertwined. Hormones control our inner biochemical environment, and mental peace tends to promote biochemical peace. Because we can't always control what goes on outside our bodies, I'll describe some ways to have greater control over what goes on within.

MEDITATION

Studies have shown that meditation can effectively decrease stress hormones such as cortisol. Some methods of meditation are extremely elaborate—for example, those of Chinese Daoism or Tibetan Buddhism. It is useful to keep in mind that these practices were developed by monks and nuns, people who had little else to do but meditate. In the modern world, most of us must fit meditation into already overloaded schedules. Fortunately, even very simple forms can help set the body into healing mode.

Realistic expectations are critical. Meditation is not, as sometimes advertised, instant ecstasy. On the contrary, progress is usually gradual, but if you persist, one day you are likely to realize that your practice has changed your life, including your relation to your hormones. (Those who want to take meditation further will find more information in the Resources section at the end of this book.) It took me about a year of regular sitting before I noticed any effects from my practice. Once I got to this point, however, I started to notice more and more benefits in rapid succession.

Many give up on meditation because they are told they must spend at least thirty minutes once, or even twice, a day. This is a fallacy; even a few minutes a day makes a difference. As with exercise, some meditation is better than none. You'll advance more, however, if you can attend an occasional retreat for a few days.

What counts in meditation is what goes on in your mind, not the externals. If you want, you can burn incense, bow to a religious image, sit cross-legged in half- or full-lotus, but you don't have to do any of these things. Meditation is a major avocation for some, but there is no need to compete with the macho meditators who boast of how many consecutive hours they can sit without moving. Just as you can exercise for physical well-being without being a serious athlete, you can meditate for calm and self-understanding without it being your main interest in life.

For most, meditation is not about attaining an exotic altered state of consciousness. Quite the contrary, it is about getting to know all your thoughts better, even your most trivial and ordinary ones. Most are surprised to discover what actually goes on in their minds from moment to moment. In Buddhism this is referred to as "monkey mind," comparing the restless movements of the mind to monkeys jumping from branch to branch. Don't worry if you cannot keep perfect focus when you meditate—no one can.

Some feel more anxious when they first start to meditate, but this fades if you stick with it. If you are a very restless person who needs to be on the go all the time, sitting meditation may not be congenial for you. If so, you can try one of the forms of moving meditation, such as tai chi, qi gong, or yoga.

One of the benefits of meditation is learning to relax without dependence on outside distractions. As Americans we tend to deal with distressing situations and thoughts by using external stimulation to push them out of consciousness. TV, video games, iPods, and cell phones are favorite devices to do this. With constant distraction, we never come to terms with our inner discomforts and so never develop resources for coping with them. The most effective way to deal with painful thoughts or sensations is to let yourself feel them. This may sound too pat to you—as I confess it did to me, until an experience that I will now relate to you.

More than a decade ago, I was staying at a Buddhist temple called Wat Phananachat in remote Thailand, near the Cambodian border. We awoke at 3:30 A.M., which was actually easy because it was already bright daylight. A few minutes later we began a session of group chanting and meditation. Breakfast, the only meal allowed, was eaten in the outdoor kitchen, after which we dispersed to isolated huts to spend the day in solitary meditation. Late in the afternoon we assembled again for a brief work period.

During one of my first work details, I was assigned to carry water. Huge recycled oil drums were used; filled with water each weighed over 100 pounds. Two monks carried them propped between their shoulders. The day before when I had seen others carrying water in this fashion, I thought it looked quaintly archaic. Trying it myself was another matter. As I walked, the 100 pounds suspended on the thin pole dug into my shoulder, while my bare feet landed on sharp pebbles and were bitten by tiny, but ferocious, red ants. The person ahead of me was a monk who had been in the monastery for several years. After a few steps, the monk, without even turning to look at me said, "I sense some tightness. Don't fight the pain; accept it and let yourself feel it." This sounded to me like pseudo-oriental mumbo jumbo, and my first reaction was irritation. But since I had nothing better to do, I tried it. When I directly focused my attention on the pain in my shoulder, I was astonished to discover that it actually did become more tolerable.

Another event a few days later brought home this lesson for me. This time the work detail consisted of helping clear jungle with machetes and shovels. Though I am proud of my manual dexterity, for example in palpating internal organs without causing discomfort, I am completely useless with a machete. So I mainly watched others in the vain hope of improving my technique. In the work area was a pit with many small stumps next to it. Suddenly the Abbott, Ajahn Passano, slipped and fell partly into the pit so that his back twisted and landed on a sharp stump. I stood by helplessly because it happened so fast. The sudden fall must have been an acute shock as well as extremely painful. As I watched Ajahn's face, however, I was astonished to discover that he did not show the least distress, merely a momentary clouding of his eyes followed a second later by a slight smile. Without any comment, he stood up and went back to work. Had this happened to me, I would have been jumping around and loudly ventilating my distress, needing to calm down before I could return to my previous activity. Seeing that Ajahn's serenity did not desert him convinced me that meditation can really increase pain tolerance.

Now I make no great claims for myself here. I still would rather avoid having to carry 100 pound objects, and I certainly don't like falling down. Nor do I turn down local anesthetic when I go to the dentist. What has changed is that, while I still don't like pain—who does?—since then I have been less afraid of it.

COPING WITH PAIN

It is not pain per se, but the brain's reaction to it that makes us miserable. The mental effort we automatically make to fight pain, and our anger that we have pain at all, contribute to the distress; it is these that mediation can alter. This is what I learned in Thailand. I do need to clarify that I absolutely do not agree with those who feel that pain should be endured as some sort of lesson. When I see patients with pain, I do my best to provide safe relief. I still think the best thing to do with pain is to take it away. But I do recommend that if pain is more than an occasional part of your life experience, you should consider meditation as a way to decrease its power over you. Meditation and medication are not mutually exclusive.

Migraine sufferers particularly may benefit from meditation. I had migraine from childhood, though as is often the case, it was never diagnosed. After I'd meditated for several years, I realized that I no longer had attacks. Instead, when I felt one coming on—if you are a migraine sufferer, you'll know what this feels like—I could somehow mentally avert it. Although it still surprises me when it works, it always does. I even remember my last migraine—it was in 1990.

The sidebar explains a technique, variously called insight meditation or vipassana, that is the most helpful for pain.

To show how this works, let's suppose you had a run-in with your boss. He or she criticized your work unfairly and would not listen to your explanation. Worse, it was PMS week and you had to dash into the ladies' room to hide your tears. For the rest of the day, the rebuke from your boss and your embarrassment over your lack of emotional control plays over and over in your head. Later, when you have a chance, try going to a quiet place and meditating. As the memories of these events arise, simply label them. If you remember starting to cry, you might label that "sad," "hurt," or "embarrassed"—depending on

MEDITATION FOR PAIN CONTROL

Sit in a comfortable meditation posture either on a chair or cushion. For meditation to be effective, your spine must be straight.

Breathe from your diaphragm. It should feel as if the air is going all the way down to your pelvis.

Concentrate on the rising and falling of your abdomen as you breathe slowly in, then out. To help focus, you can say to yourself "in," then "out," as you breathe.

When a thought arises, simply note the thought, stay with it, and when it wanes, gradually return your focus to your breathing.

Instead of getting involved with the thoughts and emotions that arise, you can label them with simple terms such as "worry," "anger," "pain," "boredom," "happiness," and so on.

That's more or less it. Just do it for a predetermined length of time on a regular basis and see what happens.

what you feel at the moment of recall. Although no one believes it will work until they try it, this simple practice greatly reduces the distress evoked by unpleasant sensations and thoughts. Over time, you will discover that negative feelings fade more rapidly than before.

PRAYER

Religious faith has been shown time and time again to be a powerful health-enhancer. Prayer can be an alternative to meditation, or you can do both. Though they are not quite the same, both can help you remain calm in the face of hormonal storms.

Some prefer to use prayers they have already learned as part of the religious tradition to which they belong. Others feel uncomfortable with standard prayers, perhaps from unpleasant experiences in childhood or because they feel that they do not express their personal spiritual beliefs. What's important is that the prayer feel natural for you. You do need to say prayers for them to work, but you do not need to say them out loud. The simple, four-part prayer provided in the following sidebar can be adapted by anyone, whatever their concerns or beliefs. It can be as long or as short as you like. I recommend that it become as much a part of your daily treatment regimen as medication.

No matter how long it has been since you have prayed, or even if you never have consciously, this simple method can help bring serenity.

HOW TO CULTIVATE FORGIVENESS

Research suggests that the ability to forgive increases life expectancy, and I believe that it can affect hormonal health as well. Forgiveness does not mean accepting hurts and injuries, but it does entail letting go of anger and bitterness and recognizing that the person with whom you are angry is human and suffers also. Letting go does not mean that it is okay that something bad happened to you. It means that you recognize that angry or bitter feelings, however warranted, mainly harm yourself. Though no scientific studies have been done, it is my experience that bitterness aggravates hormonal vulnerabilities. Part of healing your hormones is letting go of prior traumas.

For many women who are hormonally vulnerable, their greatest

THE FOUR-PART HEALING PRAYER

One: Identify yourself and give an address to which your prayer is to be sent. This may be to Jesus, Jehovah, St. Jude, Buddha, Guanyin, Isis, or to any other sacred being. (The address does not need a zip code.) Equally, it can be addressed to an abstract principle, such as the One, the Dao, Peace, or universal harmony. The purpose of the address is to open up a channel connection you to the sacred. The being you are about to call upon already knows that you need his or her help.

Two: State your problem and let yourself simply be with what is troubling you—without feeling that *you* have to solve it at this moment. That to which you are praying knows what is on your mind and has heard the same worries billions of times.

Three: Express the sort of help you need. My own view is that prayers work best when used to facilitate what you can do for yourself. I don't discount the possibility of miracles, but I don't plan on them either. Sometimes, though, as when someone you love has a serious illness, it is entirely appropriate to ask for help from outside yourself. If you are not sure what sort of help might solve your problem, just keep the problem in your awareness for a while. The being or principle to which you are praying knows better than you what you need; that is why you are praying.

Four: Give thanks for the help you are going to receive.

bitterness is toward their own bodies. All of us have such feelings to some degree. No one likes every part of their body. Part of healing is to own these parts of oneself. If you are hormonally vulnerable, it is almost impossible not to feel frustrated at your own biochemistry. Yet, blaming your body gets you nowhere.

Theravada, the oldest branch of Buddhism and the one closest to the Buddha's original teachings, developed a powerful method for letting go of angry feelings called *metta*, or loving kindness, meditation. There is actually nothing specifically Buddhist about this simple, but profound practice. You sit in a comfortable meditation posture and after calming and centering yourself, think of someone whom you have only neutral feelings about. This is actually quite hard because we almost always feel some degree of like or dislike. When you have this person in mind, one then mentally send waves of love out to him or her. Next, you repeat the process for someone you like, then someone you love. This strengthens your positive feelings. Then comes the hard part: You picture someone you mildly dislike and, finally, someone you strongly dislike. To them too you send loving feelings. You can also picture unhappy events in your own life and send love to them as part of your life. The purpose of this meditation is to develop your positive thoughts and to help you let go of your negative ones. It can help you realize that even your enemies have their own difficulties. It is also useful for improving your relationship with your body. Start with a part you feel neutral about, perhaps your hand, go to one you like, perhaps your nose, then one you dislike, perhaps your tummy or thighs. Women are often quite harsh in judgments of their bodies and this may help to loosen these unproductive aversions.

Metta meditation can help you become aware of your changing states of mind. You may discover that when you are having PMS, it is much harder to send out loving thoughts both to yourself and to others. You don't need to try to change these feelings directly, just accept them and let them pass out of your mind when you are ready.

Meditation is, of course, not a substitute for medical treatment. For example, if you have PCOS with cystic acne, sending out loving thoughts to your ovaries and skin will not cure your condition. Nor will it make you actually like having acne; what it will do is decrease the power that negative thoughts hold over you. This, in turn, frees up your energy to seek out effective treatment.

USING THE POWER OF IMAGES FOR QUICK RELIEF

It is hard to prevent spirituality from becoming separate from daily life, something to which we can give attention only during church services, meditation retreats, yoga classes, and the like. Much as we try to maintain a mindful connection with something greater than ourselves throughout each day, it's hard to do so. Like everyone else, I tend to get caught up in the routine aggravations of a day at work, such as trying to get a lab to fax a missing report or hassling with an insurance company. When frustrations arise, few of us can head for church, a meditation retreat, or even go for a walk in the woods. To help deal with difficult moments, whether hormonal or not, there are simple practices that take almost no time and can be deployed in almost any situation.

Meditation, especially vipassana, discussed above, can help at such moments, but another, even simpler, way is to draw on the power of sacred images and objects. Nearly all religions use the inspiriting power of art to awaken our sense of the spiritual. Indeed, until the last three centuries, virtually all art was religious, and could only be seen in religious monuments, museums, or the homes of the wealthy. Now it is available to all, either as printed reproductions or even stored in high-tech form, such as PDA, iPod, or cell phone.

The choice of image is entirely personal. What I find most calming are Chinese landscapes, calligraphy, or Buddha images. For others it may be pictures of Jesus, Mary, Mother Theresa, a menorah, a phrase from the Qur'an, or a sacred word or symbol. Images that bring a sense of meaning or calm need not be specifically religious; millions look at pictures of loved ones for comfort in difficult moments.

Not only pictures but small objects can be used as a quick way to center yourself. Fingering strands of beads is a technique used by many religious traditions to help focus the mind on the sacred. Amulets worn as pendants are similarly used. There is a tendency to dismiss such practices as materialistic or superstitious. Though they may be both at times, they are much more because they bring the sense of touch into play to help connect to the sacred—just as pictures do with sight and music does with hearing.

SPIRITUAL HEALING IN A SCIENTIFIC CULTURE

Spiritual healing is no more a cure-all than is medication or surgery. One of the impediments to spiritual healing is that it is so often presented as a substitute for medical approaches. Much of this stems from regrettable self-interest on the part of alternative practitioners who are not medically licensed and, therefore, cannot prescribe medication. On the other side, physicians vary in their attitudes toward nonmedical healing. Although many are sympathetic, they do not have experience applying it to their medical practice. My view, as I hope I have made evident, is that *both* medical and spiritual approaches have value and that each can help in ways the other cannot.

Throughout this book, I have been candid about the weaknesses of the health care establishment. Spiritual healing has become an establishment too, and it also has weaknesses. The following sidebar itemizes some of them.

EIGHT MYTHS THAT BLOCK SPIRITUAL HEALING

- Faith is incompatible with science.

- You can't combine alternative with conventional treatment.

- Spiritual healing methods can cure anything. When they don't work, it is your fault because you did not have enough faith.

- Prayer is only for those who go to church regularly.

- Only standard prayers work.

- Meditation is mysterious and exotic.

- Meditation will give you *instant* relief from stress.

- Meditation works only if you do it for long periods every day.

- Don't question the teaching of _____. (Fill in the blank: your guru, spiritual adviser, and so on).

AN END TO HORMONAL PESSIMISM

It's easy, if you are hormonally vulnerable, to feel unfairly singled out. Sometimes it's tempting to give way to feelings of helplessness and bitterness because what seems so easy for others is so difficult for you. No one's life is trouble-free, however. Over the decades I've been practicing medicine, I've heard the private concerns of thousands of people, women and men both. This taught me at first hand that there is no one—no matter how smart, how educated, how rich, how happily married, how beautiful—who does not have something to overcome.

In writing this book, I've done everything I could to show women troubled by hormonal misery the way back to a happy and fulfilling life. I hope I've convinced you not to give up. For some hormonally vulnerable women, a few lifestyle changes, a simple herb, or a medication may solve everything. For others, the road is long and winding. But whether the road is short or long, it is there. My more than twenty years helping women with hormone problems has proved to me that there is a solution for virtually every hormonally vulnerable woman.

A Note to the Reader Regarding Medications and Laboratory Results
Medicine abounds in esoteric words and symbols. To make matters worse, many technical terms have synonyms and multiple abbreviations. Though I have done my best to be consistent, I thought that clarifying some potentially confusing matters at the outset would be helpful.

Medication Names Prescription drugs typically have both a brand name and a generic name. In medical journals, only generic names are acceptable in order to avoid appearing to endorse a specific product. I have followed this practice only partially; for the sake of clarity, I have used the name that is most familiar. Thus "Viagra" instead of sildenafil. When brands differ in important ways, I have also used the brand name when discussing these differences, for example, Vivelle and Climara. To distinguish brand from generic names, I have followed standard medical usage in which brand names are capitalized and generic in lower case, for example, Aldactone, which is the brand name, and spironolactone, which is generic.

My use of brand names is for clarity, not for commercial endorsement. When I feel a particular product has advantages, I say so directly. I have done research or consulted regarding some of the products I mention and usually indicate this in the text. When I make recommendations, I base this on what my experience suggests is best in a particular situation.

Drug doses These are most often stated in milligrams, (mg), but sometimes in grams (g) or micrograms (µg or mcg). These differences are important because misinterpretation of units could result in a thousand-fold error (1 g = 1000 mg or 1,000,000 µg). Though I've been specific about doses, because it is critical to safe and effective therapy, I definitely do not advise self-dosing with prescription drugs. Final dose decisions must be made in consultation with a physician experienced with that medication.

Laboratory test results Test results are stated in units. Most ignore these; for example, an estradiol result of 80 pg/mL is generally referred to simply as "80." The problem is that not all labs use the same units.

A BILL OF RIGHTS
FOR WOMEN WHO ARE
HORMONALLY VULNERABLE

FROM FAMILY MEMBERS, FRIENDS, AND OTHERS:

- Extra consideration during times of hormonal chaos.

- Respect and accommodation for your special needs at this time, such as dietary limits, time for extra rest, quiet, and less overtime.

- Be sure to keep up your side: Explain when and why you are feeling out of sorts, apologize if you have lost your temper, show your appreciation by doing extra things for others once you are feeling better.

FROM HEALTHCARE PROFESSIONALS:

- Respectful treatment without condescension from all health care providers.

- Have your prior and present hormone-related problems carefully listened to without any being dismissed as unimportant.

- Be treated as an individual socially, biologically, and spiritually.

- Have adequate testing to clarify your problem—but be spared unnecessary testing.

- Have your test results explained to you clearly.

- Receive specific guidance on how to best cope with any medical condition so that it does not impose limits on your abilities and happiness.

- Receive an explanation of what is likely to happen with your condition in the future.

- Have all reasonable options for treatment be presented so that you can choose what is best for yourself.

- Be able to talk to a medically knowledgeable person in your doctor's office regarding your medications and possible side effects.

- Have medication carefully adjusted until it is right for you, no matter how many changes are needed.

- Have regular monitoring to be sure your treatment continues to meet your individual needs.

- Be kept abreast of new developments that might suggest ways to make your treatment safer and more effective.

- Have your treatment adjusted in response to changes in your body and your life.

The same estradiol level of 80 pg/mL might be reported as 800 pg/dL or 0.8 ng/dL. For this reason, I have indicated the units in discussing interpretation of lab results. If the numbers on your lab report differ markedly from those I mention, first check the units to see if those in your laboratory's report are different. If they are, since doing the conversions can be confusing, you may want to ask your doctor to clarify matters.

RESOURCES

THE HORMONE HELP CENTER

This is my own website: www.hormonehelpNY.com. Included are a question and answer feature and an online newsletter for which you can sign up. Information about my New York City practice is included.

BOOKS

Benson, Herbert, and Miriam Z. Klipper. *The Relaxation Response.* New York: HarperTorch, 1976. Meditation without mystification.

Bratman, Steven M.D., and David Kroll, Ph.D. *The Natural Health Bible,* 2nd ed. New York: Three Rivers Press, 2000. Comprehensive coverage of vitamins and supplements, with critical reviews of evidence regarding effectiveness and safety.

Jahnke, Roger. *The Healer Within: Using Traditional Chinese Techniques to Release Your Body's Own Medicine.* San Francisco: HarperSanFrancisco, 1999. A sound, somewhat detailed treatment by someone with real knowledge.

Kaptchuk, Ted J., O.M.D. *The Web That Has No Weaver: Understanding Chinese Medicine.* New York: Contemporary Books/McGraw-Hill, 2000. The author studied for an extended period in China and has written one of the few English-language books that accurately describes Chinese Medicine—theoretical rather than practical.

Vasant Lad. *The Textbook of Ayurveda.* Albuquerque: Ayurvedic Press, 2001. A detailed presentation of traditional Indian medicine by a leading practitioner.

Maleskey, Gale, Kittel, Mary, and the Editors of *Prevention for Women: The Hormone Connection.* Emmaus, PA: Rodale, 2001. I was an adviser for this publication and can testify to how carefully it was produced. Definitely worth consulting, but the advice tends to be somewhat general.

Pert, Candice B., Ph.D. *Molecules of Emotion: The Science Behind Mind-Body Medicine.* New York: Scribner, 1999. What science has learned about hormones and the brain by one who made some of the most important discoveries.

Redmond, Geoffrey, M.D. *The Good News About Women's Hormones.* New York: Warner, 1995. While most is superseded by the present book, covers some additional topics, such as problems of adolescence and pituitary disease.

Sheehy, Gail. *The Silent Passage: Menopause.* New York: Pocket, 1998. The first book to honestly describe the experience of menopause. Useful for experienced aspects but not current medically.

Skelly, Mari. *Women Living with Fibromyalgia.* Alameda, CA: Hunter House Publishers, 2001. Excellent coverage of this common and difficult chronic pain syndrome.

Speroff, Leon, M.D., and Marc A. Fritz, M.D. *Clinical Gynecological Endocrinology and Infertility,* 7th ed. Philadelphia: Lippincott Williams & Wilkins, 2005. The standard text, with an immense amount of detail. The writing is highly technical, and some matters stated as fact—for example, that menopause does not cause depression—are more questionable than the book admits.

The Staff of *Resolve* with Diane Aronson. *Resolving Infertility: Understanding the Options and Choosing Solutions When You Want to Have a Baby.* New York: HarperResource, 1999. Comprehensive and balanced. The book is good to start with if you have concerns about fertility.

Thatcher, Samuel, M.D., Ph.D. *PCOS: The Hidden Epidemic.* Indianapolis: Perspectives Press, 2000. A detailed treatment by a true expert.

Warga, Claire, Ph.D. *Menopause and the Mind.* New York: Free Press, 1999. Detailed coverage of how menopause affects cognitive function. An antidote to the common medical denial of these distressing effects of estrogen deficiency.

Wallach, Edward C., M.D., and Esther Eisenberg, M.D., M.P.H.: *Hysterectomy: Exploring Your Options.* Baltimore: Johns Hopkins University Press, 2003. A balanced guide to decision making if you have uterine problems.

Weschler, Toni, M.Ph. *Taking Charge of Your Fertility: The Definitive Guide to Natural Birth Control, Pregnancy Achievement, and Reproductive Health,* rev. ed. New York: HarperCollins, 2002. All you need to know about your own fertility.

Vliet, Elizabeth Lee, M.D. *Screaming to be Heard: Hormonal Connections Women Suspect, and Doctors Still Ignore,* rev. ed. New York: M. Evans, 2001. Covers many of the conditions I do, with a somewhat different approach, based on the author's background in psychiatry.

Weiss, Andrew. *Beginning Mindfulness: Learning the Way of Awareness.* Novato, CA: New World Library, 2004. A useful guide to getting started in a meditation practice.

ORGANIZATIONS

Professional Societies

These organizations have websites; many include sections in lay language for non-physicians. Their position statements can be useful summaries but sometimes shy away from taking a clear stand on controversial issues.

American Association of Clinical Endocrinologists: www.aace.com
American College of Obstetrics and Gynecology: www.acog.org
Androgen Excess Society (The professional society for PCOS and related conditions.): www.androgenexcesssociety.org
International Society for the Study of Women's Sexual Health: www.isswsh.org
Endocrine Society: www.endo-society.org
North American Menopause Society: www.menopause.org
Society for Sex Therapy and Research: www.sstarnet.org

Lay and Advocacy Organizations

American Hair Loss Association: www.americanhairloss.org
Two other useful sites for alopecia are www.thebaldtruth.com and www.hairsite.com.
CARES Foundation (Adrenal hyperplasia): www.caresfoundation.org
HS-USA (Hidradenitis Suppurativa): www.hs-usa.org
Polycystic Ovary Syndrome Association: www.pcosupport.org
Resolve (Infertility): www.resolve.org

Medical information online—some comments:

The Internet has made medical information available to the general public that was previously hidden away in medical libraries. Overall, it has been a good thing—I find my patients are far better informed when they first see me than was the case in the pre-Web era. It is a mixed bag, however. Some information is sound; much is not. It can be hard to decide what to believe. A problem with disease descriptions is that often only severe forms are described, creating unnecessary fear in those who have mild versions.

The least reliable parts of the Web are chat rooms and other individual posts. They simply represent one person's view, which may be anything from scientifically rigorous to off-the-wall. I suggest being very skeptical of unsubstantiated statements by individuals. If such posts raise issues important to you, I suggest printing out the relevant pages and bring them with you when you visit your doctor.

The ultimate site for medical information is Medline, the database of the National Library of Medicine database. It contains abstracts of several hundred million articles. Keep in mind that only summaries are given and that not all research reports turn out to be correct. For access: www.hcbi.nlm.nih.gov/entrez/query.fegit or simply type entrez pubmed in your browser.

The NIH National Center for Complementary and Alternative Medicine has a useful website: http://NCCAM.gov

Commercial product websites:

Eve's Garden and Good Vibrations. Both are excellent woman-friendly sources for lubricants and other sexuality-related products. Websites: www.evesgarden.com and www.goodvibes.com

Drugstore.com. A source for medications online. A prescription is required. A convenient place to check prices in order to be sure your local pharmacy is not overcharging. This site is reliable, unlike spam drug sites, which may sell counterfeit medications. If the price seems too good to be true, it is.

Mi Fine Skin. The best moisturizers that I have found; these will not exacerbate acne. Produced by a dermatologist colleague, Beno Michel, M.D. Website: www.mifineskin.com

Toppik Sells products to help conceal alopecia, and it may help you to feel more comfortable in public while you wait for treatment to help. Website: www.toppik. com

ACKNOWLEDGMENTS

Writing a book is an arduous task, no matter how many times you have done it before. When the health of readers is at stake, every effort must be made to achieve both clarity and accuracy; I hope I will be judged to have achieved both. While any inadequacies in the present work are mine, whatever merits it possesses would not have been possible without the help of many who have educated and guided me over the years. Though I have not avoided criticizing the medical establishment when I felt it necessary, I must pay tribute to one of its great virtues: the unselfish sharing of hard-won knowledge. Much medical teaching is done without remuneration or career advancement, simply because the possessor of healing knowledge has a humane obligation to pass it along to others. So many have helped me along the way that choosing whom to acknowledge within the limitations of space and memory has been most difficult.

If writing a book is an arduous task, so is being around the person writing it. For putting up with me and actually keeping me cheerful, primary credit must go to my wife, Mingmei Yip. Herself a writer whose considerable talents are a source of pride to me, Mingmei read through the entire manuscript and made invaluable suggestions.

My agent, Susan Crawford, not only found the best possible home for the book, but also kept me inspired by her enthusiasm for the project and her conviction that it offered something of unique value to the millions of women challenged by their hormones. Judith Regan, my publisher, drew upon her acute sense of the reading public to make vital suggestions as to organization and emphasis. I could not have dreamed of a better editor than Cassie Jones, who quickly and meticulously went through the manuscript and always found time to communicate. Her assistant, Tammi Guthrie, was always ready to help keep the process running smoothly.

My practice manager, Michelle Vrenko, tirelessly attended to the thousand and one details that needed to be addressed while I was writing.

I have been fortunate to have had many outstanding teachers and colleagues without whom I would not have the knowledge and skills that I draw upon throughout each day in my practice. Here I must first mention Wilma Bergfeld, M.D., one of America's leading dermatologists, with whom I had the privilege of collaborating during my nearly ten years at the Cleveland Clinic. It was from Wilma that I first learned about female hair loss, its relationship to hormones, and its emotional impact. Without her knowledge and inspiring example, I would never have been able to develop treatments for this disturbing condition.

During my specialty training, Jennifer Bell, M.D., taught me to recognize the subtle effects of hormones on development, skills that provide valuable clues to what hormones are doing.

My good friend Walter Futterweit, M.D., wrote the first book on PCOS that succeeded in making sense of the plethora of seemingly contradictory research on this trying condition. His book helped me greatly when I began to study this disorder. Through his work with the Polycystic Ovary Syndrome Association and the Reproductive Medicine Committee of the American Association of Clinical Endocrinologists, Dr. Futterweit has been an effective advocate for women with PCOS and their doctors; with his encouragement I have become active in both organizations. Walter is a model of the physician who is both scholar and gentleman. His practical advice was invaluable when I decided to move my practice back to New York City.

Much information of vital importance appears in medical journals late, if at all. For this reason, informal conversations with well-informed colleagues are essential to keeping one's own knowledge on the cutting edge. Of particular value for me have been my conversations with Richard Derman, M.D., not only a good friend, but also one of the world's most erudite specialists in women's health. I always feel smarter after a conversation with Richard. Others from whom I have learned much in conversations at conferences include Raquel Arias,

M.D.; Andrew Kaunitz, M.D.; Sandra Leiblum, Ph.D.; Dan Mishell, M.D.; Michael Perelman, Ph.D.; Raymond Rosen, Ph.D.; Lee Shulman, M.D.; and Michelle Warren, M.D.; Jean Fourcray, M.D., Ph.D. has set an example for me and others in her concern for drug safety.

Samuel Thatcher, M.D., Ph.D., another friend, is notable both for his enthusiastic interest in human ovarian biology and his humane concern for women with ovarian dysfunction. I particularly recall a conversation in front of a hotel elevator during which we stayed up until 4:00 A.M. talking about ovaries and what happens to them in PCOS. If I had PCOS and wanted to get pregnant, he'd be my doctor.

Norman Mazer, M.D., involved me in the first controlled studies on use of testosterone to restore sex drive in women. While we have not always agreed, I have found our conversations immensely stimulating.

In the area of alternative medicine, I have learned much from Fredi Kronenberg, Ph.D.; Michael Balick, Ph.D.; and Kenneth Zysk, Ph.D. A special privilege was participating in two conferences organized by Ruth-Inge Heinze, Ph.D., on shamanism and alternative healing; these exposed me to a rich diversity of ideas and viewpoints undreamt of in the halls of orthodox medicine. Elizabeth LaBlanc read and commented on an important section.

One special friend whom I must mention is John Deri, M.D., an extraordinary psychiatrist now in San Francisco whose complete command of both the philosophical and practical underpinnings of his profession continually amazes me. I have learned much from him.

Sonia K. Guterman, Ph.D., read several portions and offered helpful suggestions.

In closing, I want to offer tribute to several of my mentors who are, to my great sorrow, no longer in this incarnation. All I can do now is acknowledge my debt to them. I first came to know Albert Grokoest, M.D., when he was my preceptor in third year internal medicine at Columbia University College of Physicians and Surgeons. Ironically nicknamed "Shorty" because of his great height, Albert touched the lives of thousands. He was an early and tireless advocate of seeing the patient as a human being with a disease rather than simply an intellectually challenging mass of disordered physiology. My clinical training in the often cold atmosphere of a great teaching hospital would have been an even greater challenge had I not had Albert's example of standing up for each patient as a unique human being.

Akira Morishima, M.D., was one of my teachers in pediatric endocrinology. Having been educated in Japan, Kary easily became irritated with the tendency of American students to ask questions instead of listening. I quickly discovered that if I was willing to keep my mouth shut for a while, Kary would teach me an enormous amount. When he had some time free, he would call me into his office and give me what amounted to an hour's private lecture on the basics I needed to know: thyroid disorders, pubertal development, genital abnormalities, and many other vital topics.

Lester Soyka, M.D., recruited me for my first faculty position as Assistant Professor of Pharmacology and Pediatrics at the University of Vermont College of Medicine. Les quickly became a good friend and supported my activities tirelessly. From him I learned much of the clinical pharmacology that has been so valuable to me as an endocrinologist. He was a model of the physician-scientist. While always humane in his approach, he upheld scientific rigor, not only in research but also in treatment decision-making. He had a knack for clarifying complex medical issues.

In the early 1980s, O. Peter Schumacher, M.D., brought me to the Department of Endocrinology at the Cleveland Clinic where he was chair. My years at that outstanding institution were invaluable ones. I was in daily contact with many superb physicians in diverse disciplines and learned as much there as in all my preceding years. Pete fostered my interest in female hormonal problems, which then became my primary focus. His open-mindedness toward medical theories that others considered unorthodox set an example to me. Pete recognized, as many doctors do not, that in treating patients with poorly understood problems, one needs to consider every possible approach to helping them. I miss his cheerful manner, his booming voice, and his unique way of working out complex medical problems.

In my expressions of gratitude, I must go back to the beginning and credit my mother, Marian White, who stimulated my early interest in biology, at first by regularly bringing me to the American Museum of Natural History and later by teaching me to dissect frogs and various other creatures. In nutrition she was far ahead of her time in preparing meals only with natural, healthy foods.

A final factor in the writing of this book must also be acknowledged: Samadhi Cushions of Karme Choling in Barnet, Vermont. Through some odd karma, I find sitting for many consecutive hours in a chair to type intolerable, and I would not have been able to complete this book without the support of these excellent meditation cushions.

INDEX

acanthosis nigricans (ACN), 332
Accutane, 284–86
ACN (acanthosis nigricans), 332
acne, 276–87
  Accutane for, 284–86
  case study, 276–77
  conventional treatments, 282–83
  hormonal treatment for, 285–86. *See*
    also testosterone control
    treatments
  hormones triggering, 277–79
  HS and, 286–87
  ongoing, 6–7
  oral antibiotics for, 283
  oral contraceptives and, 280–81, 299
  secret of controlling, 280–81
  skin care for, 283–84
  testosterone and, 277, 278–79,
    280–81
  tests identifying reasons for, 288–89
  topical preparations for, 282–83
  treating promptly, 280
  why dermatologists can't treat, 278
Actonel (risedronate), 421, 422
Actos (pioglitazone), 336
acupuncture, 117, 160, 390
adhesions, 140
adrenal hyperplasia, 291, 294
aging, hormones and, 11–12. *See also*
  hormone therapy (HT); menopause

Alesse, 57, 79, 80
alopecia. *See* hair loss (alopecia)
alternative medicine/approaches, 17.
  See also spiritual practices;
  supplements
  acupuncture, 117, 160, 390
  fasting/detoxification, 118–19
  heart disease and, 390
  massage therapy, 117–18, 137, 148,
    152, 379
  for menopause, 391–94, 411–13
  overview, 389–91
  thyroid and, 390
Alzheimer's disease, 376–77
American (Wisconsin) ginseng, 115
anabolic steroids, 28, 35, 203–4, 209
Androcur. *See* cyproterone acetate
  (CPA, Androcur)
AndroGel, 192, 202, 203, 205
androgen blockade, 287
androgen deficiency syndrome, 200
androgenic alopecia, defined, 240. *See*
  also hair loss (alopecia)
androgenic disorders, 227, 293, 295,
  299, 300, 306. *See also* acne; hair
  loss (alopecia); hair, unwanted
  (hirsutism)
androgenicity, 66
androgens, 35, 37, 68
androstenedione, 35, 294

anovulation (no period), 55–56, 57, 323, 325, 344
antiandrogens, 68, 308, 325
antidepressants
  case studies with, 82–83, 94, 96
  deciding about, 123–24, 125–26
  hair growth and, 268
  hormonal treatment and, 95, 372, 408
  for hot flashes, 394–95
  pain management with, 137, 147–48
  PCOS and, 341
  for PMS, 82–83, 97, 122–26
  reducing pleasure, 170, 182–83
  sex drive and, 170, 213
  sexual arousal time and, 221
  side effects, 124–25
  SSRIs, 123–26, 147, 213, 221
  testosterone acting as, 219
Avandia (rosiglitazone), 336
Avodart, 306–7

benzoyl peroxide (BP), 282
bicalutamide (Casodex), 305–6
bill of rights, 442–43
biochemical self-understanding, 15
birth control. See also oral contraceptives
  to avoid, 76–77
  "being careful" method, 61
  condoms, 60–61
  Depo-Provera, 76–77
  diaphragms, 60
  injectable, 75, 76–77
  IUDs, 75–76
  natural family planning, 61
  patches, 68, 69, 74–75, 281
  vaginal rings, 75
black cohosh, 114, 116, 381, 391
bleeding, heavy, 56–58
blood clots (DVTs)
  Diane-35 and, 79
  estrogen and, 355, 377
  hormone therapy and, 351, 355, 377

oral contraceptives and, 62–63, 65, 70, 254, 304
bodily discomforts, 9
body hair. See hair, unwanted (hirsutism)
bone density
  calcium and, 418, 419, 420, 422–23
  constant flux of, 418–19
  estrogen and, 30–31, 55, 419, 420–21
  osteopenia/osteoporosis treatments, 420–21
  preventing osteoporosis, 418–23
  soy products and, 394
  test for, 420, 422
  vitamin D and, 418, 422–23
Boniva (ibandronate), 421, 422
botanicals. See specific botanicals; supplements
breast cancer
  breast pain and, 141
  case study, 358–59
  CPA and, 304
  estrogen and, 32, 33, 142, 252, 351, 383, 401, 421
  Evista and, 421
  hormone therapy and, 351, 353–55, 360, 361, 387, 401, 414
  HT treatment risk, 354, 355
  the pill and, 67
  progestins and, 351, 353, 354, 404, 409
  soy products and, 391–92
  testosterone and, 195–96
  TriEs and, 401
  WHI findings, 354–55
breast(s)
  development, 29
  pain, tenderness, 9, 14, 27, 80, 141–42
  size, pill and, 69
bupropion. See Wellbutrin (bupropion)

calcium (Ca), 113
  best form of, 422–23
  losing, 55, 241, 419

low estrogen and, 56
magnesium and, 114
osteoporosis and, 418, 419, 420,
    422–23
requirements, 423
taking, 56, 116, 418, 422–23
vitamin D and, 56, 418, 422–23
calcium channel blockers, 158–59,
    182–83
cancer. *See also* breast cancer
endometrial, 56, 170, 323–24, 340,
    391, 403, 404, 408, 409, 414
progesterone protecting against, 55,
    56, 170, 324
carbohydrates, 108–9, 259
Casodex (bicalutamide), 305–6
Celecoxib, 145
chaste tree/berry. *See* vitex (chaste tree
    or chaste berry)
chloasma (melasma), 70
cholesterol
lipid profile, 333
menopause and, 414
PCOS and, 195, 310, 331, 332, 333,
    334–35, 337
progestins affecting, 66
soy products and, 391, 392
synthetic testosterone affecting, 37
testosterone and, 195, 196, 201
chronic daily headaches, 153
chronic fatigue
cause, 116
fibromyalgia and, 143, 379
herb for, 115
pain and, 134, 143, 379
PMS and, 11, 15, 115
Cialis, 208, 212, 213, 221
comfort foods, 109–10
condoms, 60–61
contraceptives. *See* birth control; oral
    contraceptives
COX-2 inhibitors, 145–46
CPA. *See* cyproterone acetate (CPA,
    Androcur)

cramps
abnormal cycles and, 53
anovulation (no period) and, 92, 323
hormones causing, 9
in legs, 70
menstrual, 51, 53, 131, 136–38,
    144–46, 148, 323
normal, vs. pathological pain, 132,
    138
PMS symptoms, 89
relief from, 120, 144–46, 148
cyproterone acetate (CPA, Androcur),
    79, 280, 304–5

Dalkon Shield, 76
Dalton, Dr. Katharina, 84, 85, 109,
    113, 120–21, 408
deep venous thrombosis. *See* blood clots
    (DVTs)
dementia, 376–77
Depo-Provera, 76–77
depression
Accutane and, 285
acne causing, 279
antidepressants for, 122–23
case study, 93–94
cortisol levels and, 295
CPA and, 304–5
exercise and, 102
menopause/estrogen and, 369,
    370–74, 428
pain and, 147
PCOS and, 311, 316, 321, 340–41
PMS and, 91
postpartum, 93
professional help for, 374
Provera causing, 139
sex drive/sexuality and, 183, 187
sleep deprivation and, 378–79
St. John's wort (hypericum) for, 116
testosterone and, 200
Desogen, 72, 75, 78, 80, 81, 281, 299
dexamethasone, 295, 299
dexamethasone suppression test, 295

DHEA, 293–94
DHEA-S, 35, 250, 289, 293–94
DHT (dihydrotestosterone), 36,
    243–44, 258, 298, 299, 306
diabetes
  blood pressure and, 333
  cause of, 330
  complications, 330–31
  dysmetabolism and, 321
  glucose intolerance test and, 333
  hemoglobin A1c test and, 333
  insulin resistance and, 329–31
  juvenile diabetes mellitus (DM), 328,
    329, 330
  menopause and, 339, 414
  normalizing insulin levels, 335–37
  PCOS and, 311, 313, 316, 321, 333,
    337
  reversing, 335
  sexual interest and, 183
  weight control and, 333, 337
diagnosing hormonal vulnerability
  abnormal cycles, 53
  heavy bleeding cause, 56–58
  importance of physical exams, 30
  PMS, 91
  test limitations, 30
Diane-35, 79, 304, 305
disease hang-up, 15
diuretics, 111, 120. See also
    spironolactone
doctors
  author background/perspective,
    21–25
  disease hang-up of, 15
  feelings, objectivity and, 20–21
  why ignore vulnerability, 14–15
  your bill of rights for, 442–43
dong quai, 114–15, 393–94
DUB (dysfunctional uterine bleeding),
    56–58
DVT. See blood clots (DVTs)
DXA tests, 420, 422
dysesthesia, 134, 249, 377–78

dysfunctional uterine bleeding (DUB),
    56–58
dysmetabolism (dysmetabolic
    syndrome), 317, 321, 331–32,
    333, 334–35, 339

Effexor (venlafaxine), 126, 394–95
eleutherococcus (Siberian ginseng),
    115
emotional symptoms, 6, 8
endocrinology, yin-yang of, 37–38
endometrial cancer, 56, 170, 323–24,
    340, 353, 391, 403, 404, 408,
    409, 414
endometrial hyperplasia, 57, 408
endometrial polyps, 57
endometriosis, 51, 138–39, 146
endometrium
  biopsy of, 57, 324, 340, 408
  defined, 353
  estrogen effect on, 323–24
  hyperplasia (excessive thickening) of,
    57, 408
  during menstrual cycle, 48, 51
  MPA and, 324
  pill effects on, 74, 76, 146, 324
  progesterone effect on, 57, 146, 170,
    353, 404
  thickening of, 30, 51, 146
  thinning of, with pill, 74
erythromycin, 282, 283, 287
escitalopram. See Lexapro
    (escitalopram)
estradiol, 27, 32
  creams, 412
  doses, 410
  fluctuations in, 224
  forms of, 398–99, 402
  gel, 398
  hair/alopecia and, 244, 250, 289
  as main estrogen form, 32, 352
  patches, 156, 398, 411, 415
  pills, 398, 399–400, 401, 407, 416
  safety of, 355

test results, 441–43
vaginal insertion, 399, 402
estriol, 27, 32, 352, 401, 412
estrogen. *See also* estrogen treatment
  adverse effects of, 6, 33–34
  biochemical description, 26–27
  blood clots and, 355
  bone density and, 30–31, 55, 419,
    420–21
  brain functioning and, 31
  breast cancer and, 32, 33, 142, 252,
    351, 383, 401
  breast development and, 29
  compounded preparations, 400–401
  deficiencies, 55
  defined, 352
  dementia and, 376–77
  effects of, 6, 30–31, 33–34
  estradiol. *See* estradiol
  fluctuations in, 6, 7, 94–95
  forms of, 27
  for hair health, 244–45, 252
  hair loss and, 13, 243, 244–45, 249,
    252, 308–9
  heart disease and, 6, 55, 252
  hormone therapy (HT) with, 357–61.
    See also estradiol; estrogen
    treatment
  instability, 94–95
  intravaginal, 402–3
  kinds of, 32
  liver functioning and, 31
  main type of, 32
  measuring levels of, 32
  in men, 31
  natural/bioidentical, 400–401,
    411–13
  objective vs. subjective description,
    26–27
  premature menopause and, 388
  progestins combined with, 404–5,
    416, 417
  pros/cons of, 33–34
  safety of, 355

scorecard, 33
sex comfort and, 207–8
sex drive and, 169–70, 175
transdermal forms, 400, 401
vasodilatation from, 31
estrogen patches, 121
  benefits of, 121, 398, 407
  as best estrogen form, 398, 415
  case studies with, 94, 151, 382–83
  dosages, 405–6, 407
  explaining to partner, 216
  menopause and, 397
  migraines and, 68, 156
  problems with, 411
  quality levels guide, 415
estrogen treatment, 396–417. *See also*
    estradiol; Premarin
  best forms of, 398–99, 415–16
  calcium/vitamin D supplements
    during, 56
  dosages, 405–6, 407, 409–11
  forms of, 398–99
  gels, 415–16
  low levels, treatment, 55–56
  menopause and, 357–61, 388,
    396–97
  minimizing risks, 413–14
  natural/bioidentical, 400–401,
    411–13
  negative results from, 405–6
  neutral results from, 405–6
  oral contraceptives and, 55–56,
    65–66, 252, 396–97
  pills, 399–400, 416
  progestins combined with, 404–5,
    416, 417
  quality levels guide, 415–17
  starting, 405–6, 407
  worst forms, 400, 416–17
  youthful vagina with, 402–3
estrone, 27, 32, 352, 398, 401, 412
Eulexin, 305, 306
evening primrose oil, 114, 381, 391
Evista (raloxifene), 361, 421

exercise
    periods and, 54, 55
    PMS and, 102

facial blemishes. *See* acne
facial hair. *See* hair, unwanted
    (hirsutism)
fasting, 107, 118–19
fasting insulin, 333, 336, 337, 338
feverfew, 159
fibroids (uterine myomata), 57–58, 139
fibromyalgia
    characteristics of, 142–43, 379
    chronic fatigue and, 143, 379
    hyperesthesia and, 134
    menopause and, 379
    treatment for, 143, 148
5–alpha-reductase inhibitors, 36, 252,
    258, 306–7
fluoxetine. *See* Prozac (fluoxetine)
food. *See* nutrition
Fosamax (alendronate), 421, 422
FSH (follicle-stimulating hormone), 48,
    53, 289, 370, 397

ginseng, 115
glitazones, 325, 336–37, 344

hair
    caring for, 261–63
    health, estrogen and, 244–45, 252
    testosterone and, 268–69
    unwanted. *See* hair, unwanted
        (hirsutism)
hair loss (alopecia), 13, 230–64
    all over body, 240
    alopecia areata, 240–41, 242, 248
    alopecia totalis, 240
    alopecia universalis, 240
    androgenic, defined, 240
    case study, 230–31
    causes, 13
    clues to hormonal causes, 245
    concealing, 263

DHT and, 36, 243–44, 258, 298,
    299, 306
diagnosing, 232, 238–40
estrogen and, 13, 243, 244–45, 249,
    252, 308–9
ethnicity and, 233–34
hope for, 263–64. *See also* hair loss
    treatment
hormonal (HA), 242–43, 245,
    246–47, 248
hormonal pessimism and, 246
hormones and, 243–44
medical establishment and, 238
oral steroids and, 241
psychotherapy and, 234
scalp biopsy for, 250
sex drive improvement vs., 199–200,
    307–8
statistics of, 13
subjective feeling of, 232–35
telogen effluvium (TE), 240, 247–48,
    256
from testosterone, 190–91
testosterone and, 195, 243, 246, 249,
    251–52
tests for, 250, 288–89
thyroid and, 241–42
warning signs, 232
weird scalp sensations (dysesthesia)
    and, 134, 248–49
why dermatologists/endocrinologists
    can't treat, 239
hair loss treatment, 251–64. *See also*
    testosterone control treatments
alopecia areata, 240–41
author background/perspective,
    235–37
Avodart, 306–7
concealment, 263
duration of, 257
estrogen, 252–54
expectations, 256–57
5–alpha-reductase inhibitors, 36,
    252, 258, 306–7

hair care, 261–63
hair extensions/additions/wigs,
    260–61
herbs, 258
with limited/no effect, 257–59
metformin, 258–59
minoxidil (Rogaine), 255–56, 258,
    259, 268
Nioxin, 259
nutrition, 259
oral contraceptives, 252–54, 309
Propecia, 298, 306–7
Proscar, 298, 306–7
testosterone protection, 251–52, 253
transplants, 260
hair, unwanted (hirsutism), 265–75
cause of, 266
common places for, 270
cream to inhibit growth, 272–73
cultural outlook (trichophobia), 265,
    267–68, 269
electrolysis for, 273, 274
ethnicity and, 268–69
ingrown hairs, 272
laser for, 273–74
local removal of (depilation), 271–72
medication for, 274–75
normal/abnormal hormones and,
    269–70
peach fuzz, 268
reasons for, 266–68
removal of, 265–66
requiring medical attention, 270
shaving, 266, 271–72
testosterone and, 268–69
tests identifying reasons for, 288–89
treatment for, 270–75. See also
    testosterone control treatments
Vaniqa (eflornithine) for, 272–73
headaches. See also migraines
chronic daily, 153
common misdiagnoses for, 153
tension, 152
heart disease

alternative medicine and, 390
COX-2 inhibitors and, 145
dysmetabolism and, 321, 331
estrogen and, 6, 55, 252
hormone therapy and, 349, 350–51,
    355–56, 360, 361, 387, 388
oral contraceptives and, 62–63
PCOS and, 311, 321, 331, 337–38
progestins and, 355, 406, 409
soy products and, 391–92
spironolactone and, 303
testosterone and, 196
Viagra and, 211
vitamin E and, 113
weight control and, 337
WHI hazard ratios, 354
Hidradenitis Supporativa (HS), 286–87
hirsutism. See hair, unwanted
    (hirsutism)
hormonal contraception. See birth
    control; oral contraceptives
hormonal pessimism
baselessness of, 4
defined, 86
end of, 439–40
hair loss and, 246
pain perspective and, 132
PCOS and, 314
perimenopause/menopause and, 380,
    384
pervasiveness of, 86–87
PMS and, 86, 87, 98
signs of, 87
hormonal vulnerability
bill of rights, 442–43
defined, 4
diagnosing. See diagnosing hormonal
    vulnerability
as end-organ response issue, 29–30
medical work-up for, 16. See also
    tests
in men, 38
overcoming, 15–16
overview, 3–5

hormonal vulnerability (*continued*)
  range of, 13–14
  symptom examples, 3–4, 6–7
  what it's like, 13–14
  why doctors ignore, 14–15
  women who have, 12–13
hormones. *See also specific hormones*
  aging and, 11–12
  biochemical descriptions vs.
    subjective experience of, 26–27
  common symptoms caused by,
    8–10
  defined, 5–6, 28
  fluctuations in, 6, 7
  functions of, 28–29
  knowledge about, 6
  learning from, 19–20
  levels of, 29
  looks and, 10–11
  measuring levels, 39–40
  mechanics of, 29–30
  moods and, 11
  purpose of, 6
  responses to, 29
  specialists understanding, 7
  triggering migraines, 155
  ways of looking at, 26
  word origin, 7
hormone therapy (HT). *See also*
    estrogen treatment
  balance sheet, 387
  blood clots (DVTs) and, 351, 355,
    377
  breast cancer and, 351, 353–55, 360,
    361, 387, 401, 414
  case studies, 381–83
  deciding about, 383–87
  defined, 352
  heart disease and, 349, 350–51,
    355–56, 360, 361, 387, 388
  minimizing risks, 413–14
  possible risks, 350–55
  progesterone, 403–4
  what you need to know, 361–62

WHI studies. *See* Women's Health
    Initiative (WHI)
hot flashes/night sweats, 365–67
HS (Hidradenitis Supporativa),
    286–87
hyperesthesia, 133–34
hypericum (St. John's wort), 116
hyperplasia
  adrenal, 291, 294
  endometrial, 57, 408
  thecal cell, 339
hypothalamic amenorrhea, 50, 54, 55
hypothalamus, 28, 48, 50, 365

immune system enhancers, 115–16
ingrown hair removal, 272
insulin
  diabetes and. *See* diabetes
  discovery/background of, 329–30
  dysmetabolism and, 317, 321,
    331–32, 333, 334–35
  functions of, 28
  low-carb diets and, 327–28
  normalizing levels of, 335–37
  PCOS and, 195–96
  testosterone and, 298
  tests, 333
insulin resistance (IR)
  natural history of, 330–31
  normalizing insulin levels and,
    335–37
  PCOS and, 329–30
irregular periods, 47
  abnormal cycles and, 53
  anovulation (no period) and, 55–56,
    57, 323, 325, 344
  causes of, 48–49, 50
  heavy bleeding, 53, 56–58
  importance of, 55
  normal variation vs., 52–53
  PCOS and, 323–24
  replacing progesterone from,
    324
  stress and, 54

irritable bowel syndrome (IBS), 133, 134, 140–41
IUDs, 75–76

Ketoconazole (Nizoral), 306

lactic acidosis, 336
lesbian women
  gender identity of, 38
  hair loss and, 234–35
  sex drive/sexuality, 168, 169, 221–22
leuprolide (Lupron), 58, 126–27
Levitra, 208, 212, 213, 221
Levlen, 80
Levlite, 80
Lexapro (escitalopram), 125, 126
Loestrin 1/20, 57, 79
Lo/Ovral, 80
l-phenylalanine, 115, 382
Lunelle, 75
Lupron (leuprolide), 58, 126–27

magnesium (Mg), 114, 116, 159–60
massage therapy, 117–18, 137, 148, 152, 379
mastalgia, 141
medications, 441. *See also* antidepressants; *specific medications*
  acne preparations, 282–83
  antidepressants, 122–23
  dosages, 441
  lipid-lowering, 337–38
  for normalizing insulin levels, 335–37
  for PMS, 119–26
  sensitivity of, 14
  tranquilizers, 121–22
  for unwanted hair, 274–75
meditation, 20, 103, 137, 152, 160, 430–35, 436–37, 438
melasma (chloasma), 70
men
  hormone fluctuations in, 95
  lacking sex drive, 221

sexual desires of, 220
testosterone levels, 36, 168
menopause
  affecting periods, 50
  alternative treatments for, 389–94, 411–13
  assessing your, 384–87
  black cohosh and, 391
  blood tests, 370
  case studies, 381–83, 411–13
  cholesterol and, 414
  deciding about, 383–87
  defined, 352
  depression and, 369, 370–74, 428
  diabetes and, 339, 414
  dong quai and, 393–94
  dysesthesia and, 377–78
  dysmetabolism and, 339
  early, 388
  estrogen and. *See* estrogen treatment
  estrogen-progestin combinations, 404–5, 416, 417
  fibromyalgia and, 379
  hormonal pessimism and, 380, 384
  hormone therapy for. *See* hormone therapy (HT)
  hot flashes/night sweats, 365–66
  joint/muscle pain in, 379–80
  mental faculties and, 375–77
  mood swings, 368–70
  nonhormonal medications, 394–95
  oral contraceptives and, 396–97
  PCOS and, 339–40
  pregnancy and, 396–97
  premature, 388
  progesterone and, 403–4, 406–9
  sex and, 207–8, 368
  sleep disturbance in, 378–79
  soy products and, 391–93, 394
  symptoms summary, 363–64
  terminology, 352–53
  testosterone and, 207–8
  vaginal changes, 367–68
Menostar patch, 407, 410, 415, 421

menstrual cycle(s). *See also* irregular
   periods; periods; PMS
   (premenstrual syndrome)
   abnormal, 53
   changes in, 9
   cramps, 51, 53, 131, 136–38,
      144–46, 148, 323
   duration of, 48
   hormonal activity during, 48–49, 51
   hormonal vulnerability symptoms, 9
   main events, summary, 51
   myths, 46
   normal, process, 47–49
   PCOS and, 339–40
   purpose of, 47
   starting point, 49
   stress and periods, 54
   tracking, 49
   variations, 49–52
Merina, 76
metabolic syndrome. *See* dysmetabolism
   (dysmetabolic syndrome)
metformin
   as hair treatment, 258–59, 320–22
   normalizing insulin levels, 298, 313,
      327, 334, 335–37
   PCOS and, 325, 335–37, 342, 343,
      344
   pregnancy, PCOS and, 325, 343, 344
   weight loss and, 327, 334
Middle Way Medicine, 16–18
migraines. *See also* headaches
   case study, 150–51
   characteristics of, 154–55
   coffee/caffeine and, 159
   hormones triggering, 155
   medication to stop, 157
   natural treatments for, 159–60
   oral contraceptives and, 68, 80,
      154–55, 156
   pain remedies for, 151
   as particular headache type, 152
   preventative treatment for, 158–59
   relief from, 156–60

treating hormonal cause of, 156–57
   why neurologists can't treat, 158
minerals. *See* supplements
minocycline, 283, 287
minoxidil (Rogaine), 255–56, 258, 259,
   268
Mircette, 65, 67, 68, 69, 73, 75, 78,
   80–81, 156, 254, 299, 397
moods/mood swings. *See also*
   depression
   botanicals for, 114, 116
   common drags on, 101
   CPA and, 304–5
   estrogen affecting, 33, 368–71, 372
   exercise and, 102
   fasting and, 118
   food affecting, 109
   hormones and, 11, 13
   hormones vs. antidepressants and,
      372
   menopause and, 368–70, 371, 385,
      386
   oral contraceptives and, 14, 66–67,
      76, 78, 79, 80, 397
   pain and, 131, 379
   progesterone and, 45, 121, 408
   progestins and, 66–67, 417
   semen affecting, 178
   sleep deprivation and, 101, 147
   spironolactone and, 120
   testosterone and, 200
morning after pill, 71
multiple vitamins, 112–13

natural family planning, 61
Neurontin (gabapentin), 395
night sweats, 365–67
Nioxin, 259
Nordette, 68, 79, 80
NSAIDs
   defined, 120
   pain relief from, 143–46
nutrition
   carbohydrates, 108–9, 259

comfort foods, 109–10
fasting and, 107, 118–19
frequent meals, 106–7
hair loss and, 259
low-carb diets, 108, 327–28, 340–41, 342
PMS and, 97, 106–11
salt intake, 110–11
soy products, 108, 391–93, 394
vegetarian diets, 107–8
water and, 110–11
NuvaRing, 75

opioids, 143, 146, 183
oral contraceptives
acne and, 280–81, 299
alternatives, 300, 397
anovulation treatment with, 57
bleeding extra with, 68
blood clots and, 62–63, 65, 70, 254, 304
brands of, 64–65, 77–81
breast size and, 69
choosing, 62, 65–67
contraindications, 63, 154–55, 397
controlling periods with, 72–74, 303, 324
cost of, 81
with CPA, 304
CPA and, 304–5
dex test and, 295
dosages, 65–66
estrogen and, 55–56, 65–66, 252
hair and, 252–54, 309
heart disease and, 62–63
inability to use, 300, 397
ingredients/mechanics of, 63–64
melasma (chloasma) and, 70
menopause and, 396–97
migraines and, 68, 80, 154–55, 156
moods/mood swings and, 14, 66–67, 76, 78, 79, 80, 397
morning after pill, 71

pain/cramp management with, 136, 137, 138, 146
PCOS and, 313
progestins and, 35, 37, 66–67
quality levels of, 77–81
reining in testosterone, 298, 299
restoring period regularity, 55
rumors about, 67
safety of, 62–63
sex drive and, 69, 183–84
solving pill difficulties, 67–70
treating HS, 287
weight and, 68–69, 80
Ortho-Cyclen, 68, 72, 74, 78, 80, 81, 281, 299
Ortho Evra patch, 68, 69, 74, 281
Ortho-Novum 1/35, Ortho 7-7-7, 79
Ortho Tri-Cyclen, 23, 74, 78, 80, 281, 299, 300
Ortho Tri-Cyclen Lo, 78
Ovcon 35, 67, 78, 80

pain. *See also* cramps; fibromyalgia; headaches; migraines
adhesions, 140
antidepressants reducing, 147–48
approaches to, 137
breast, 9, 14, 27, 80, 141–42
chronic fatigue and, 134, 143, 379
diagnosing, 135
dysesthesia, 134
eliminating cause of, 135, 137
endometriosis, 51, 138–39, 146
fibroids (uterine myomata), 57–58, 139
hormones causing, 133
hyperesthesia, 133–34
internal, severity of, 132–33
irritable bowel syndrome (IBS), 91, 133, 134, 140–41
management approach, 135–36
in menopause, 379–80
nature of, 131–32
non-hormonal causes, 134

pain. (*continued*)
  other internal, 140–41
  pelvic, 136–38
  peritoneum, 140
  processing, 133–34
  during sex, 9, 207–8, 368
  weird sensations and (dysesthesia),
    134, 249, 377–78
pain relievers, 143–49
  antidepressants, 137, 147–48
  COX-2 inhibitors, 145–46
  natural, 148–49
  NSAIDs, 143–46
  opioids, 143, 146, 183
  oral contraceptives, 136, 137, 138,
    146
paroxetine. *See* Paxil (paroxetine)
patches. *See also* estrogen patches
  birth control, 68, 69, 74–75, 281
  estradiol, 156, 398, 411, 415
  testosterone, 201, 202
Paxil (paroxetine), 125, 126, 395
PCOS. *See* polycystic ovary syndrome
  (PCOS)
PDE-5 inhibitors, 211–13. *See also*
  Viagra
pelvic region changes, 9
perfectionism recognition, 104–5
perimenopause, defined, 352. *See also*
  menopause
periods. *See also* menstrual cycle(s);
  PMS (premenstrual syndrome)
  controlling when/if have, 47, 72–74,
    303, 304
  exercise and, 54, 55
  infrequent but heavy/prolonged, 56
  irregular. *See* irregular periods
  not getting. *See* anovulation (no
    period)
  nutrition and, 54–55
  pain during, 136–38
  predictability of, 45–47
pill, birth control. *See* oral
  contraceptives

pioglitazone, 336
PMDD (premenstrual dysphoric
  disorder), 83. *See also* PMS
  (premenstrual syndrome)
PMS (premenstrual syndrome)
  benefits of, 87–88
  case studies, 82–83, 92–94
  causes, 13
  challenges of, 85
  diagnosing, 91
  history of, 84–87
  hormonal cause, 83
  hormonal pessimism toward, 86, 87,
    98
  hyperresponsive nervous systems and,
    13
  as legal defense, 84–85
  month-long irritation from, 91–92
  new name for, 83
  other causes of symptoms, 90–91
  progesterone and, 34, 35, 120–21
  recognition of, 85–87
  symptoms, 88–90
  Total PMS, 91–92, 93–95, 113
  true feelings exposed during, 87–88
  when it happens, 90–92
  without periods, 92
PMS treatment, 96–128
  acupuncture, 117
  antidepressants, 82–83, 97, 122–26
  carbohydrates, 108–9
  comfort foods, 109–10
  consistent habits, 100–101
  diuretics, 111, 120
  estrogen patches. *See* estrogen patches
  exercise, 102
  fasting/detoxification, 118–19
  four-point comprehensive plan, 97,
    98–99
  frequent meals, 106–7
  herbs (botanicals), 97, 114–17
  insight, 103–4
  last resort, 126–27
  leuprolide, 126–27

lifestyle, 97, 99–106
managing expectations, 105–6
massage therapy, 117–18
nutrition, 97, 106–11
overview, 96–97
perfectionism recognition, 104–5
prescriptions, 97, 119–26
progesterone, 120–21
psychotherapy, 106
salt intake, 110–11
self-awareness, 99–100
setting priorities, 104–5
soy products, 108
stress reduction techniques, 102–3.
    See also spiritual practices
supplements/herbs, 97, 111–16
timing of activities, 101–2
tranquilizers, 121–22
vegetarian diets, 107–8
water and, 110–11
polycystic ovary syndrome (PCOS), 49,
    310–45
ACN and, 332
after menopause, 339–40
anovulation (no period) and, 323,
    325, 344
author background/perspective,
    314–18
case study, 312–13
causing irregular, absent periods, 50
confusion of, 314–15
cysts, 318–20
defined, 315
depression and, 340–41
dysmetabolism and, 317, 321,
    331–32, 333, 334–35
heart disease and, 311, 321, 331,
    337–38
hormonal pessimism and, 314
irregular periods and, 323–24
long-term maintenance, 337–38
medical establishment and, 315–17
metformin and, 325, 335–37, 342,
    343, 344

with normal insulin levels, 332–34
nutrition and, 327
oral contraceptives and, 80, 313, 325
overview, 310–12
pregnancy and, 341–44
progesterone and, 323–24
puzzle of, 313–14
slender, 329
symptoms/diagnosis, 56, 311, 313,
    320, 321–22
testosterone and, 195, 320–22
unwanted hair and, 269
weight and, 325–29, 342
prayer, 435, 436
pregnancy
Accutane and, 281, 284, 286
amenorrhea preventing, 54
avoiding pelvic surgery before, 140
CPA and, 305
estrogen, hair and, 243, 244, 253
estrogen and, 30, 32, 33, 406
excessive weight loss/exercise
    preventing, 54
fibroids and, 58, 139
5–alpha-reductase inhibitor risk, 258,
    306–7
hair fullness during, 243
menopause and, 396–97
menstrual cycle and, 46, 47, 48,
    111
migraines during, 159
PCOS and, 311, 312, 313, 321, 323,
    325, 336, 341–44
postpartum depression and, 93
preventing. See contraceptives; oral
    contraceptives
progesterone and, 34–35, 170,
    352
reducing endometriosis risk,
    138–39
saw palmetto risk, 258
slender women and, 54, 329
testosterone blockers and, 301–2
testosterone treatment and, 210

Premarin
  breast cancer risk and, 353, 354
  coronary heart disease and, 355
  cream, estradiol vs., 402
  doses, 410
  horse-source, 351, 352, 383, 400
  negative reviews of, 401, 416–17
  as poor pharmaceutical, 416–17
  vegetable-based, 383
  WHI study, 351, 353, 354
  as worst estrogen, 400
premenstrual syndrome. See PMS
    (premenstrual syndrome)
Premphase, 417
Prempro, 351, 353, 354, 355, 377, 417
prescriptions. See medications
Proactiv, 282
progesterone
  adverse effects of, 6, 34
  best form of, 416
  creams, 34, 408–9
  deficiencies, 55
  defined, 352–53
  endometrial cancer and, 323–24
  functions of, 6, 34–35
  in HT regimen, 403–4
  irregular periods and, 323–24
  menopause and, 403–4, 406–9
  natural, 35, 56, 324, 352, 406, 416
  PCOS and, 323–24
  PMS and, 34, 35, 120–21
  pregnancy and, 34–35
  problems with, 406–8
  quality levels guide, 416, 417
  reducing cancer risk, 55, 56, 324,
    353, 404
  safety of, 355
  sex drive and, 170
  synthetic. See progestins
  word origin, 34
progestins
  breast cancer and, 351, 353, 354,
    404, 409
  cholesterol and, 66

  defined, 35, 352–53
  estrogen combined with, 404–5, 416,
    417
  heart disease and, 355, 406, 409
  in HT regimen, 403–4
  oral contraceptives and, 35, 37,
    66–67
  risks of, 352–53, 354–55
  worst forms, 417
prolactin, 48, 50, 53, 170–71, 289
Prometrium, 35, 56, 324, 352, 406,
    407, 416, 417
Propecia, 298, 306–7
Proscar, 298, 306–7
prostaglandins, 27, 136, 144, 146
Provera. See also Depo-Provera
  breast cancer and, 353, 404
  causing PMS, 35, 121, 406
  for endometriosis, 139
  heart disease and, 355, 406
  for infrequent periods, 56, 324
  as poor pharmaceutical, 417
  side effects, 35, 121, 351, 353, 355,
    406
Prozac (fluoxetine), 122, 124, 125–26,
    395
pseudofolliculitis barbae (PFB), 272
psychotherapy
  hair loss (alopecia) and, 234
  for PMS, 106
  sex problems and, 185–86, 187,
    222–23
pyridoxine (B/S16/S0), 113

resources, 445–48
Retin A Micro, 283
Rezulin, 336
rosiglitazone, 344

safety, of treatment, 18–19
saliva tests, 42, 295–96
salt intake, 110–11
scalp biopsy, 250
Seasonale, 72, 254

selective serotonin reuptake inhibitors (SSRIs), 123–26, 147, 213, 221

self-care, 429. *See also* spiritual practices

serotonin, 28, 122–23, 126, 170

17 hydroxyprogesterone (17 OHP), 294

sex
  happiness and, 178–79
  keeping comfortable with, 208–9
  learning what feels good, 179–81
  lubrication/moisture for, 207, 208–9, 368
  medical role in, 165, 166
  menopause and, 207–8, 368
  normal amount of, 167–68, 172
  pain during, 9, 207–8, 368
  prerequisites for, 171
  public openness to, 164
  testosterone and. *See* testosterone, for sexuality
  thoughts, energy/pleasure from, 219
  what men want, 220

sex drive/sexuality
  anger and, 185
  antidepressants and, 170, 213
  anxiety and, 175
  case studies, 172–73, 174–76, 185, 186
  change, in long-standing relationships, 217–18
  Cialis/Levitra and, 208, 212, 213, 221
  clues to underlying problems, 187
  common hormonal turnoffs, 183
  common nonhormonal turnoffs, 184
  deeper problems, 185–86, 187
  estrogen and, 169–70, 175
  female sexual dysfunction (FSD) and, 166, 190
  hair loss vs., 199–200, 307–8
  herbs for, 213
  hormones and, 166–67, 168–69, 183
  male dysfunction treatments, 221
  marriage well-being and, 175–78, 220
  medications taking away, 182–84
  men lacking, 221
  normal amount of, 172–73
  oral contraceptives and, 69, 183–84
  PDE-5 inhibitors and, 211–13
  progesterone and, 170
  prolactin and, 170–71
  psychological treatment for, 223
  quick fix, 222–23
  between relationships, 218–20
  self-doubt about, 173–74
  sex therapists and, 186–88
  taking the initiative, 174–76
  testosterone and. *See* testosterone, for sexuality
  unmet expectations, 165–66
  vaginal changes and, 367–68
  Viagra and, 211–13, 214, 221, 223, 368, 441

sex steroids, 28. *See also* estrogen; progesterone; testosterone

sex therapists, 186–88

SHBG (sex hormone-binding globulin), 290, 299

skin/hair changes. *See also* acne; hair loss (alopecia); hair loss treatment; hair, unwanted (hirsutism); testosterone control treatments
  common symptoms, 9
  PCOS and, 320–22
  reversing, 194–95
  testosterone causing, 163, 194–95, 198–99

sleep deprivation
  menopause and, 378–79
  mood/depression and, 101, 147, 378–79

soy products, 108, 391–93, 394

spiritual practices, 137, 390, 427–40
  cultivating forgiveness, 435–37
  fasting and, 118–19
  images for quick relief, 437–38

spiritual practices, (*continued*)
  medical modalities and, 16–17, 96, 103
  meditation, 20, 103, 137, 152, 160, 430–35, 436–37, 438
  Middle Way Medicine and, 16–18
  myths blocking spiritual healing, 439
  overcoming negativity, 103
  overcoming pessimism, 439–40
  overview, 24, 427–30
  pain and, 137
  PMS and, 101–2
  prayer, 435, 436
  in scientific culture, 438–39
  self-awareness, PMS and, 99–100
  self-care, 429
  stress reduction techniques, 102–3
  timing of activities and, 101–2
spironolactone, 119–20
  for alopecia, 237, 252, 302, 309
  controlling testosterone, 298, 300–301, 302
  as diuretic, 111, 120
  names of, 441
  ovulation restoration and, 325
  for PMS, 97, 111, 119–20
  pregnancy and, 343
  side effects, 19, 302–3
  for skin recovery, 199, 277, 280, 285, 302
SSRIs (selective serotonin reuptake inhibitors), 123–26, 147, 213, 221
steroid receptors, 29
St. John's wort (hypericum), 116
stress
  periods and, 54
  reduction techniques, 102–3. See also spiritual practices
supplements
  American (Wisconsin) ginseng, 115
  black cohosh, 114, 116, 381, 391
  botanicals, 114–16, 391–93
  calcium. See calcium (Ca)
  choosing, 116

dong quai, 114–15, 393–94
eleutherococcus, 115
  during estrogen treatment, 56
  evening primrose oil, 114, 381, 391
  hypericum (St. John's wort), 116
  immune system enhancers, 115–16
  l-phenylalanine, 115, 382
  magnesium (Mg), 114, 116, 159–60
  multiple vitamins, 112–13
  for PMS, 97, 111–14
  pyridoxine (B/S16/S0), 113
  safety of, 116–17
  vitamin D, 56, 418, 422–23
  vitamin E, 113, 116, 142, 394
  vitamins and minerals, 112–14
  vitex, 114, 116, 142, 390, 394, 407
syndrome X, 331

tamoxifen (Nolvadex), 142, 358–59
Tazorac, 283
telogen effluvium (TE), 240, 247–48, 256
tension headaches, 152
Testim, 202, 205
testosterone
  acne and, 277, 278–79, 280–81
  adverse effects of, 6, 36, 195, 227–28
  blockers. See testosterone control treatments
  compounded preparations, 201–2
  controlling. See testosterone control treatments
  for depression, 200
  DHT and, 36, 243–44, 258, 298, 299, 306
  for energy, 200
  facial/body hair and, 266–67, 268–69
  female vs. male levels, 36
  fluctuations in, 7, 95, 292
  functions of, 6, 36
  gels, 192, 201–6, 207, 215, 216, 218
  hair loss from. See hair loss (alopecia)
  heart disease and, 196

levels of, 35, 266
in men, 36, 95, 168, 266
as mixed blessing, 227
for mood, 200
as most problematic hormone, 36
negative effects of, 190–91, 194–96
overview, 227–28
pharmaceutical forms of, 37
production glands, 35
pros/cons of, 229
questions to consider, 199
safety of, 194–97
skin/hair changes from, 163, 194–95,
    198–99
transdermal application, 192, 195,
    201, 206–7
vaginal rings, 207
vulnerabilities, 198–200
wrong ways to use, 197
yin-yang of, 37–38
testosterone, for sexuality, 201–24
appropriate dosing, 204–6
benefits of, 163
changes in long-standing
    relationships, 217–18
effects of, 192–94
estrogen and, 207–8
gels, 192, 201–6, 207, 215, 216, 218
happiness and, 178–79
ill-advised old approaches, 189–91
lesbian women and, 221–22
limited libido enhancement, 219–20
medication as quick fix, 222–23
menopause and, 207–8
pain during sex and, 207–8
patches, 201, 202
postponing, indicators, 210, 211
reasons for, 217
between relationships, 218–20
research results, 191–92
sex drive and, 168–69, 176, 178–79,
    209–11, 307–8
taking initiative and, 174
telling partner about, 214–17

vulnerabilities and, 198–200
when unlikely to help, 188
women responding to, 193–94
women vs. men, 168–69
wrong ways to use, 197
testosterone control treatments,
    297–309. See also spironolactone
background on, 297–98
blocking testosterone, 300–307
Casodex (bicalutamide), 305–6
CPA (Androcur), 79, 280, 304–5
5–alpha-reductase inhibitors, 36,
    252, 258, 306–7
Ketoconazole (Nizoral), 306
lowering testosterone in blood,
    299–300
overview, 298–99
pregnancy and blockers, 301–2
sex drive and, 307–8
unsafe blockers, 306
testosterone research
ill-advised old approaches, 189–91
safety, 194–97
sex drive effects, 191–94
testosterone tests, 288–96
androstenedione, 294
dexamethasone suppression test, 295
DHEA and, 293–94
DHEA-S and, 35, 250, 289, 293–94
fluctuations in, 291
forms of testosterone tested, 290
normal levels, 291–92, 293
pitfalls in interpreting, 293
saliva tests, 42, 295–96
17 hydroxyprogesterone (17 OHP),
    294
total and free testosterone, 289, 290,
    293
unorthodox tests, 295–96
value/validity of, 292–93
tests. See also testosterone tests
accuracy of, 39–40
acne, 288–89
bone density, 420, 422

tests. (*continued*)
  dysmetabolism, 333
  estradiol, 250
  false positives, 40
  hair loss (alopecia), 250, 288–89
  hirsutism, 288–89
  hormonal vulnerability and, 41–42
  hormone levels, 16, 39–40
  importance of physical exams, 30
  interpreting, 7
  lab pitfalls, 39–41
  reading lab results, 441–43
  saliva, 42, 295–96
  thyroid, 41, 241, 289, 422
thecal cell hyperplasia, 339
thyroid
  alternative medicine and, 390
  cysts, 319
  hair loss, 241–42
  tests, 41, 241, 289, 422
timing of activities, 101–2
Total PMS, 91–92, 93–95, 113
tranquilizers, 121–22
treatment, 38. *See also specific*
      disorders, treatments
  Middle Way Medicine and, 16–18
  plan ingredients, 17
  safety of, 18–19
  trusting different approaches, 17–18
Tri-Levlen, 80
trimethoprim-sulfa, 287
TSH tests, 41, 241, 242, 289, 422

unwanted hair. *See* hair, unwanted
      (hirsutism)
uterine myomata (fibroids), 57–58, 139

Vagifem, 402
vagina
  changes in, 9, 367–68

common hormonal symptoms in, 9
  youthful, with estrogen, 402–3
vaginal rings
  estrogen, 399
  NuvaRing contraceptive, 75
  testosterone, 207
Vaniqa (eflornithine), 272–73
vasodilatation, 31, 211
vegetarian diets, 107–8
venlafaxine. *See* Effexor
      (venlafaxine)
Viagra, 211–13, 214, 221, 223, 368,
      441
vitamins. *See* supplements
vitex (chaste tree or chaste berry), 114,
      116, 142, 390, 394, 407
VTE (venous thromboembolism), 70

water and salt, 110–11
weight, 9
  contraceptive effectiveness and, 69
  cultural misconceptions about,
      235–36
  gaining, 68–69
  getting pregnant and, 342
  losing, 327–28
  oral contraceptives and, 68–69, 80
  PCOS and, 325–29, 342
Wellbutrin (bupropion), 125, 126, 182,
      213
Women's Health Initiative (WHI)
  breast cancer findings, 354–55
  defined, 353
  hazard ratios, 251–54
  important facts about, 357
  study overview, 350–55

Yasmin, 67, 68, 72, 77–78, 80, 81,
      254, 281, 299, 300
yin-yang nature, 37–38, 298